RESEARCH FOR THE
HEALTH PROFESSIONAL

Research for the Health Professional

A Practical Guide
Second Edition

Diana M. Bailey, EdD, OTR, FAOTA
Associate Professor
Boston School of Occupational Therapy
Tufts University
Medford, Massachusetts

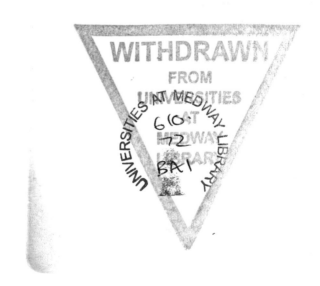

F. A. DAVIS COMPANY • Philadelphia

F. A. Davis Company
1915 Arch Street
Philadelphia, PA 19103
http://www.fadavis.com

Printed in the United States of America

Last digit indicates print number: 10 9

Publisher: Jean-François Vilain
Editor: Lynn Borders Caldwell
Production Editor: Jessica Howie Martin
Cover Designer: Steven Ross Morrone

As new scientific information becomes available through basic and clinical research, recommended treatments and drug therapies undergo changes. The author and publisher have done everything possible to make this book accurate, up to date, and in accord with accepted standards at the time of publication. The author, editors, and publisher are not responsible for errors or omissions or for consequences from application of the book, and make no warranty, expressed or implied, in regard to the contents of the book. Any practice described in this book should be applied by the reader in accordance with professional standards of care used in regard to the unique circumstances that may apply in each situation. The reader is advised always to check product information (package inserts) for changes and new information regarding dose and contraindications before administering any drug. Caution is especially urged when using new or infrequently ordered drugs.

Library of Congress Cataloging-in-Publication Data

Bailey, Diana M., 1942–
    Research for the health professional : a practical guide / Diana
  M. Bailey.—2nd ed.
     p. cm.
  Includes bibliographical references and index.
  ISBN 0-8036-0151-4 (pbk.)
  1. Medicine—Research—Methodology. I. Title.
  [DNLM: 1. Research Design. 2. Data Collection—methods. 3. Data
Interpretation, Statistical. 4. Writing. 5. Publishing. W 20.5
B154r 1997]
R850.B35 1997
610'.72—dc21
DNLM/DLC
for Library of Congress   96-36840
                                    CIP

Foreword

Fear and lack of understanding are by far the two most common barriers facing the beginning researcher. How can we as educators help our students overcome these barriers? This was obviously the question facing Diana Bailey when she decided to write *Research for the Health Professional*.

This book's greatest strength is its unique skill-oriented approach, which helps the reader apply research theory in a practical manner. Numerous worksheets provide incentive to study and learn and a method for testing ideas. Discussion of potential pitfalls and stumbling blocks, and boxed asides of actual occupational and physical therapy literature provide valuable learning tools by illustrating important points clearly and succinctly.

Since occupational and physical therapy practitioners must develop their research skills to substantiate theory and practice and to validate their services, both students and practitioners will find this book extremely helpful in meeting that challenge.

Susan B. O'Sullivan, EdD, PT
Associate Professor
Department of Physical Therapy
University of Lowell
Lowell, Massachusetts

Preface to the Second Edition

One is always pleased to be asked to prepare a second edition and, indeed, I have been thrilled with the response to *Research for the Health Professional: A Practical Guide.* There was clearly a need for a practical, hands-on, straightforward workbook on research for students and clinicians. However, there was one recurring suggestion for change: "Please spend more time on qualitative research." So that is what I have done in the second edition.

Material on the process, methods, and techniques for qualitative research has been threaded throughout the book. In Chapter 4, the naturalistic method is introduced with a description of its idiosyncratic features. Data collection methods have been expanded in Chapter 7 to include methods that are par-

ticularly suited to qualitative research. Chapters 9 and 10 are devoted to qualitative designs and techniques for analyzing data gleaned from naturalistic studies. The final additions, presented in Chapter 12, are some suggestions for writing qualitative studies. The worksheets and boxed examples have been expanded to include qualitative styles of research.

My intent is still to lead the investigator through the research process in a step-by-step manner while pointing out potential problems. I hope the new material will prove helpful and that the book will remain useful to students writing a thesis and clinicians launching a research project.

Diana M. Bailey, 1996

Preface to the First Edition

This book is intended for students who are conducting research projects or writing theses and for clinicians who are considering doing research in their clinics. It is not meant to be a comprehensive text on research. Instead it gives a brief and simple overview of the research process, leading the reader in a logical, step-by-step sequence through each stage while providing an opportunity to try out ideas on worksheets at the end of each chapter. For those who have previously taken courses in research and statistics, this book may prove to be a memory-jogger, guiding you through the various steps. Those who have not done research before, and those who are taking their first course in research, will need to use a more detailed text alongside this one.

The manual is designed to be a hands-on working tool containing useful tips on managing potential pitfalls, together with worksheets at each step in the sequence. Readers are expected to move in and out of the process at various points along the way. Although many people enter the research cycle at the question identification stage, some find themselves entering at other points and are comfortable moving backward and forward in no particular sequence. This is possible in the manual because each step is designed as a self-contained unit and can be tackled individually.

The original notion for the book came after I had been asked by working therapists to run workshops to refresh their memories and help them get started on research in their clinics. Typically, these clinicians had completed a thesis or a research project in school and had been working for several years. They were now ready to pursue clinical research but had forgotten some procedures or had lost sight of the larger issues.

Because therapists are usually able to sit down to read professional literature only after a full day's work, this book was kept brief and straightforward, outlining a logical sequence of steps to be followed in designing and implementing a project. Similarly, students studying research for the first time are sometimes apt to lose sight of the greater picture, or even the point of their own projects. The ordering of the information in this book may help them stay on track.

I have included numerous examples from the literature in physical therapy and occupational therapy, which are presented in boxed format. This information was boxed so that if you do not wish to interrupt the flow of the narrative, you may skip the boxes and come back to them later. If you enjoy illustrations sprinkled liberally throughout a text, you may prefer to read the boxes as you go along. Often the box gives a brief outline or one small portion of a study in order to make a point; you are encouraged to look up the article in its entirety for a greater understanding of the material.

Because I wanted this book to be utilitarian and pragmatic, I have included a list of stumbling blocks at the end of each chapter. The stumbling blocks include things that are likely to go wrong—and are usually things that have gone wrong for me! The purpose is to give the inexperienced researcher some warning of potential pitfalls so that they may be avoided.

Another feature of the book is the collection of worksheets at the end of each chapter. I have developed these over several years while teaching courses in clinical research and providing workshops for working therapists. I hope you will feel comfortable writing directly on these sheets. If you complete all the worksheets, you will have done much of the work needed for the design and writing of your project. Making the results of the project known to colleagues via a published article—the ultimate goal for most clinical researchers—will be greatly facilitated if you fill in the worksheets as you go along.

Finally, I hope this workbook will assist and guide you through the research maze and, above all else, that you will enjoy yourself as you go. My aim is to make research enticing and to encourage therapists to give it a try. In Horace's words from *Odes*, Book IV, "He who has begun has half done. Dare to be wise; begin!"

Diana M. Bailey, 1991

Acknowledgments

Thanks to the following reviewers for their suggestions for the second edition:

Bette R. Bonder, PhD, OTR, FAOTA
Professor and Chairwoman
Department of Health Sciences
Director
Center for Health Sciences and Human
  Services
Cleveland State University
Cleveland, Ohio

Debra J. Byram, MA, OTR
Assistant Professor
Occupational Therapy Department
University of North Dakota
Grand Forks, North Dakota

Christine K. Malaski, MS, OTR
Instructor and Level II Fieldwork
  Coordinator
Occupational Therapy Department
St. Ambrose University
Davenport, Iowa

Terrie L. Nolinske, PhD, OTR, CO
Associate Professor
Department of Occupational Therapy
Rush University
Chicago, Illinois
and
President
Consultants in Professional Development
Oak Park, Illinois

Otto D. Payton, PhD, PT, FAPTA
Professor of Physical Therapy
Virginia Commonwealth University
Richmond, Virginia

Donna Redman-Bently, PhD, PT
Professor and Director
Physical Therapy Program
California State University–Northridge
Northridge, California

Barbara A. Schell, PhD, OTR, FAOTA
Associate Professor and Department Chair
Occupational Therapy Department
Brenau University
Gainesville, Georgia

Louise R. Thibodaux, MA, OTR, FAOTA
Associate Professor
Occupational Therapy Department
University of Alabama at Birmingham
Birmingham, Alabama

Thanks also to the reviewers of the first edition for their insights and useful suggestions:

Bette R. Bonder, PhD, OTR, FAOTA
Associate Professor and Chair
Department of Health Sciences
Cleveland State University
Cleveland, Ohio

Leonard Elbaum, PT
Associate Professor
Physical Therapy Department
Florida International University
Miami, Florida

Patti Maurer, PhD, OTR
Chair, Department of Occupational
  Therapy
Virginia Commonwealth University
Richmond, Virginia

Terrie L. Nolinske, MA, OTR, CO
Assistant Professor
Department of Occupational Therapy
Rush Presbyterian St. Luke's Medical
  Center
Chicago, Illinois

Otto D. Payton, PhD, PT
Director, Graduate Studies
Department of Physical Therapy
Medical College of Virginia
Virginia Commonwealth University
Richmond, Virginia

Louise R. Thibodaux, MA, OTR, FAOTA
Assistant Professor and Director
Graduate Curriculum Development
Division of Occupational Therapy
University of Alabama at Birmingham
Birmingham, Alabama

With heartfelt thanks to:
   Sharan Schwartzberg for valuable assistance and for lightening my work load so that this book could be written—and for introducing me to Jean-François
   Jean-François Vilain and Lynn Borders Caldwell for guiding me through the process and making it fun along the way

Contents

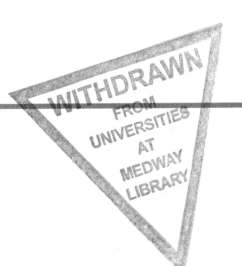

10 *Analyzing Qualitative Data*   **158**

11 *Final Preparation Before Implementing the Research Plan*   **180**

12 *Reporting Results and Drawing Conclusions*   **190**

13 *Writing and Publishing*   **209**

Appendices   **234**

Index   **273**

Illustrations

Tables

Introduction

What Is Research?

Research can be fun, exciting, and fascinating. Often a student who is required to write a research thesis starts out appalled by the idea, yet comes to enjoy the challenge and ends up feeling proud of the results. Great satisfaction can be derived from completing this exacting, often complex, and always stimulating process.

Unfortunately, some people put off attempting research because of preconceived notions. For a few, the word *research* conjures up pictures of statistics, rats, and mazes. In fact, research is any activity undertaken to increase our knowledge; it is the systematic investigation of a problem, issue, or question. This may mean reviewing all the literature on a given topic and drawing new conclusions about that topic, manipulating certain variables to see what happens to other variables, or merely searching in an organized manner for relationships between characteristics or entities.

Two means of discovering and using knowledge are inductive and deductive reasoning. In using deductive reasoning, one accepts or believes a general principle, then applies that principle to an individual case. For example, based on anatomical and physiological information and the resulting theory concerning exercise and joint wear, a therapist may believe that arthritic patients will benefit from receiving short treatment sessions as frequently as possible. Conse-

quently, he or she or will treat the next arthritic patient 5 days per week for 15- to 20-minute sessions.

In using inductive reasoning, one accepts or believes a finding about an individual and then applies that belief to all similar individuals, assuming that it will be true for all. For example, if a therapist finds that a specific arthritic patient benefits more from short treatment sessions given five times per week than from longer treatment sessions given twice per week, he or she may be inclined to treat all subsequent arthritic patients five times per week.

The problem with deductive reasoning is that, although the principle is usually true, there may well be exceptions. The problem with inductive reasoning is that the individual upon whom you have based the principle may be the exception, so that the principle will probably not apply to all other cases that follow. This is an inherent problem with the case study approach, which uses inductive reasoning. To compensate, researchers often try to have as many cases as possible in their research samples, in order to increase their chances of developing real principles.

Research Is a Challenge

Research in the health sciences is ͻ easy undertaking. Human behavior tremely complex and, therefore, dif isolate and to measure. Because working in the health field, there is the added complication that the clients who are the subjects of our research are, by definition, not functioning optimally. Some clients may not want to participate in research studies; numerous ethical issues need to be considered in doing research on human beings. And last, research takes time and other resources that busy clinicians may not have.

Categorizing Research

There are several ways to categorize the basic types of research. For example, research may be pure or applied, experimental or descriptive, clinical or laboratory. Figure 1 describes these three categories.

Estimating Time Needed to Complete a Research Project

Therapists often ask, "How long will it take to complete a research study?" or "How long must I spend at it each day or week?" In my experience in advising graduate occupational therapy students in their thesis preparation and writing, it takes them an average of 6 months to 1 year. This includes conceptualizing the issue to be studied, carrying out the project, and writing the study. Students are usually not carrying a caseload of clients and are not tied to a 40-hour work week; however, they do have classes to attend, and often they are working full-time on an affiliation.

In my experience, research being conducted by therapists in the clinic tends to take longer—about 1 year to 18 months—with some time spent on the project each week. Of course, different phases of the research demand more or less input. For example, if a new treatment approach is being investigated, the therapist must adhere to the number and length of treatment sessions stipulated in the research protocol and put time into preparation and record keeping. Reading the literature and writing the results may be done in one's own time and on a less precise schedule. The therapist working from 9 to 5 should plan on reading and writing in the evening and on weekends. Few clinical situations afford therapists enough free time during the day to do the extra work required to complete a research study. Figure 2 depicts the amount of time I took to complete a study conducted in a nursing home while I held a full-time teaching position. I investigated changes in speech patterns of chronic schizophrenic patients following a program of sensory stimulation. The hypothesis was tested using a pre-test and post-test design with an experimental group and a control group.

Steps in the Research Process

It is useful to remember that research is a circular process. The researcher starts with a question in mind, goes through the investigative stages, and ends up with an answer

A. **Pure**	**Applied**
Abstract and general, concerned with generating new theory and gaining new knowledge for the knowledge's sake.	Designed to answer a practical question, to help people do their jobs better.
B. **Experimental**	**Descriptive**
Manipulating one variable to see its effect on another variable, while controlling for as many other variables as possible and randomly assigning subjects to groups.	Describing a group, a situation, or an individual to gain knowledge which may be applied to further groups or situations, as in case studies or trend analyses.
C. **Clinical**	**Laboratory**
Performed in the "real world" where control over variables is quite difficult.	Performed in "unreal" or laboratory surroundings that are tightly controlled.

FIGURE 1   Description of categories of research.

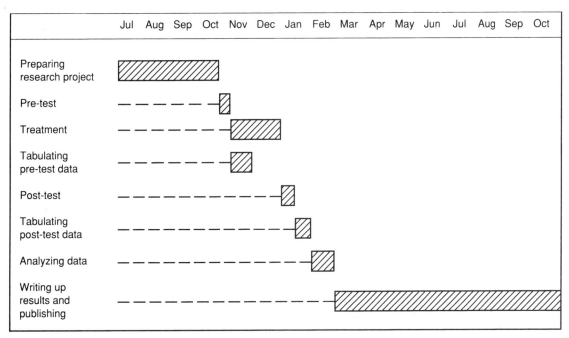

FIGURE 2 Time chart for conducting a research study.

to the question. More often than not, further questions arise during the analysis and interpretation of the data, leading to yet more research ideas.

There are different points of entry into the research process. Some people enjoy starting afresh at the question identification stage; others may happen upon some study results that they question and feel they would like to investigate for themselves. Still others enter at various phases along the way. Whatever the entry point, the steps required to complete a research project follow a logical sequence:

1. Identify a problem that needs to be solved or a question that needs to be answered.

2. Review the existing writing on that issue.

3. Formulate a question or hypothesis about the problem based on the reading.

4. Design a procedure that will address the question or hypothesis.

5. Carry out the procedure.

6. Collect and interpret the findings.

7. Publish the answer to the question so that others may benefit from the identified knowledge.

We will go through this process step by step, exploring each step and offering practical hints on how to get over the hurdles that frequently present themselves. Worksheets at the end of most chapters will help you complete each step of your study. If you persevere, you will be able to carry out a research project from its inception to publication by working your way through this manual.

The beginning chapters discuss how to formulate a research question or problem, how to review the literature, and how to refine the subject by developing background material and establishing parameters for the study. Next, we examine the process of deciding on a research method and explore various research designs. Chapters on collecting and analyzing quantitative and qualitative data are followed by a chapter on reporting the results and drawing conclusions from the findings. Finally, we consider in detail how to prepare the study for publication or for thesis format.

Identifying a Topic

Where Do Research Topics Come From?

Research topics usually come from the work environment; for most therapists, that means the clinic or other patient settings. You may have found you often ask yourself and your coworkers clinically based questions such as: "I wonder why this patient with hemiplegia made more gains than that patient with hemiplegia?" "What did I do differently, that Mr. Smith complies with his home program but Mr. Brown doesn't?" "Would a behavioral approach or a sensory integrative approach work better for that group of retarded clients?" "When I use this particular type of group treatment, there seems to be more response from the patients. I wonder why?" "Why do we always do it this way? What if we tried . . . ?"

Professional literature is another source of research topics. Reading about other people's treatment programs or ideas may trigger questions in relation to your own treatment. You may see something in other people's findings or recommendations that doesn't agree with your clinical experience. Or you may identify gaps in the literature that make it difficult to answer your specific questions (Box 1–A).

Perhaps you have read a fascinating study that has particular significance for you and decide that you would like to replicate it, either just as it is or with modifications based on your own interests. Replication is an excellent way to learn and to practice the scientific inquiry process (Boxes 1–B and 1–C).

Clinical practice, the literature, and conference presentations are all legitimate sources of research topics. Keep these things in mind when deciding on a topic:

- Choose an area of study that fascinates you. Research is a lengthy, sometimes tedious business with many pitfalls. If you aren't excited about your topic to begin with, you most certainly won't be by

---

Box 1–A

Four physical therapists noticed that "clinical literature *suggests* that lumbar lordosis, pelvic tilt and abdominal muscle function are related to each other" (emphasis mine). They further noted that "experimental evidence . . . demonstrating the relationship of abdominal muscle 'strength' . . . , lordosis and pelvic tilt has not been published." This led to their conducting an experimental study to examine if such a relationship really does exist; in fact, they found "that the three items are not related during normal standing." They conclude: "This study demonstrates the need for re-examination of clinical practice based on assumed relationships. . . ."

(Walker, Rothstein, Finncane, & Lamb, 1987, pp. 512, 516)

Box 1-B

Middlebrook (1988) replicated a thesis study that had been conducted to see if certain functional movement patterns would elicit a hemodynamic response. The original study was conducted on college students who were in the 18- to 22-year age range. Middlebrook was interested to see whether similar findings would exist in an older population, and repeated the study using subjects in the 60- to 80-year age range.

the time you finish. If you lose the drive to find the answer to your question, it is almost guaranteed that you won't finish the study.

- Keep it simple. It is tempting to add some "juicy" subquestions to see whether they can be answered at the same time; however, this may result in your not knowing which variables are responsible for which changes. It is usually better to try to answer one question at a time.

- Do a pilot study to iron out the kinks before starting the main study. A pilot study is a smaller version of the main study and will allow you to see if there

Box 1-C

In *Two Approaches to Improving the Functional Performance of a Head-Injured Adult,* the efficacy of two occupational therapy approaches—functional and transfer of training—was examined. Rabideau's study (1985) examined which of the two treatment approaches is more effective in rehabilitating functional performance of cognitively impaired head-injured adults. In 1989, Loftus replicated the study, holding all variables constant except for the cognitive level of functioning of the subjects. She hypothesized that the results would be different based on her clinical experience with adults with head injury. Hence Loftus was changing a variable in a study because her knowledge and experience told her that the study results would change if the degree of symptoms in the subjects was different.

are any problems in the design. (Pilot studies are described in Chapter 9.) Such a study can save innumerable headaches later and prevent the feeling that you would have done a host of things differently had you known then what you know now.

- Keep writing things down to clarify your thinking—the question, variables, definitions, methods. Whenever you have a brainstorm about your project, take a minute to write it down.

Ending up with a researchable question is undoubtedly a difficult task, and people go about it in different ways. However, most people go through several common stages, including:

- Having an idea
- Thinking about the idea
- Discussing the idea with colleagues
- Checking in the literature to see if it makes sense
- Deciding exactly what goals are to be achieved through the research
- Defining the questions more precisely to formulate the hypothesis

Identifying a Reasonable Question

Identifying a reasonable question may well be the most difficult step in the research process. What makes a question reasonable? By "reasonable" we mean that the study will be related to one's profession, will serve some useful purpose, will add to the profession's body of knowledge, and will be "doable." This means that it will be possible to convert it into a research design, there will be an instrument to measure the variables, and the subjects and other resources needed will be available. To be reasonable and researchable, a question must have the following attributes:

- A rationale or *theory base.* How will this study add to the body of knowledge of the profession? Does it fall into an existing treatment approach (e.g., developmental, behavioral, biomechanical, rehabilitative) so that it will add to the theoretical base of the approach? The project is more useful to clinicians if it is

---

Box 1-D

Parker and Chan (1986) studied stereotyping among occupational and physical therapists because they felt that their study would have importance in those therapists' ability to work together effectively as a team.

---

based on a theory with which they are familiar and through which they can refine their treatment.

- There must be *significance* to your question. Will anyone care whether you answer this question? Will you be proud of the contribution of knowledge you have made to your profession? This is the "so what" of the study. When you describe your study to someone and he or she asks, "So what?" can you give a valid answer (Boxes 1–D and 1–E)? Try to think about possible outcomes of your study to be sure that your work will be worthwhile. Although experienced researchers sometimes engage in philosophical research where the benefit of the study is not immediately apparent, it is better for the beginning researcher to engage in studies in which clear implications exist that either the clients or the program will benefit as a result (Box 1–F).

- What *variables* will you be studying? A variable is any attribute or characteristic that can vary, such as diagnosis, age, heart rate, elbow flexion, and self-

---

Box 1-E

Physical therapists compared the reliability and validity of four instruments that have been used for a similar purpose: to measure lumbar spine and pelvic positions (Burdett, Brown, & Fall, 1986). They felt it would be useful to know if one instrument was more reliable and appropriate than the others, so that therapists could select the best tool. If there was no difference, then such issues as expense, ease of use, and convenience for patients could be considered in selecting an instrument.

Box 1-F

In a survey following a therapeutic work program for adults with head injury (Lyons & Morse, 1988), it was found that a greater percentage of clients than that reported by other prevocational programs were participating in occupational activities at follow-up. The activities, counseling, scheduling, and other components of the vocational program under study were clearly of benefit to head-injured clients.

---

esteem. Can your variables be identified and measured? Some variables are easy to identify, particularly visual ones such as height, dressing skills, or grip strength as measured on a dynamometer. Others, such as nonverbal communication, professionalism, and schizophrenia, are more difficult to identify and characterize. Some variables are easy to measure (e.g., joint angles, weight, heart rate), whereas others require complicated measuring instruments (e.g., job satisfaction, sense of mastery, altruism, dysphasia).

Variables may be expected to change and be measured in some studies but may be held constant or unchanging in others, and the same variable may be changeable in one study but held constant in another. For example, task attention may be measured in 9-, 10-, 11-, and 12-year-olds in one study, and in another, a group of 12-year-olds may be tested for a relationship between reading comprehension and level of attention. Age would be a changing variable in the first study and would be held constant in the second.

Many studies look for relationships between variables (i.e., Is this variable related to that one? If so, how?). Other studies look for a cause-and-effect relationship between variables (i.e., If this variable is changed, does it have an effect on that one? If so, what effect?). For example, Nelson (1989) was trying to determine whether there was a relationship between therapists' professionalism and their self-esteem. She was conducting correlational research. Konrad (1994) wanted to see if patients with "rheumatoid arthritis . . . [could] benefit from ultrasonic treatment of their hands" (p. 157). She was engaging in experimental research. (These research designs are explained in Chapter 5.)

- What *resources*, such as money, time, computer use, and statistical assistance, will you need to carry out the project, and are those resources available to you? For instance, if answering the question you have in mind will require extensive statistical analysis, do you have the services of a statistician at hand?

- What *subjects* will you need to carry out the project, and are those subjects available to you? It is invariably more practical for clinicians to include in their studies patients or clients at their own facility rather than to try to locate certain types of patients, such as those with a specific diagnosis, who may be found only at other facilities. Using patients you can easily reach greatly increases the chance of the project being completed.

The Purpose of the Study

Setting the specific research aims and objectives for your research is most important and should be done early in the process. Clarifying your goals will help you establish a hypothesis. What do you want your project to achieve for your clients, your program, or the profession (Box 1–G)? What do you think might be changed for the better, according to your results? Stout (1988), for example, thinks that occupational therapists have skills and knowledge useful in planning chil-

---

Box 1–G

In a multicase study described in the *American Journal of Occupational Therapy* (Giles & Clark-Wilson, 1988), the purpose was to improve the washing and dressing skills of four adults with brain injury. All were heavily dependent on others in their personal hygiene. The authors were investigating the benefits of a specific treatment approach that they hoped would assist other patients.

---

dren's playgrounds and that if they participate in this activity, more playgrounds will be accessible and available for children with disabilities.

The Hypothesis

What is your hunch about the possible outcome of your research? The answer to this question will help you formulate the hypothesis. The hypothesis may or may not be supported at the end of the research, but it is important to postulate what may happen. The purpose of the hypothesis is to suggest new experiments and new ways of looking at clinical practice, and it is the tool that is used to guide the research process. Some examples of hypotheses from the occupational and physical therapy literature follow.

- There is no significant correlation between grip strength and hand function in the normal population.

- The dominant hand has a different pattern of correlation between strength and function than does the nondominant hand.

- Guided visual imagery is effective in treating patients with psychosomatic, psychogenic, or chronic somatic disorders.

- The Trager Psychophysical Integration Method improves the chest mobility of patients with chronic lung disease.

- Prior knowledge influences the automatic and voluntary postural adjustments of healthy and hemiplegic subjects.

- Age influences prosthesis use in subjects with above-knee amputation.

- There is a positive relationship between the self-esteem of female therapists and their attitudes and behaviors toward professionalism.

- Occupational health promotion is a viable practice area for occupational therapists.

- Chronic psychiatric patients live out unsatisfying patterns of maladaptive behavior characterized by:

    Poor balance of work, leisure, activities of daily living, and sleep.

Poor planning for the future reflected in use of time.

Dissatisfaction regarding use of time.

As you can see, the hypothesis is the essence of a research study. All the variables that will be studied are mentioned, together with the expected effect of the interrelationships of those variables. Formulating hypotheses will be discussed in more detail in Chapter 3.

Stumbling Blocks

When problems in carrying out your research begin to look insurmountable and overwhelming, enlisting a colleague to work with you on the project can be an enormous help. My guess is that far more studies are completed that have two or more researchers than those that have one. When the inevitable problems get one person down, there is someone else who still has the energy to deal with them, enabling the project to move forward. Although it is heartily recommended that you work with a colleague, it may be more difficult to find a question that interests both of you and meets all the criteria.

Talking with others about your ideas for a research topic is an excellent idea, but be sure it does not prevent you from actually getting started. Everyone has his or her own "pet" theory about how the project should be carried out, what variables should be measured, and which book should be read to enlighten you on the topic. Listening to and acting on some of these ideas can be most helpful in shaping your research, but it will also present conflicting opinions. At some point, you must decide if you have had enough input from colleagues, family, and friends. At this point, the project must be designed and you must "go with it," or you will never get started. This does not mean that you cannot make minor changes as you go along, if compelling reasons arise.

WORKSHEETS

Jot down questions that have arisen from your clinical practice or discussions with your colleagues. Choose questions about which you are very curious and to which you would love to know the answer.

Look over your list and decide which question interests you the most. Rank your questions in order of fascination.

Write the number 1 question here:

Answer these questions about your chosen topic:

Why does it excite you?

Do you *really* want to know the answer? Why?

Is it a simple question, or does it have several parts? If so, list the parts:

Is it possible to do a "mini" study on this question, or on a part of it, to see if it is feasible?

Is there an obvious theory base for this question? If so, name it here:

Write a paragraph on the major points of the theory:

In your opinion, does this question address a significant problem? If so, answer the question "So what?" here:

What variables will you be studying? List them here:

At first glance, does it appear to you that you will be able to find a way to identify and measure those variables?

Take a stab at identifying types of measuring instruments for as many variables as possible:

Guess what resources you might need to study this question:

Time

Money

Equipment

Computer

Statistician

Fellow therapists

Other

What types of subjects will you need to study this question?

Are these people available to you?

Repeat this investigation process for your second identified question, and so on, until you find the most favorable. Remember that your question must be reasonable and researchable.

If you encounter what appear to be insolvable problems with each question, don't despair. This is probably because you are not yet familiar with the variety of methodological options available to you in the research process. Read on; in subsequent chapters you may find methods you can use to solve some of these problems.

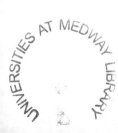

References

Burdett, R.G., Brown, K.E., & Fall, M.P. (1986). Reliability and validity of four instruments for measuring lumbar spine and pelvic positions. *Physical Therapy, 66*(5), 677–684.

Giles, M.G., & Clark-Wilson, J. (1988). The use of behavioral techniques in functional skills training after severe brain injury. *American Journal of Occupational Therapy, 42*(10), 658–665.

Konrad, K. (1994). Randomized, double blind, placebo-controlled study of ultrasonic treatment of the hands of rheumatoid arthritis patients. *European Journal of Physical Medicine and Rehabilitation, 4*(5), 155–157.

Loftus, S.K. (1989). *Two approaches to improving functional performance of a head injured adult: A replication.* Unpublished master's thesis, Tufts University, Medford, MA.

Lyons, J.L., & Morse, A.R. (1988). A therapeutic work program for head-injured adults. *American Journal of Occupational Therapy, 42*(6), 364–370.

Middlebrook, J.A. (1988). *The effect of functional movement patterns on hemodynamic responses in older individuals.* Unpublished master's thesis, Tufts University, Medford, MA.

Nelson, B.J. (1989). *Self-esteem and professionalism in female occupational therapists.* Unpublished master's thesis, Tufts University, Medford, MA.

Parker, H.J., & Chan, F. (1986). Stereotyping: Physical and occupational therapists characterize themselves and each other. *Physical Therapy, 66*(5), 668–672.

Rabideau, G. (1985). *Two approaches to improving the functional performance of a head injured adult.* Unpublished master's thesis, Tufts University, Medford, MA.

Stout, J. (1988). Planning playgrounds for children with disabilities. *American Journal of Occupational Therapy, 42*(10), 653–657.

Walker, M.L., Rothstein, J.M., Finncane, S.D., & Lamb, R.L. (1987). Relationship between lumbar lordosis, pelvic tilt, and abdominal muscle performance. *Physical Therapy, 67*(4), 512–516.

Additional Reading

Berger, R.M., & Patchner, M.A. (1988). *Planning for research: A guide for the helping professions.* No. 50 in the Sage Human Services Guide Series. Newbury Park, CA: Sage Publications.

Boer, M.R., & Gall, M.D. (1973). Selecting and defining a research problem. In Hubbard, A.W. (Ed.): *Research methods in health, physical education, and recreation.* Washington, DC: American Association of Health and Physical Education Research.

Depoy, E., & Gitlin, L.N. (1994). *Introduction to research: Multiple strategies for health and human services.* St. Louis, Mosby Year Book.

McLaren, H.M. (1973). So you want to conduct a clinical study. *Physiotherapy Canada, 25,* 219–224.

2

Reviewing the Literature

Now that you have explored some research questions and found one that you would like to answer, the next step is to review what has been written about your topic. Many novice researchers ask, "Why is this necessary? Why can't I just start in on my project?" There are several reasons:

1. Perhaps someone has already researched your question, or one just like it, and the answer is already published. You certainly would not want to waste your time and that of your subjects by repeating what has already been accomplished.

2. Perhaps someone has tried to investigate your question or one very similar and met with insurmountable problems (e.g., not finding a test instrument sensitive enough to measure one of the crucial variables or not being able to control enough of the intervening variables to have confidence in the results). This information would be useful before embarking on a similar project.

3. Perhaps someone has investigated your question or a very similar one, but not in the same way that you intend to investigate it. You may plan to use slightly different methods or subject characteristics. You would, however, want to benefit from the information that could be gleaned from the previous study.

4. Someone may have already studied one component of the topic, and you can build on that research, saving yourself time and energy.

5. You will wish to place your study in context with similar studies, so that the reader will know how to perceive your work.

6. It is a good idea to place the study within the theoretical base in which the topic falls (e.g., biomechanical or behavioral theory), again for the reader's benefit, as well as for your increased understanding of the topic.

7. It will be reassuring to find reasons in the literature to suggest why the study you propose will address the problem and how your study is capable of solving the problem or answering the question.

8. It is probable that while searching the literature, you will find evidence that will prompt you to change your question. It may need a different emphasis; you may decide to look for a correlational effect rather than a cause and effect; you may refine the sample; and so on.

9. There are strongly held impressions in any profession about various areas of practice, things with which most clinicians would agree. However, impressions are not good enough as the basis for research, and documentation of these beliefs through the literature is

---

Box 2–A

In studying the temporal adaptation of chronic psychiatric patients, therapists reviewed literature in the areas of use of time in the "normal" population and in the chronic psychiatric population, including the human drive to explore and to master the environment, purposeful activity and the productive use of time, the environment and demographics of people similar to those in the sample, and methods of measuring temporal adaptation.

---

always needed (see Walker, Rothstein, Finncane, & Lamb, 1987, cited in Box 1–A).

So you can see that a thorough review of written material on the proposed topic of study is essential if the researcher is to design a relevant, original, helpful, and timely research study. In addition to articles and books that pertain strictly to your chosen subject, it is important for you to read related material and to be well versed in the whole topic being studied. Some examples of such reading are given in Boxes 2–A, 2–B, and 2–C. From these examples you can see that breadth of reading is as important as depth of reading in preparing an effective research proposal.

How to Do a Literature Search

You are likely to find material relevant to your topic in journals, books, and govern-

---

Box 2–B

Another example would be the study on the effect of technological aids on the exploration behavior of adults with severe physical and cognitive impairments (Einis & Bailey, 1990). It was necessary to explore literature on the range of available technological aids, other populations using technological devices to improve exploration behavior, and the literature on exploration behavior per se.

Box 2–C

For a study in *Physical Therapy* regarding prosthetic use by elderly patients with dysvascular above-knee and through-knee amputations (Beckman & Axtell, 1987), the literature survey included statistics on the whole population, followed by those in the elderly population who are undergoing amputations; conditions commonly leading to amputations; review of the literature concerning whether or not to fit elderly amputee patients with a prosthesis, including such topics as costs versus benefits, physical limitations, motivation, training time, and the likelihood of patients using the prostheses upon discharge; and finally, an overview of studies describing functional outcomes of prosthetic use by elderly people. Additionally, the authors stated that they had limited their literature search to the past 15 years because of recent changes in surgical procedures and rehabilitation care and improvements in prostheses.

---

ment documents. Because much of the material relevant to occupational and physical therapy is found in the medical, social, educational, anthropological, psychological, and engineering sciences, the best place to locate material is in institutional libraries, such as those found in universities, postgraduate medical centers, training institutions for health care professionals, and other institutions of higher learning. Although this may cause problems for the clinician who is isolated geographically, frequently material can be found through the public library by using the services of interlibrary loan. However, this service may require a wait of several weeks before the receipt of material.

Once a well-stocked library and a helpful librarian have been located, it is necessary to decide whether you will do a hand search or a computer search of the literature. For a hand search, the following will be used:

1. The card catalog (usually computerized) and reference books to find relevant books on your topic

2. U.S. government documents for relevant government writings

3. The indexes and abstracts to find relevant articles in journals

The Card Catalog and Reference Books

There is a card (or computerized entry) in the library catalog for every item housed in the library, except for individual journal articles. There are three cards or entries for every item, filed by author's last name, by title, and by subject. If you are aware of leading authorities in your topic area, such as A. Jean Ayres in the area of sensory integrative techniques or Signe Brunnstrom in kinesiology, you can look up in the catalog or call up on the computer those authors' names and review titles to find appropriate books. If you are not aware of experts in the field, the subject index/database should be used to find appropriate books or journals. Unfortunately, searching for books by subject can be somewhat frustrating if you are not aware of how the subject terms are chosen. An important point to keep in mind is that the catalog/database makes use of a specialized vocabulary, sometimes quite unlike the terms used in everyday language. Here are some examples:

Everyday Language	*Catalog/Database Language*
Films, movies	Moving pictures
Abstract art	Art, abstract
Vietnam War	Vietnamese conflict

A two-volume list of Library of Congress subject headings is usually kept near the catalog, to assist one in finding the right words for a topic.

There are several reference books that might be helpful for investigating a topic in general rather than trying to find something specific to a health field. *Books in Print* and *British Books in Print* are huge tomes containing every book currently available. Each consists of four separate volumes, one each for authors, subjects, titles, and publishers. Incidentally, the 1995 to 1996 *Books in Print* lists occupational therapy as a subject and contains 165 entries. Physical therapy lists 197 entries. Other useful reference books are the *Annual Reviews,* which are published in specific content areas and which exist in such fields as psychology and physiology.

U.S. Government Documents

Select libraries around the country are depositories for U.S. government publications. This collection is arranged by the Superintendent of Documents' classification scheme and is updated monthly. It lists publications issued by all branches of the U.S. government, including congressional, department, and bureau publications. Issues are indexed in separate volumes for authors, titles/key words, subjects, and series or report titles. The type of documents likely to be useful to therapists include amendments to the Medicare law, Public Law 94-142 Equal Educational Opportunities, the Report of the President's Commission on Mental Health, and laws concerning Americans with disabilities and architectural barriers.

Journal Indexes and Abstracts

A hand search of hard copy indexes and abstracts requires that the subject terms be isolated unless the authors of specific articles are known. The volumes are organized by subject and sometimes by author, and are often bound 1 year at a time. It is necessary to define the subject being researched carefully in order to locate relevant articles because terminology can be specific to the field and can vary from field to field (e.g., one index may use the term "adolescent," whereas another uses "teen" or "teenager"). The following are the most useful hard copy indexes for therapists:

1. *Index Medicus,* which contains entries from the major medically related journals around the world (approximately 4680 of them) and which is updated monthly. Entries from the *American Journal of Occupational Therapy* and *Physical Therapy* are included in the *Complete Index Medicus.* However, the *American Journal of Occupational Therapy* is not included in the *Abridged Index Medicus,* so be sure to specify to the librarian which version you want. There is an accompanying volume of Medical Subject Headings to assist in locating subject terms.

2. Professional journals of the major health fields also have their own indexes. The *American Journal of Occupational Therapy* is indexed by subject and author and is cumulative from 1972 to 1983 and annual thereafter. *Physical Therapy* is also indexed by subject and author annually. These in-

dexes are generally available only in the libraries of universities with training programs in those specific professions.

3. The *Cumulative Index to Nursing and Allied Health Literature* lists more than 125 allied health journals, including occupational, physical, and speech therapy and 12 other rehabilitation disciplines. It includes related books, book chapters and audiovisuals, has a subject heading list, is updated monthly, and is available in yearly hard copy editions from 1956 to the present.

4. Three other indexes that are likely to be helpful for therapists are the *Resources in Education (RIE),* the *Current Index to Journals in Education (CIJE),* and the more recent *Exceptional Child Educational Resource (ECER).* The *RIE* abstracts educational research reports (from 1975) by subject, author, and institution, and most reports are available on microfilm. The *CIJE* and *ECER* abstract articles in education and education-related journals by subject, author, and journal content and are companions to the *RIE.* A thesaurus of terms accompanies these indexes.

5. *Psychological Abstracts* is an index that contains abstracts of books, journal articles, technical reports, and scientific documents concerning psychology. It started in its present form in 1927. It uses a classified arrangement with author and subject indexes and has cumulative indexes by year. A companion volume provides a thesaurus of psychological index terms. Figure 2–1 shows an example of what would be found in looking up the entry for cognitive ability. The major terms used for cognitive ability are "cognitive functioning" and "intellectual functioning," but the narrower terms "mathematical," "reading," "spatial," and "verbal" ability also are found. The book suggests that the reader may be interested in the related term "ability." The numbers are used for entering these terms on the computer, should one be doing a computer search.

6. *Sociological Abstracts* includes abstracts from some sociology books and from sociological and social science

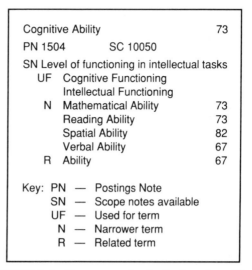

FIGURE 2–1 Thesaurus entry for the term "cognitive ability" in the *Psychological Abstracts.*

journals in various languages. There is a classified arrangement of abstracts with access by subject terms; however, some feel that the subject headings are poorly defined and thus find this index difficult to use.

7. *Dissertation Abstracts* can be another useful source of research studies and the hard copy can also be handsearched. One problem with using dissertations as reference material is that if you come across a study that is relevant to your project and decide that you would like to review the study in its entirety, you must either send away for a paper copy of the dissertation, which may cost from $20 to $35, or find a library that has microfilm copies of dissertations. However, the *Dissertation Abstracts* volumes themselves contain comprehensive abstracts of the studies, which may be sufficient for your purposes. The volumes are divided into two major categories: sciences/engineering and humanities/social sciences. Other indexes and abstracts useful for therapists are listed in Appendix A.

Because most indexes and abstracts are bound 1 year at a time, you need to look through several volumes of the same index, depending on how far back in time you wish to search. How far back to look is something for careful consideration. If the subject is rapidly developing and a great deal is currently being written about it (e.g., acquired immune deficiency syndrome [AIDS], the plight of the homeless, or Alzheimer's disease), then 2 to 5 years may be sufficient to give you a great deal of material on the most up-to-date thinking. If the subject has been developed over many years (topics such as the development of personal values or carpal tunnel syndrome) and has remained fairly stable in content since the original work, it may be wise to go back to the time of most plentiful writing on that topic, sometimes as many as 20 or 30 years, to find the classic works. If one or two articles or books are constantly referred to in more recent works, they are probably the classic and important writings related to that topic. It would be well to read them for a more thorough grasp of the topic.

Computer Searches

For speed and thoroughness, you may decide to conduct a computer search of the literature, requiring a facility that has that capability. University libraries, public libraries, and some medical facilities have access to on-line computer searches of journal indexes. The following are the major databases of interest to health professionals:

1. MEDLINE is the database derived from *Index Medicus* and provides access to more than half a million entries, recognizing some 13,000 subject headings. Medically oriented articles from occupational and physical therapy journals are included in MEDLINE. Again, some occupational therapy material is not contained in the abridged version. The volume of *Medical Subject Headings* contains codes for quicker computer searching.

2. CINAHL is the computerized version of the paper indexes of the same name and is also available on CD-ROM. The database features 200,000 records covering 1982 to the present. Therapy students and practitioners find this an extremely well-organized and useful database.

3. The Reliable Source for Occupational Therapy is a recent on-line information system with a bibliographic database called OT BibSys. OT BibSys is a comprehensive listing of literature and audiovisual material on occupational therapy together with some directly related literature in rehabilitation, education, psychiatry, psychology, health care delivery, and administration. Material is international, although less than 1 percent of it is in foreign languages. All of the actual material is contained in The Wilma L. West Library in Bethesda, Maryland. The earliest items date from the 1890s; however, literature is covered up to current material.

4. ERIC is the database of the Educational Resources Information Center and is formulated from the *RIE, CIJE,* and *ECER* paper indexes. There is an accompanying thesaurus of ERIC terms to make searching easier.

5. PsycINFO, derived from the *Psychological Abstracts* hard copy, uses a content classification scheme that divides the field of psychology into 16 major categories and 64 subcategories. It is a well-organized and popular computerized database.

If you have to pay for the time you spend on line, it is important to do some preparation before you actually get logged on to the computer. This entails having the research question well thought out and having the terms (sometimes called descriptors or key words) identified. The terms come from the thesaurus that accompanies each index (Box 2–D). If you cannot find the topic under one

---

Box 2–D

In a study on therapist attrition from occupational therapy (Bailey, 1990), terms were identified by the researcher as "employee turnover," "personnel turnover," "career mobility," "job involvement," "career change," "tenure," and "occupational aspirations." These terms were found in the thesauruses accompanying the *Index Medicus* and the *Psychological Abstracts.* As mentioned previously, different indexes and abstracts use different terms to identify similar subjects. For example, one index used the term "employee turnover," whereas another used "personnel turnover."

heading, try finding it under another. It is quicker to look through the list of terms in the accompanying thesaurus than to rack your brain for possible alternative words.

There is quite a range of costs for computer searches, depending on the database used and the facility where the search is performed. Sometimes there is a special price offer for use of specific databases during a given week, which will cut the cost dramatically (Boxes 2–E and 2–F).

Selecting the database to be searched (e.g., MEDLINE or ERIC) will depend on which field you think will contain material relevant to your project, such as medicine, sociology, or education. Once the terms are entered, the computer will scan all the material in that database for articles keyed in with those words for as far back as you wish. Terms can be crossed with one another, so that you receive only those articles keyed in with both

terms (e.g., arthritis and joint protection). You can ask for three or four terms to be listed for each article but are likely to get very few responses if you are this specific. It is often simpler and more cost effective to have only titles printed out at first, so that the items that appear most promising can be selected before asking for an abstract.

You will be paying for the amount of time the computer is actually on line—that is, searching and producing material. Thus, it is well to be prepared ahead and not to be thinking out terms and alternative strategies while logged on to the computer. If you are not paying for the search, these considerations need not constrain you, of course, and people tend to spend many an hour happily scanning through databases in their quest for relevant material. Some find it addictive and have a difficult time knowing when to stop!

Locating Articles and Books

Once a list of articles and books has been generated from the hard copy or computer search, the abstracts need to be reviewed to see if they appear relevant to the study. You must then go to the book stacks, the periodical room, or the government documents depository to find the items. If an article is only peripherally related to your topic, you can jot down the relevant points together with the complete reference while you are in the li-

---

Box 2–F

In 1992, a search on schizophrenic patients' use of time cost $32 in total and yielded 204 titles, 27 of which were actually related to the topic. This search was conducted on MED-LINE and PsycINFO and took 8 minutes logged on to the computer. A search on the same topic in the *Mental Health Abstracts* produced six articles, only one of which was relevant, for a cost of $2.40. A final search of this subject in the *Sociological Abstracts* cost $6.70 and produced an additional eight articles, of which two were useful. Preparation for the search on schizophrenic patients' use of time was about 1 hour because this was a difficult subject to pin down.

Box 2–E

The search on attrition described in Box 2–D was conducted on the MEDLINE, PsycINFO, and ERIC databases in 1989. The MEDLINE search took 5 minutes on line and cost $3.75. Using the terms "occupational and physical therapists," "social workers," "personnel turnover," and "career mobility," 84 titles were generated, of which 10 looked relevant and were printed with abstracts. Of these 10 articles, three were located, and one was eventually used in the publication. In the PsycINFO search on the same topic, the terms "occupational, physical, and speech therapists;" "social workers;" "psychologists;" "nurses;" "mobility;" "tenure;" "employee turnover;" "career change;" and "job involvement" were used. The search took 5.25 minutes on line, cost $5.58, and generated 82 titles. Nineteen of those titles appeared relevant and were abstracted. Of these, 15 were located, and five were actually used in the article. In the ERIC search, the terms "occupational, physical, and speech therapists;" "social workers;" "nurses;" "turnover;" "career change;" and "occupational mobility" were used to generate 57 titles. The relevant 15 were abstracted, seven were located, and four were eventually used. This search took 2.5 minutes on line and cost $3.02. Preparation for the search by finding useful terms in the thesauruses, took about 30 minutes.

brary. However, it will probably be preferable to make copies of the most pertinent articles or to check out the most relevant books so that it is possible to study them at your leisure.

Organizing the Material

Some people feel comfortable organizing their literature finds directly on their computers, and there are now several programs that make this a simpler task. However, many of us still find index cards useful in keeping information manageable and retrievable. Many people find the 5″ × 8″ size most useful. Take a package of these cards to the library and jot down information from the peripheral articles and books directly on the cards, a separate card per article or book. Cards on the more important or complicated articles of which you made copies can be completed at your convenience at home. Arrange the information in the same way on each card. Figures 2–2 and 2–3 illustrate how cards may be completed.

It is helpful to add at the top of the card the more specific subject area within the general research topic, such as those mentioned in Box 2–G. Cards can then be grouped by subject areas, which will make recording the material easier. When more than one subject area is mentioned in an article or book, it is possible to cross-reference and to have a card in each section for that article or book. At the end of the most useful articles, the ones most

relevant to the topic, be sure to peruse the reference lists. These can be a most useful source of additional reading.

Those who prefer to organize the information from their literature search directly on the computer may choose to use a simple coding program to cross-reference materials. This is an efficient way to organize material because the file can eventually be used to construct the actual literature review section of the article. The only time it may be inconvenient to work directly on a computer is when you are in the library taking notes on articles that are only peripherally related to your topic.

As soon as you have read and prepared cards or computerized notes on all the articles and books, you are ready to write the review. Start by reviewing the subject headings at the top of the index cards and putting them in a logical sequence (Box 2–H). In this way, the reader is carried through a progression of topics pertinent to the study. By the end of the literature review, the reader should understand why the project was being undertaken.

> Berger, R.M. & Patchner, M.A.
> Planning for research: A guide for the helping professions.
> #50 in Sage Human Services Guide Series.
> Newbury Park, CA: Sage Publications   1988
> A comprehensive description of the planning stages for a research project:
>   Finding the question
>   Stating the purpose
>   Stating the significance
>   Deciding on the design

FIGURE 2–3   Sample card completed for a book.

> Decision to fit the elderly with prostheses
> Beckman, C.E. & Axtell, L.A.
> Prosthetic use in elderly patients with dysvascular above-knee and through-knee amputations.
> Physical Therapy, 67(10), 1510-1516   1987
> Contains a thorough review of literature on whether to fit the elderly with prostheses
> Includes:
>   Costs versus benefits
>   Physical limitations
>   Motivation
>   Training time
>   Likelihood of patient using the prosthesis
> Plus, an overview of studies describing functional outcomes of prosthetic use by elderly.

FIGURE 2–2   Sample card completed for an article.

> **Box 2–G**
>
> If a researcher were trying to identify factors related to prosthetic candidacy in elderly people, likely subject headings might include "Types of prostheses," "Incidence and causes of amputation in elderly people," "Decision to fit the elderly patient with prosthesis," "Physical limitations and motivation factors," "Costs versus benefits," "Training procedures," and "Functional outcomes."

Box 2-H

If you were writing the review of the study concerning prostheses mentioned earlier, it would be logical to order the subjects in the following way:

1. Causes and incidence of amputation in elderly people
2. Types of prostheses
3. Decision to fit the elderly patient with a prosthesis
4. Costs versus benefits
5. Physical limitations and motivation
6. Training procedures
7. Functional outcomes

Next, concentrate on one group of cards at a time. Look for common themes that run through the various authors' papers, and make a note of the themes on a separate card. If a sole author makes a point you would like to include, mark it. Now look at these themes and important points. Do they fall into a logical sequence? Do they flow from one to the other, making the progression of ideas you want to convey to the reader? Write these ideas down in sequence and see if any steps are left out. If so, add them in your own words. When you are satisfied that you have stated the important issues about this topic in a clear, concise manner, add the authors' names whose ideas you have cited, together with the year of publication, in parentheses, after each idea. You are now ready to move on to the next major subject area of your literature review and to repeat the process.

It is a real challenge to write a literature review well. Try to avoid starting every sentence with "Smith (1988) says . . ." or "Brown (1989) feels that. . . ." Read through some literature sections in published articles to get some ideas for imaginative ways to start sentences and ways to incorporate several authors' ideas and findings in one or two sentences. There are space constraints in journals, so you will not be able to devote many paragraphs to the literature summary. In fact, you will probably read many more articles and books than you will be able to include. Restrict yourself to the most important and convincing work on the points you wish to make. Refer to the articles listed in Appendix B for well-written literature reviews.

The format used to cite references is most specific, and each journal has a required format. Styles will be addressed in detail in a later chapter of this book in the section on publishing an article.

How Long Should the Literature Review Be?

The length of a literature review varies greatly, depending on the type of document being produced. For the student writing a thesis, the literature review should be comprehensive and should demonstrate that all literature relevant to the study has been examined and that the most important material has been analyzed. All literature should be examined that explains the problem, suggests why your study is appropriate to it, describes your study's capability for solving the problem, and relates to any other studies that have attempted to solve the problem. Consequently, a thesis literature review may typically run from 20 to 40 pages.

The literature review for a journal article, on the other hand, tends to be brief and to the point. This is because space constraints are imposed by journal editors, and there is often a requirement that an entire article be kept within five to seven printed pages. The *Publication Manual of the American Psychological Association* (1994) offers helpful guidelines for what to include in the background or literature review section of a journal article (Box 2–I).

Completing the literature review is a major step in the right direction. It does not have to be written in final form at this stage of the project, of course, but it is certainly a potential hurdle, and it is a good idea to get the writing accomplished as soon as possible. You are now ready to refine your research question and to develop the background material for your study, based on what you have read.

Stumbling Blocks

By including all the reference information immediately as you prepare index cards, you will save yourself time and trouble when you

Box 2–1

"Discuss the literature but do not include an exhaustive historical review. Assume that the reader has knowledge in the field for which you are writing and does not require a complete digest. A scholarly review of earlier work provides an appropriate history and recognizes the priority of the work of others. Citation of and specific credit to relevant earlier works is part of the author's scientific and scholarly responsibility. It is essential for the growth of cumulative science. At the same time, cite and reference only works pertinent to the specific issue and not works of only tangential or general significance. If you summarize earlier works, avoid nonessential details; instead, emphasize pertinent findings, relevant methodological issues, and major conclusions. Refer the reader to general surveys or reviews of the topic if they are available.

"Demonstrate the logical continuity between previous and present work. Develop the problem with enough breadth and clarity to make it generally understood by as wide a professional audience as possible. Do not let the goal of brevity mislead you into writing a statement intelligible only to the specialist."

(American Psychological Association, 1994, pp. 11–12.)

What are the major factors contributing to attrition from occupational therapy?
    Articles on attrition from nursing, physical therapy, speech and audiology, social work, psychology, other health care fields.
Possible factors:
    Poor pay
    Stress on the job
    Lack of career mobility
    Lack of part-time work
    No job available in geographic area
    Lack of autonomy in practice

FIGURE 2–4   Sample card for use when searching the literature.

may be straying too far afield or have forgotten the major issues, I glance at this card and it gets me back on track.

If during a computer search you cannot find any sources or very few sources relevant to your topic, there are several possibilities for what may be happening:

1. Your topic does not make sense. No one has written in this area because it is not logical and there is nothing there to research.

2. You are looking in the wrong database (e.g., you are looking in medicine and should be looking in vocational services).

3. You have chosen virgin territory; nothing has been done in your area. That is very exciting—go ahead!

Because many people find writing literature reviews a tiresome task and one that they put off as long as possible, promptness is definitely the best policy and possibly the only policy that will ensure the completion of the article. Besides, it is easier to write a review with the material fresh in one's mind and while inspiration is still present. I have encountered many budding authors whose only stumbling block to having an article completed was the literature review. Usually the researcher had done all the reading and taken all the notes but could not quite get around to writing the review.

are ready to organize the reference list. This is the moment when it is common to find that you have:

- Lost the article
- Returned the book
- Loaned the article to someone else
- Spilled coffee on the volume number

When you are immersed in piles of journals or computer printouts, it is common to lose sight of the topics being sought and to get sidetracked into other interesting areas. I find it helpful to have in front of me a card containing my research question and a list of the major areas for which I am searching, as illustrated in Figure 2–4. When I feel as if I

WORKSHEETS

Locate a convenient library.

Visit the library and familiarize yourself with the following:

> Card catalog
> Reference librarian
> Reference section
> Periodical room
> List of periodicals/journals stocked by that library
> Location of copying machines
> Location of nearest depository of government documents

Write your research question and main subject areas on an index card, as well as here:

Decide if you wish to do a hand search or a computer search:

_____ Hand Search   _____ Computer Search

HAND SEARCH

If you decide on a hand search, decide which indexes and abstracts are the most appropriate for your subject (a conversation with the reference librarian might be helpful).

List the indexes and abstracts you plan to use:

COMPUTER SEARCH

If you decide on a computer search, decide on the database most appropriate for your subjects (discuss with the librarian) and peruse the thesaurus for terms.

Database: *Database:*

Terms: Terms:

If you do not have access to database searching yourself but must go through a librarian:

Discuss the search with the librarian (costs, methods of payment, if you can search alone, mailing time if the librarian will be doing the search for you) and arrange a time for the search.

When the search has been carried out, review the list of titles and abstracts generated by the computer and check off those you wish to locate.

FOR HAND OR COMPUTER SEARCH

Find books, articles, or dissertation abstracts and complete index cards on peripheral subjects at the library.

Make copies of important articles or abstracts. Take these home, together with books you need.

Complete index cards on all data sources, or enter information on a computer.

Decide on specific subject areas. List here:

Subject A:

B:

C:

D:

E:

Group index cards according to specific subject areas.

Store cards in a safe place until you are ready to write your literature review.

Write your literature review as soon as you have located and read all the items on your literature search list.

References

American Psychological Association. (1994). *Publication manual of the American Psychological Association* (4th ed.). Washington, DC: Author.

Bailey, D.M. (1990). Reasons for attrition from occupational therapy. *American Journal of Occupational Therapy, 44*(1), 23–29.

Beckman, C.E., & Axtell, L.A. (1987). Prosthetic use in elderly patients with dysvascular above-knee and through-knee amputations. *Physical Therapy, 67*(10), 1510–1516.

Einis, L.P., & Bailey, D.M. (1990). Case Report—The use of powered leisure and communication devices in a switch training program. *American Journal of Occupational Therapy, 44*(12), 931–934.

Walker, M.L., Rothstein, J.M., Finncane, S.D., & Lamb, R.L. (1987). Relationship between lumbar lordosis, pelvic tilt, and abdominal muscle performance. *Physical Therapy, 67*(4), 512–516.

Additional Reading

Berger, R.M., & Patchner, M.A. (1988). *Planning for research: A guide for the helping professions.* No. 50 in Sage Human Services Guide Series. Newbury Park, CA: Sage Publications.

Currier, D.P. (1984). Chapter 3: Literature review. In *Elements of research in physical therapy* (pp. 34–50). Baltimore: Williams & Wilkins.

Hall, M. (1987). Unlocking information technology. *American Journal of Occupational Therapy, 41*(11), 722–725.

Harter, S.P. (1986). *Online information retrieval: Concepts, principles and techniques.* Orlando, FL: Academic Press.

Haynes, R.B. (1986). How to keep up with the medical literature: Part IV. How to store and retrieve articles worth keeping. *Annals of Internal Medicine, 105,* 978–984.

Marshall, J.G. (1985). How to choose the online medical database that's right for you. *Canadian Medical Association Journal, 134,* 634–640.

McCarthy, S. (1988). *Personal filing systems: Creating information retrieval systems on microcomputers.* Chicago: Medical Library Association.

Oyster, C.K., Hanten, W.P., & Llorens, L.A. (1987). Chapter 1: Foundations of health science research. In *Introduction to research: A guide for the health science professional* (pp. 1–16). Philadelphia: J.B. Lippincott.

Payton, O.D. (1994). Chapter 10: The library as a tool. In *Research: The validation of clinical practice,* (3rd ed.). (pp. 201–216). Philadelphia: F.A. Davis.

Stein, F., & Cutler, S.K. (1996). Chapter 5: Review of the literature. In *Clinical Research in Allied Health and Special Education* (pp. 151–173). San Diego, CA: Singular Publishing Group, Inc.

Williams, R., Baker, L., & Marshall, J. (1992). *Information searching in health care.* Thorofare, NJ: Slack.

3

Refining the Question and Developing the Background

As a way of refining the research question and developing the background, I find it helpful to start writing about the project at this juncture. Information from the literature search is still fresh in my mind, and most of the literature findings will be incorporated into the early parts of the written article. Writing the initial sections as work progresses also makes preparation for publication easier when that time comes.

Problem

The heart of the study is the problem statement, from which all other elements will flow. This is the reason for undertaking the study; it is the problem or question that caught your interest in the first place—the issue you wanted to solve in your clinical practice. After reviewing what has been written about the topic, you should be able to write about the problem comprehensively. Is it a problem for many clinicians/educators/administrators? Have others identified it and tried to do something about it? Were their attempts successful or unsuccessful? What will you do differently in your attempt to solve the problem? Or are you merely trying to gather more data about it? (Box 3–A)

We are usually driven to action such as carrying out research by identifying something that is wrong or something that needs attention, or by old ideas or methods that are no longer adequate. The paragraph stating the problem you intend to address should be brief and to the point. Tell the reader what is wrong, what has failed, what is missing, what current ideas are presumed true that you wish to challenge, or what program needs to be scrutinized. Write two or three sentences about the problem, and read it to a colleague. If he or she misses the point, try again. Listen to yourself as you read. Is this really the problem you want to do something about? (Box 3–B)

Background

Once you are satisfied with the wording of the problem, you are ready to address the background of your study. The background answers the questions, "Why is this problem of concern?" "Why is it of theoretical interest?" Based on your reading, you should mention why other people think the problem is important and needs work. Opinion as well as fact can be given in the background material when it relates to the importance of the

Box 3-A

Moncur states the underlying problem for her study:

A consensus currently exists among rheumatologists. . . and physical therapists that physical therapy should be an integral part of the treatment program of the patient with arthritis. The ability of the physical therapist to provide appropriate care to those who suffer with this group of chronic diseases has been questioned recently. In 1982, the National Arthritis Advisory Board (NAAB) reported that, because of severe budgetary restraints, the education of health care professionals in rheumatology was limited severely. The NAAB suggested that nursing and allied health professionals do not have adequate rheumatology training programs and depend on an informal process in clinical practice to learn to treat patients with arthritis.

Moncur talks of others' attempts to determine the adequacy of classroom and clinical exposure of physical therapists to rheumatology, then states that her approach to the problem is "to investigate what skills physical therapists and [rheumatologists] believe an entry-level physical therapist should have to treat [arthritis] patients."

(Moncur, 1987, p. 331)

Box 3-B

"Occupational therapists and health administrators have long been concerned about the shortage of occupational therapists. . . . Recently, the shortage has become critical, . . . and there is increasing pressure to boost the number of therapists practicing in the field. . . .

"The attrition of occupational therapists from the work force is a major contributor to the shortage, and retention is of primary importance in keeping a viable number of therapists practicing. . . .

"The purpose of the present study was to identify why occupational therapists are leaving the field, so that we can take the necessary steps to change certain conditions that affect occupational tenure."

(Bailey, 1990; p. 23)

problem (e.g., a certain senator may believe that a national health scheme is of primary importance; you can quote him or her if it lends credence to your problem statement).

In preparing this section of your article for publication, try to make it interesting to readers. It should capture their attention and leave them agreeing that the problem is important and worthy of investigation. If readers are not captivated by this section, they may not read any further.

If, during your literature search in government publications, you found general statistics related to your topic, now is the time to use them. More often than not, these types of data offer additional background information about the problem but do not have direct bearing on the specific clinical situation under investigation. For example, if the central problem concerns insufficient subsidized health care for the poor, statistics on how many poor people there are in the United States, and the dollar amount of the poverty line as defined by the government, may be included in the background. However, the study itself might be concerned specifically with Medicaid as a partial solution to the problem. In another example, you might be studying the specific issue of falls experienced by elderly persons that result in fractured femurs. In this case, it would be useful to mention the number of falls by elderly persons each year, the cost of medical treatment for these traumatic events, and the percentage of elders who are unable to return to their homes as a result of the fall.

Purpose

A clear statement of the purpose of the study should follow the background material.

Box 3-C

The purpose of Keating, Matyas, and Bach's study was stated clearly in the abstract:

The aim of this study was to evaluate whether postgraduate physical therapy students studying manipulation could learn to accurately produce specific forces during palpation of an intervertebral joint.

(Keating, Matyas, & Bach, 1993, p. 38)

Box 3-D

In a study of shoulder pain and subluxation after stroke, Zorowitz and colleagues stated their purpose thus:

> The present study was conducted to determine whether shoulder pain after stroke is related to shoulder subluxation, age, limitations in shoulder range of motion, and severity of upper extremity motor impairment. The results may clarify not only the etiologies, but also possible treatment rationales of shoulder pain after stroke.

(Zorowitz, Hughes, Idank, Ikai, & Johnston, 1996, p. 195)

Some editors prefer that the purpose be nearer the beginning of the article, in which case you can insert it immediately after the problem statement and before the background. The purpose should tell the reader what you hope to accomplish regarding the problem by carrying out your study. Be clear about this by starting the sentence, "The purpose of the research was. . . ." Then describe your intentions. The purposes of various studies are illustrated in Boxes 3–C, 3–D, 3–E, and 3–F. At this point in your article, the reader should be able to understand what you intend to accomplish with your project and will later be able to judge

---

Box 3-E

Williams, Agho, and Holm conducted a survey on the perceptions of computer literacy among occupational therapy students. The purpose of their study was to:

> (a) describe entry-level occupational therapy students' opinions about computer technology, (b) compare students' perceptions of their current and desired knowledge of computer applications in occupational therapy, and (c) examine the relationship among opinions about computer technology, current and desired knowledge of computer applications, and the number of semesters of computer technology courses completed (i.e., level of computer literacy).

(Williams, Agho, & Holm, 1996, p. 218)

Box 3-F

A review of the literature regarding perceptual-motor deficits in alcoholic patients has its purpose stated clearly in the beginning of the article:

> A literature search on perceptual-motor dysfunction in alcohol abusers was conducted for the following reasons: (a) to determine what evidence links alcohol abuse with perceptual-motor dysfunction, (b) to examine the possibility that perceptual-motor function can be improved through rehabilitation programs for alcoholics, and (c) to determine whether perceptual-motor dysfunction of alcohol abusers is related to deficits in activities of daily living and is therefore relevant to occupational therapists.

(Van Deusen, 1989, p. 384)

---

whether your methodology is likely to achieve it.

Significance

Another section of the article that can be written as a result of the literature review is the significance of the study. The significance elaborates on what your study will do to affect the problem and why your study is important. It tells what makes your purpose worth pursuing. There are many ways to address a problem—why did you choose your particular purpose? This section will justify your search. For example, there may be other studies addressing the issue, but you have a different purpose in mind (e.g., a group of individuals may have been overlooked by other studies, and you wish to address their needs). The significance paragraph says that your study is appropriate for the research problem and that some important benefits will occur if you do it. This is the answer to the question, "So what?" It gives you the chance to provide a persuasive, rational response (Box 3–G).

In writing these four sections, the problem, background, purpose, and significance, you have engaged in expansive thinking. Ideas have been global and far-reaching. Now is a good time to pull back into microscopic thinking and ask yourself, "How

---

Box 3–G

In the study of physical therapists' competence to treat arthritic patients mentioned in Box 3–A, the author feels that her study is significant because:

> The competencies identified in this study should assist academic planners in defining clearly their curricula and in preparing the entry-level physical therapist to treat patients with rheumatic disease. Clinicians may use these competencies to measure their ability to manage treatment of their patients who suffer from arthritis.

(Moncur, 1987, p. 338)

Box 3–H

Gaebler and Hanzlik state that

> the purpose of the . . . study was to provide more rigorous methodological control related to the healthy preterm infants' experience and maturation while studying the effects of stroking and perioral and intraoral stimulation on these infants.

The researchers' hypotheses were that

infants in the experimental group, compared with infants in the control group, would

1. participate in more nipple and partial nipple feeds during the course of their hospitalization
2. score higher on the Revised-Neonatal Oral Motor Assessment Scale (R-NOMAS) on the 3rd and 5th days of testing relative to their initial score
3. be discharged earlier from the hospital
4. demonstrate a greater average nutritive intake during the first 5 min of tested feedings on the 3rd and 5th days.

(Gaebler & Hanzlik, 1996, pp. 185–186)

---

would I go about achieving all this? Is it feasible?" This will give you a glimpse at methodology, the reality of how you will accomplish your purpose. Different methods for conducting studies are discussed in later chapters.

Research Question or Hypothesis

As a result of the writing that has been done so far, the original research question or hypothesis should have become clearer. This is the time to refine and reshape it. For example, what may have started out as the global question, "What causes therapists to leave physical therapy?" now becomes the hypothesis, "Physical therapists are leaving their practice because of disillusionment with the field, low pay, and lack of promotional opportunities." Rework your hypothesis until it contains all the variables you wish to study and puts them in a relationship with one another that is supported by the literature. They may have a cause-and-effect relationship; that is, one variable causes something else to happen. Or they may merely be correlated; that is, if one happens, the other is more (or less) likely to happen in its presence. Boxes 3–H, 3–I, and 3–J show some examples of hypotheses.

You will note that the example in Box 3–H takes a positive approach to the hypothesis, stating that there will be a difference between the infants in the experimental and control groups in terms of their feeding abil-

ities. This is known as a directional hypothesis. The last two studies, however, use the null hypotheses or nondirectional format, stating that there will be no connection between grip strength and hand function, and so on, and that there will be no difference

---

Box 3–I

Ball's thesis investigated pinch and grip strength related to performance on a specific hand function test. He tested the null hypotheses:

1. There is no significant correlation between grip strength and hand function in the normal population.
2. There is no significant correlation between pinch strength (lateral, 2 point tip, 3 point tip, 2 point pad, 3 point pad) and hand function in the normal population.
3. Dominant hands will have a different pattern of correlation between strength and function than nondominant hands.

(Ball, 1986, p. iii)

Box 3–J

A study to examine the effort made by subjects engaged in purposeful and nonpurposeful activities tested the following null hypotheses:

That there would be no significant difference between jumping with a rope and jumping without a rope on each of the following dependent variables:

- pulse rate increase from baseline to cessation of jumping,
- duration of jumping,
- ratings on each of the three factors of the Osgood Semantic Differential,
- activity preference.

(Bloch, Smith, & Nelson, 1989, p. 27)

---

between jumping with a rope and jumping without a rope on certain characteristics. Whether you choose to pose your hypothesis in the directional or nondirectional format will depend on your clinical experience and the outcome of the literature review. If most of the material leaned in a specific direction, it would be appropriate to frame your hypothesis in that direction. If the material was noncomittal, it would be appropriate to use a null hypothesis.

Whether the hypothesis is directional or of the null type will have implications for the type of statistics used in the data analysis.

For example, if you are comparing two statistically different variables such as measurements of grip strength and hand function with a *t* test, a null hypothesis would indicate that you should use a two-tail test of significance, whereas a directional hypothesis would indicate that you should use a one-tail test of significance. This concept is discussed in greater detail in Chapter 8.

When you feel pleased with your hypothesis, go back to Chapter 1 and review the items that make a question realistic and researchable, to be sure that yours still meets the criteria. Perhaps you will find that you now need different resources or a more refined subject pool. Rework the appropriate sections of the Chapter 1 worksheets.

Stumbling Blocks

It is quite common for the researcher to confuse the problem, purpose, and significance of a study. Remember:

- The *problem* is the larger issue that others have tried to do something about.
- The *purpose* is what you hope to accomplish as a result of your small contribution to the larger problem.
- The *significance* is the importance of your particular study and what it will do to help solve the larger problem. It is the "So what?" of the study.

PROBLEM STATEMENT

What is the general topic area of your project?

What is the specific problem you plan to address?

- Is there something wrong?
- Does something need attention?
- Is something missing?
- Do old ideas need revising?
- Do old methods need revising?
- Has something failed?
- Is there a program that needs revising?

Relate your problem statement to a colleague.

Did he or she understand it?

Is this really the problem you want to do something about?

BACKGROUND

Look at your problem statement:

Give at least three reasons why your problem is important and valid—to you, to society, to your profession.

    1.

    2.

    3.

Specify at least two concrete examples of the problem:

    1.

    2.

To what public statistics, political trends, or theoretical controversy does your study relate?

PURPOSE

What do you hope to accomplish regarding the problem by carrying out your project?

Will you:

- Change something?
- Understand something?
- Interpret something differently?

Write the purpose of your study here:

Read through your purpose. Can the reader now understand what you intend to accomplish through your project? How you are going to help solve the problem?

If doubtful, restate your purpose, beginning:

"The purpose of this study is. . . ."

SIGNIFICANCE

Why is your study important? To whom is it important other than yourself? (Note that here you do not deal with the importance of the problem, but rather with the importance of the study.)

What can happen that will be beneficial if the study is done?

What might happen if it is not done?

Write the significance section here:

Place yourself in the position of responding to someone who asks you, "So what?" about your project. What would be your persuasive, rational response?

RESEARCH QUESTION OR HYPOTHESIS DEVELOPMENT

Write your original research question here.

In searching the literature, did you find:

      A. _____ A great deal directly related to your topic?

      B. _____ Very little directly related to your topic?

      C. _____ Mostly material peripheral to the topic?

      D. _____ Nothing much at all related to the topic?

If your answer was B, C, or D, you may want to leave your topic framed as a research question. You will probably be setting the groundwork for your topic, rather than adding to an established body of knowledge.

Develop your research question, adding the variables that have surfaced during your literature search and discussions with colleagues.

If your answer was A, make a judgment about whether or not there was a "direction" for most of the literature. State the direction here.

If the answer is "yes," then write a directional hypothesis (it might help to write a complete research question first, then convert it to hypothesis/statement form).

If the answer is "no," then write a nondirectional hypothesis.

References

Bailey, D.M. (1990). Reasons for attrition from occupational therapy. *American Journal of Occupational Therapy, 44*(1), 23–29.

Ball, J.H. (1986). *Pinch and grip strength related to performance on the Jebsen Hand Function Test.* Unpublished master's thesis, Tufts University, Medford, MA.

Bloch, M., Smith, D., & Nelson, D. (1989). Heart rate, activity, duration, and affect in added-purpose versus single-purpose jumping activities. *American Journal of Occupational Therapy, 43*(1), 25–30.

Gaebler, C., & Hanzlik, J. (1996). The effects of a pre-feeding stimulation program on preterm infants. *American Journal of Occupational Therapy, 50*(3), 184–192.

Keating, J., Matyas, T., & Bach, T. (1993). The effect of training on physical therapists' ability to apply specified forces of palpation. *Physical Therapy, 73*(1), 38–46.

Moncur, C. (1987). Perceptions of physical therapy competencies in rheumatology. *Physical Therapy, 67*(3), 331–339.

Van Deusen, J. (1989). Alcohol abuse and perceptual-motor dysfunction: The occupational therapist's role. *American Journal of Occupational Therapy, 43*(6), 384–390.

Williams, A., Agho, A., & Holm, M. (1996). Perceptions of computer literacy among occupational therapy students. *American Journal of Occupational Therapy, 50*(3), 217–222.

Zorowitz, R., Hughes, M., Idank, D., Ikai, T., & Johnston, M. (1996). Shoulder pain and subluxation after stroke: Correlation or coincidence? *American Journal of Occupational Therapy, 50*(3), 194–201.

Additional Reading

Berger, R.M., & Patchner, M.A. (1988). *Planning for research: A guide for the helping professions.* No. 50 in the Sage Human Service Guide Series. Newbury Park, CA: Sage Publications.

Marshall, C., & Rossman, G.B. (1989). *Designing qualitative research.* Newbury Park, CA: Sage Publications.

4

Choosing a Research Method

You are now ready to think about the method that will be used in your research project; that is, what design you will use to answer the question you have posed. First, you must decide whether to use a qualitative or a quantitative research design. In order to make this decision, you must understand the underpinnings of each type of research.

It is generally believed that we can adopt one of two views of the world and our surroundings: that of a positivist or that of a relativist. As a way of understanding the natural sciences, scientists search for universal laws, or the "truth"; these are the positivists. Those who studied the social sciences, however, soon came to terms with the fact that there are very few common experiences among people and that a fluid, unstructured approach is necessary to understand society and individual relationships. Knowledge, in this case, is based on how the individual perceives, experiences, and understands his or her world. Scientists holding this opinion view the world in a relativistic way, asserting that there is no one "truth," but rather that there are many ways to understand people and their culture. Traditionally accepted quantitative research methods are an outcome of positivist attitudes, whereas relativist predilections have led to the development of qualitative methods.

From this proposition, it is a short step to understanding how the goals of quantitative and qualitative research will be different. The goal of the quantitative researcher is to answer a specific research question by showing statistical evidence that the data may be addressed in a particular way. Qualitative researchers try to verify or generate descriptive theory that is grounded in the data gleaned from the investigation. To achieve these goals, the two types of researchers start out in different ways. The quantitative investigator begins the study with a theory and very specific hypotheses that address one defined issue, whereas the qualitative investigator begins with research questions that may be vague and general within a study that addresses a broad topic. The questions usually change throughout the qualitative study process and the project ends by posing some specific hypotheses and grounded theory. The example in Box 4–A will help distinguish the two approaches.

The phenomena that can appropriately be studied using these two styles of research are quite different. In a study using qualitative methods, the data can be amorphous and difficult or impossible to quantify or measure. Qualitative methods lend themselves to the study of individuals or small groups of subjects; issues are typically judged from an emic, or insider's, point of view. With quantitative methods, on the other hand, data are more tangible and easier to measure; the researcher can study large groups of subjects

---

Box 4–A

Three groups of occupational therapy students were recently asked to design a study that would investigate the research question: Are therapists losing the leisure component from their treatment domains (the domains being activities of daily living, work/play, and leisure)?

One group felt that an answer could be found by asking experienced therapists to complete a quantitative survey giving percentage of treatment time spent on leisure along with some other quantitative measures. They asked therapists to respond with information about current practice and about their practice 5 years ago. They set out to answer the research question with the "truth."

A second group elected to garner opinions from therapists regarding the whole area of leisure and its use within the practice of occupational therapy. These individuals felt that it was important to investigate the whole notion of the role of leisure in treatment and that they could generate enough information to allow them to make some substantiated guesses about whether leisure was being used less in recent years. In other words, they felt that answering the assigned research question was less important than gaining sufficient data on the general topic to allow them to propose informed hypotheses.

The third group chose a mixed approach, searching treatment records for numerical data with which to answer the question, as well as interviewing selected therapists so that they could augment their data with anecdotal material. They felt it was impossible to answer the research question meaningfully with empirical methods. Nonetheless, they tried to do just that while hedging their bets with additional qualitative data.

(or sets of data) and is viewing issues from an etic, or outsider's, point of view.

Depoy and Gitlin (1994) have proposed that naturalistic (qualitative) and experimental (quantitative) designs can each be viewed on a separate continuum. The placement of a study on the naturalistic continuum would depend on the degree to which the design

> . . . involves the personal "essence" experience, and insights of the investigator, the extent to which individual "experience" vs. patterns of human experience is sought, and the extent to which the investigator imposes structure in the data collection and analytic processes. (p. 21)

An experimental study's placement on the quantitative continuum would depend on the degree of control and variable manipulation and the extent of structure imposed by the investigator.

Although I have presented the two styles of research as if they were independent, the reality is that designs may be integrated and many research projects employ a combination of both designs. Some of the reasons to take an integrated approach to designing a study are to strengthen a study so that methods complement each other and add power to the findings; to gain a comprehensive understanding of a phenomenon by uncovering different dimensions with different techniques; and to compensate for the flaws of one design with the strengths of another. Perhaps the most common reason for using both qualitative and quantitative designs is to achieve triangulation. The purpose of triangulation is to confirm information about a phenomenon and to obtain convergent validity—confidence that a finding is valid because it has been confirmed by more than one method.

Sociologists, anthropologists, and educators have been integrating qualitative and quantitative designs for many years, although it is a relatively new concept for health professionals. However, it is important to understand the basic tenets of the two methods: which purpose would best be served, what kind of data can be generated, what the researcher's activities are likely to be, and what the outcome will look like. Only when the doctrine and activities of both methods are fully grasped can the researcher become adept at using the methods independently or together. It is for this reason that, in the following chapters, quantitative and qualitative research methods are treated separately.

Qualitative Research

Whereas qualitative research used to be solely the domain of anthropology, history, and political science, in recent years other traditionally "quantitative" fields such as psychology, sociology, education, public administration, and urban planning are using qualitative methods. In fact, it seems that many fields are "moving more toward phenomenological approaches and away from experimental approaches, thus becoming less precise but more real" (Yerxa, 1991, p. 201). As part of this movement, it has become apparent that qualitative research methods and designs are useful to health professionals, among them therapists. Many now feel that there is a legitimate place in occupational and physical therapy research for qualitative methods and that there are phenomena within our fields that can usefully be studied using naturalistic methods. In studying such experiences as therapists with their clients, clients in relation to their disabilities, and the process of therapeutic interaction, our understanding can be significantly increased by conducting research that employs a naturalistic approach.

Occupational and physical therapy literature over the past few years has included qualitative studies investigating the clinical reasoning of occupational therapists (Mattingly & Fleming, 1994), motivation in chronic illness (Helfich, Kielhofner & Mattingly, 1994), interdisciplinary team meetings in health care (Crepeau, 1994), a couple's experience with and adaptation to one member's stroke (Jongbloed, 1994), occupational therapists' descriptions of their roles and boundaries (Sachs & Labovitz, 1994), the identification of helping factors in a peer-developed support group for persons with head injury (Schultz, 1994; Schwartzberg, 1994), and an ethnographic study of patient socialization to the culture of a rehabilitation hospital (Spencer, Young, Rintala, & Bates, 1995).

Features of Qualitative Research

Some features cross boundaries among different types of naturalistic designs. They are pervasive qualities that are common to many qualitative research studies.

Naturalistic Settings

Qualitative research can be described in general terms as descriptive and naturalistic, with natural settings as the sources of data. Researchers spend the bulk of their time in the field (at the site of the study), observing and talking to participants, and gathering and analyzing data. They are greatly interested in learning about the participants within the context of the participants' own world. Because understanding the culture is of overriding concern, participants are observed and spoken with in their own environment while going about their usual business. Qualitative researchers are concerned with the process as well as the outcome of their studies. What happens during the data-gathering and analysis phase of the study is crucial to the eventual theory and hypotheses that are generated.

Local Groundedness

One of the strengths of qualitative research is that the focus on naturally occurring, ordinary events in natural settings gives us a good handle on what "real life" is like for the participants in the study. This confidence in the data is assisted by local groundedness: the data have been collected in proximity to the specific situation under study, rather than through the mail or the telephone. The researcher's emphasis is on a specific case (person, place, event) embedded in its context. Thus underlying, nonobvious issues and local influences can be taken into account.

Phenomenological Perspective

Although many approaches can be grouped under the generic heading of "qualitative research," the phenomenological perspective is central to most qualitative researchers' outlook. They have a primary interest in meaning from the participant's point of view. As Glesne and Peshkin (1992) see it:

> . . . since qualitative researchers deal with multiple, socially constructed realities or "qualities" that are complex and indivisible into discrete variables, they regard their research task as coming to understand and interpret how the various participants in a social setting construct the world around them. (p. 6)

Qualitative data place emphasis on people's lived experience and are thus well suited for identifying and locating the meanings people place on the events, processes, and structures of their lives (Box 4–B). Their perceptions, assumptions, judgments, and suppositions become clear and can be placed in context in the social world around them.

Box 4–B

Helfrich, Kielhofner, and Mattingly (1994) have presented a powerful image of the vocational experiences of two individuals with bipolar disorder. To achieve the purpose of the study, to expand the current concept of volition in the Model of Human Occupation, the authors adopted a frankly phenomenological perspective when interviewing the participants to gather data.

The paper details their situations specifically from the participants' point of view, providing generous quotations from the interviewees to inform the reader of their particular ideas about their own situation.

Adopting the phenomenological viewpoint lends itself perfectly to any study in which therapists are concerned with patient's perspectives on their own life or environment, or their view of their own particular situation such as their illness and how they will cope with it. McCuaig and Frank (1991) adopted a phenomenological perspective throughout their investigation into the independent life of a 53-year-old woman with cerebral palsy, gaining such an insight into her life from her own viewpoint that they felt able to challenge professionals' assumptions concerning disability and treatment for clients similar to this woman.

Data as "Thick Description"

Geertz (1973) is credited with borrowing the phrase "thick description" when he was discussing a definition for "culture." He stated that culture can be viewed as interwoven systems of symbols and, as such, is a context within which social events, behaviors, institutions, or processes "can be intelligible—that is, *thickly*—described" (p. 14).

Qualitative data are rich and powerful with the potential for revealing complexity. These data provide "thick descriptions" that are vivid, are nested in a real context, and have a ring of truth that has strong impact on the reader (Box 4–B). They are usually collected over a sustained period of time, making them powerful for studying process (including history). Rather than gaining a one-shot view (such as is gained using the

survey method), one can see why things happen the way they do and even assess causality as it occurs in a particular setting.

Lived Experience

Because naturalistic data emphasize people's lived experience, they are well suited for identifying the meanings people place on the events, processes, and structures of their lives. As the data gathering and analysis proceed, participants' perceptions, assumptions, judgments, and suppositions become clear and can be placed in context in the social world around them.

Power of Qualitative Data

A final feature of qualitative data is their power: they are the best strategy for exploring a new area and developing hypotheses; they have strong potential for testing hypotheses; and they are useful when one needs to supplement, validate, explain, illuminate, or reinterpret quantitative data gathered from the same setting (Miles & Huberman, 1994).

Recurring Features of Qualitative Research

Although qualitative research may be conducted in dozens of ways, there are some recurring features of the methodology. A slightly modified version of a list of such characteristics by Miles and Huberman (1994) follows:

- Qualitative research is conducted through intense and prolonged contact with a "field" or life situation. These situations are typically "normal" ones, reflecting the everyday life of individuals, groups, societies, and organizations.

- The researcher's role is to gain a holistic overview of the context under study: its logic, its arrangements, its explicit and implicit rules. The researcher adopts a learner role, learning from the participants and their surroundings.

- The researcher attempts to capture the perceptions of local actors from a phenomenological viewpoint, through a process of deep attentiveness, empathetic understanding, and suspending preconceptions about the topics under discussion.

- Reading through the data, the main task is to explain the ways people in particular settings come to understand, account for, act on, and otherwise manage their day-to-day situations.

- Many interpretations of this material are possible, but some are more compelling for theoretical reasons and because they meet the goals of the particular study.

- Questioning occurs simultaneously with collecting information and making sense of it. One process drives the other and results in the reformulation and refinement of the problem and the structuring of smaller questions, which are then pursued in the field.

- Relatively little standardized instrumentation is used. The researcher is essentially the main "instrument" in the study.

- Most analysis is done with words. The words can be assembled, clustered, and broken into segments. They can be organized to permit the researcher to contrast, compare, analyze, and search for patterns and themes.

Qualitative Strategies

As more health professionals have come to embrace naturalistic research, it is useful to see what can be learned from the strategies employed by other disciplines. Some of these strategies are more useful than others for therapists. They are listed here to show some of the creative methods that investigators have used to study particular topics. Health professionals can gain some ideas for their own needs by studying how others have tackled challenging study topics.

- **Ethnography:** Ethnographies are studies that attempt to describe a culture or aspects of culture. The ethnographer's goal is to share in the meanings that the cultural participants take for granted and then to depict the new understanding for the reader (Bogdan & Biklen, 1982).

- **Ethnography of Communication:** This style of ethnography focuses on gaining an understanding of the culture by studying all forms of communication within the culture, including verbal, nonverbal, and symbolic. Communication between the cultural participants is seen as the key to understanding the culture.

- **Ethnomethodology:** This term, coined by Harold Garfinkel, refers to the subject matter researchers will investigate. That is, they will study how individuals create and understand their daily lives; how people see, explain, and describe the world in which they live. The subjects for ethnomethodologists are people in our own society rather than members of primitive tribes. Researchers in education have been heavily influenced by Garfinkel's approach.

- **Phenomenology:** Researchers in phenomenology are studying culture from the informants' own point of view, emphasizing the subjective aspects of their behavior. They attempt to understand the meaning of events and interactions to ordinary people in particular situations, trying to gain entry into the conceptual world of their subjects in order to understand how and what meaning they construct around events in their daily lives (Bogdan & Biklen, 1982).

- **Unobstrusive (Nonreactive) Research and Observer Studies:** In these types of studies, the investigator takes the role of an observer, making an effort to be unobtrusive. The goal is to gather most of the data for the study solely through observation, thus influencing the participants and environment as little as possible and gather "uncontaminated" data.

- **Participant Observation:** This research strategy builds on the observer strategy, in that the investigator does take part in the participants' world to some degree in order to obtain more data.

- **Interview Strategies:** These strategies include investigative journalism, biography, and oral history; the researcher interviews participants in order to learn about their personal experience.

- **Archival Strategies:** Archival strategies include literary criticism, historical research, content analysis, and philosophical research, in which documents and artifacts are used to gather data.

We will examine in detail four major strategies or designs that are particularly useful for the type of topics often studied by health professionals. These qualitative research designs are: ethnography, case methods, historical research, and unstructured interviews. How to conduct these particular styles of research will be described in some detail in Chapter 9. Meanwhile, the following is a brief description of some of the features of these four designs.

The Ethnographic Research Design

The attempt to describe culture or aspects of culture is called ethnography. Some anthropologists define culture as "the acquired knowledge people use to interpret experience and generate behavior." Thus, culture embraces what people do, what people know, and things that people make and use (Spradley, 1980, pp. 5, 6). Using this perspective, a researcher might think about events in the following way: "Ethnography should account for the behavior of people by describing what it is that they know that enables them to behave appropriately given the dictates of common sense in their community" (McDermott, 1976, p. 159). It has been said that an ethnography succeeds if it teaches readers how to behave appropriately in the cultural setting, whether it is among patients in a rehabilitation hospital, residents in a community residence, workers in a sheltered workshop, elderly patients in a day program, or psychiatric patients in a day treatment facility (Box 4–C).

The writing of ethnography can be seen as writing thick description, as described earlier. When culture is examined from the perspective of thick description, the ethnographer is faced with a complicated interpretation of a slice of life and an understanding of the community under study based on common sense. The ethnographer's goals are to share in the meanings that the participants take for granted and then to depict their new recontextualized understanding for outsiders.

The Case Method Research Design

Case studies in the health sciences tend to draw from other disciplines for their theoretical base and format. Anthropology, sociology, psychology, history, and business have informed the qualitative case method in occupational and physical therapy. As in other qualitative research methods, case methods can be differentiated according to their purpose and end product. Some are descriptive, some interpretive, and still others evaluative.

Other disciplines have traditionally taken a broad view of the case method, readily viewing "the case" as a naturally occurring group of people rather than as an individual. Health professionals, on the other hand, have more commonly used a single patient as the case, and have only recently begun treating groups of people as cases or units of study. This change in attitude brings health professionals more in line with the disciplines that developed ethnographic, phenomenological styles of research and allows health researchers to use these research approaches to the case method in the way they were intended (Box 4–D).

The case method, then, can be used to study individuals or groups of individuals as a unit, such as a group of patients in a nursing home, a support group for caregivers of people with Alzheimer's disease, or a group of people at an Alcoholics Anonymous meeting. Case studies can also use one depository

---

Box 4–C

A group of occupational therapists (Spencer, Young, Rintala, and Bates, 1995) conducted an ethnography into the life of a patient in a rehabilitation hospital following his spinal cord injury.

Box 4–D

Kielhofner (1979) used a case method research design to study temporality in a group of 32 mentally retarded adults living in board-and-care facilities in Los Angeles.

of documents or one particular event as a data source.

The Historical Research Design

It is interesting to note that Bogdan and Biklen (1982) have listed historical organizational case studies as a distinct type of historical study. These studies focus on a particular organization over time and trace the organization's development. Therapists could use this type of design to study, for example, the American Physical Therapy Association or one of the state occupational therapy associations. The task would be to trace how and for what reason the organization came into being, who was involved in starting the organization, what events and changes have happened over time, what it is like now, and how it came to a close (if it did).

Unstructured Interviewing as a Research Design

Although this is not found in the literature as a distinct design for naturalistic research, it is included here because of its popularity among health care researchers. It probably enjoys such popularity because it is "do-able" and convenient. When using unstructured interviewing as a qualitative research design, investigators are simply confining their data gathering to one of the many techniques available, and are using solely the analysis of that data to formulate their ideas about the participants' experience (Box 4–E).

Quantitative Research

Although there are many ways to think about and organize quantitative research designs, one of the most helpful is to divide them into the following three categories:

Box 4–E

Carpenter (1994) learned of meaningful aspects of the disability experience for people with spinal cord injuries by conducting in-depth, unstructured interviews with her participants.

---

1. True experimental designs
2. Quasi-experimental designs
3. Nonexperimental designs

As listed, these designs have decreasing levels of experimental rigor but become more and more practical when it comes to human subject research, as it is often difficult to achieve the standards required for true experimental designs because of the vagaries of human behavior.

To illustrate this, let us look at exactly what is required for each level of design. We will begin by exploring three concepts:

1. Manipulation
2. Control
3. Randomization

Manipulation

Manipulation is a sinister-sounding word that has a particular meaning in research. In research, it merely means doing something to the subjects in the study; for example, if the researcher offers a group of patients with schizophrenia a daily program of self-care activities to see if their appearance can be improved, manipulation is being provided in the form of daily self-care activities. Generally, any therapy offered to subjects in the hope that they will show improvement can be called manipulation.

In other words, the researcher is manipulating one or more variables in connection with the subjects. A variable is anything that can vary or change and therefore can be measured. In the foregoing example, the variable of self-care is being manipulated or given as treatment to see if it will have an effect on another variable, namely, the patient's appearance.

Dependent and Independent Variables

It is important to understand which variable is manipulated and which one is measured. In the previous example, the independent variable self-care is manipulated to see its effect on the dependent variable (the patients' appearance). The independent variable is sometimes called the experimental or treatment variable. The dependent variable (appearance) determines the effectiveness of the manipulation or treatment and is the item observed and measured at the beginning and end of the study.

Manipulation must be part of the methodology if the study is to qualify as a true experimental design. Thus, if the researcher does not actually manipulate a variable pertaining to the subjects, a study cannot be termed "experimental." For example, a study in which subjects are asked to complete a questionnaire and the researcher merely examines answers or variables after the fact is not experimental.

Control

The second concept that needs definition in order to understand quantitative research designs is that of control. Control refers to the experimenter's ability to control or eliminate interfering and irrelevant influences. This will allow the researcher to say that the results are due to manipulation of the variables and not to chance interferences of other variables. In the earlier example, if there were no control, it is possible that instead of the program of self-care skills, some other event in the patients' lives (such as a volunteer taking them to the store to buy new clothes) might have caused improvement in their appearance.

The researcher may be able to control some variables such as: (a) environmental influences (e.g., the amount of noise or the aesthetics of surroundings); (b) change of therapist providing the treatment (it might be important to the study that the same therapist be used so that patients become accustomed to him or her, or it might be equally important that different therapists be used to eliminate the influence of certain therapist styles); and (c) certain events in the patients' lives (such as obtaining a physician's cooperation in not changing patients' medications during the period of the study).

However, it is not possible to control all variables that may affect the study results. That is why it is usual to have a control group of subjects who experience the same day-to-day occurrences and influences as the experimental group but do not receive study treatment. By including a control group, the researcher is attempting to ensure that any helpful or detrimental event influencing the amount of change in the dependent variable (the one being measured) will happen to both groups of subjects. At the end of the study, when the dependent variable is measured for both groups, if there is greater improvement in the experimental group, the researcher can say that this was probably due to the manipulation or treatment.

There are times when it would not be ethical to withhold treatment from a group of patients in order for them to serve as a control group. Perhaps a therapist would like to know if a new form of treatment is more effective for a certain condition than the traditional treatment for that condition. In that case, the control group could receive the traditional treatment and the experimental group could receive the new treatment, and all other conditions would be held constant. This design satisfies the need for a control group as well as the ethical concern. In some cases, it may be possible to improve on this design by adding a third group that receives no treatment at all while experiencing the same day-to-day conditions. The results would be even more convincing if a group receiving one of the treatments showed more improvement than the untreated group.

It can be seen, therefore, that control is about the business of eliminating influences that are not part of the study design. The concept of control embraces elements of the third concept to be discussed—that of randomization.

Randomization

As one way of setting boundaries for the study, quantitative researchers use deductive logic to select the people who will participate in their study. They figure out whom they wish to study and set criteria for the subjects; for example, people diagnosed with chronic schizophrenia who have had multiple admissions to hospitals totaling at least 5 years and who have one or more family members available for support. These are known as subject selection criteria. The researcher now must choose a method to select a group of individuals to be in the study from among those who meet the criteria. The most useful method is randomization.

Randomization is designed to reduce the risk of systematic bias creeping into the study. This is done by (a) ensuring that the subjects are representative of the group from which they are chosen, by randomly selecting them from a population; and (b) ensuring that the experimental and control group subjects are similar, by randomly assigning subjects to groups. Randomization increases the internal validity of the study, which is the chance that we are actually changing and measuring what we think we are changing and measuring, and the external validity of the study, which is the chance that results found in subjects can be generalized to others who are similar (Box 4–F). Randomly selecting subjects from a larger group of people and randomly assigning those chosen to experimental and control groups will also reduce the chance of bias in the formation of the study groups.

Randomization has a precise meaning in research. **Random selection** means that every subject in the population concerned has an equal chance of being selected for the study sample. **Random assignment** means that those in the selected sample each have an equal chance of being assigned to either the experimental group or the control group.

The term **population** also has a specific meaning in research. It is the entire group of people or items that meet the criteria set by the researcher. Population refers to all such subjects, whereas **subpopulation** is a researcher-defined subgroup of the population. A sample is selected from the population or the subpopulation (Box 4–G). In research, a population does not necessarily refer to people but may refer to things such as records or events that are being studied (see the example in Box 4–H).

Box 4–G

In King's 1974 study of sensory integrative therapy used with patients with schizophrenia, the population of interest included all the chronic, nonparanoid schizophrenic patients in the world, while the subpopulation included all the chronic, nonparanoid schizophrenic patients residing in the Arizona State Hospital. The sample for the study was selected from this subpopulation.

If, for true random selection, every subject in the population must have an equal opportunity of being selected, merely using as subjects patients who come through your door or client records that happen to land on your desk would mean that not all subjects had the same chance of being included in the study, because all those who did not walk through your door or whose records did not land on your desk had no chance of being selected. Instead, a complete list of people or items in the population or subpopulation must be available to the researcher and a random selection made from that list. In King's case (see Box 4–G), she would have needed a complete list of all the patients in the Arizona State Hospital who met the research criteria (i.e., all those with chronic nonparanoid schizophrenia). She then could have placed all the names in a hat and picked out the required number for the study, or assigned a number to each patient and used a random number chart to select patients for the study sample. Either one is an acceptable method of random selection, but the latter is probably more practical.

Box 4–F

If I want to change and measure the performance of mentally retarded adults on their work assembly skills and I have not randomly selected and assigned the clients, it is possible that those in the experiment (as compared with other mentally retarded adults or those in the control group) may by chance have received some work-skills training in the past, have a greater degree of manual dexterity, or have some other trait in common of which I am not aware, any of which could make them better (or worse) at the study task.

Box 4–H

In studying the effects of guided visual imagery on patients with psychosomatic, psychogenic, and chronic somatic disorders, Moore (1989) reviewed patients' charts. His subpopulation was composed of all the charts of patients meeting his criteria at a specific hospital. His sample was composed of 50 charts randomly selected from the subpopulation.

A random number chart, which may be found in the back of a statistics book, lists numbers that have been generated by a computer in true random fashion. The chart may be read in any direction (up or down, side to side, diagonally) starting at any point, to produce a list of random numbers. This method is commonly used when researchers are mailing questionnaires and have access to a complete mailing list of potential subjects who meet their criteria, a population. It is simple enough to assign a number to each name, then to pick a series of numbers from the chart and to include the people with corresponding numbers in the study. For a list of names that has already been entered into a computer file, programs are available that will make a random selection straight from the database, saving the researcher a great deal of time.

The second component of randomization is that of randomly assigning the selected subjects to experimental and control groups. A complete subject sample should be selected first, then a similar process used to assign subjects randomly to the two groups. Random assignment is done primarily to ensure that the candidates in each group will be as alike (or as unalike) as possible; it also ensures that the researcher will not be tempted to assign a "good" candidate to the experimental group because it looks as if he or she will show a lot of improvement.

The point of randomization is to be sure that the sample is as representative of the population as possible and to be sure that the experimental and control groups are as similar to each other as possible. This will enable the researcher to state more confidently that the results are due to the treatment given rather than to a difference in characteristics between the two groups. It also minimizes the chance that the sample members were not typical of the population and improved because of some uncontrolled trait they held in common.

Random assignment, on the other hand, will improve **internal validity;** that is, that the experimental treatment made a difference rather than something else within the study design. It will even out the impact on the study of such things as attrition (subjects dropping out of the study), developmental maturation or practice effect having an influence on results, differences in response to testing, and regression (patients getting sicker over time).

Random selection will also ensure that the sample is as much like the population as possible and will therefore improve **external validity;** that is, that similar findings are likely if another portion of the population were to be studied. Thus, the results of your study can be more readily generalized to the population as a whole and are more useful to other therapists who would like to use your treatment method with similar patients. Remember, if random selection has not been used, the results of a study cannot be generalized to other people in the population.

Randomization is not perfect. It is based on the laws of probability, and every once in a while the improbable will happen and a source of bias will appear in a study. For example, one group may end up being composed of patients who are sicker or older than those in the other group. Also, methods must be used correctly for random selection to be effective (Box 4–I).

With the concepts of manipulation, control, and randomization in mind, we can return to the requirements for the three categories of quantitative research design: true experimental designs, quasi-experimental designs, and nonexperimental designs.

True Experimental Designs

In true experimental designs, all three of the concepts—manipulation, control, and randomization—are required. There must be an element of control, independent variables

---

Box 4–I

A classic example of poor methodology occurred in the 1969 selection of men who were to be conscripted into the army. A slip of paper with the name and month of birth for each man were put into an urn and drawn out, but the slips were not well mixed. The last slips put into the urn were of men whose birthdays fell in October, November, and December, and disproportionately more of these men's names were drawn than others. This was a case in which poor methodology had serious consequences.

concerning the subjects must be manipulated, and subjects must be randomly selected or randomly assigned to groups. The result is the classic experimental design known as cause-and-effect research that enables the researcher to say there was a good chance that the manipulation of the independent variable caused a change in the dependent variable. This method allows the researcher to compare different types of treatment and to determine which type is likely to be the most effective.

In experimental research, the researcher deliberately does something to the independent variable in one group (such as providing a self-care training program, as in our earlier example) but not to the other (no self-care program for the control group), then looks for the results of those differences on the dependent variable (patients' appearance). The dependent variable is usually measured before and after treatment so that comparisons can be made on the same group; comparisons between groups are made by measuring both "after" tests. The before and after tests are called pre-tests and post-tests.

For ease of communication with other researchers and to permit the researcher to sketch out designs quickly, a system of shorthand known as research notation was developed by Campbell and Stanley (1969). Their system will be used throughout this book. An O represents the observations or measurements that occur at pre-testing and post-testing; an R represents random assignment; and an X represents manipulation or treatment. Each study group is written or represented on a separate line, and time periods are aligned vertically. If we wished to show in research notation a design consisting of two randomly assigned groups, one with treatment and one without, and both with pre-testing and post-testing, we would show it thus:

$$R \quad O \quad X \quad O$$
$$R \quad O \qquad O$$

This is a classic experimental design and one that would be most effective in investigating the efficacy of a new treatment method. If one wanted to investigate whether a new treatment method were more effective than a traditional one, and if the two methods were better than no treatment at all, one could use the design mentioned

earlier, with a third group added. It would look like this in research notation:

$$R \quad O \quad X_1 \quad O$$
$$R \quad O \quad X_2 \quad O$$
$$R \quad O \qquad O$$

The two treatment groups would be differentiated by the use of subscripts 1 and 2.

As mentioned at the beginning of this section on quantitative designs, in human subject research it is not often possible to provide all the requirements for experimental research (manipulation, control, and randomization). Perhaps it is impossible to assign subjects randomly to different groups (Campbell and Stanley [1969] feel that random assignment is sufficient to qualify as a true experimental research design because random selection is so difficult to achieve), or it is ethically impossible to have a control group go without treatment. In these cases, it is often necessary to move to the next category—to a quasi-experimental research design.

Quasi-experimental Designs

A quasi-experimental design differs from a true experimental design in that, although it contains an independent variable that is manipulated in order to look for an effect on a dependent variable, either control or randomization is lacking. The resulting designs are still very useful to clinicians looking for validation of treatment methods and techniques. However, the researcher cannot generalize the outcome if there is no random selection, and the study is open to outside influences on the results if there is no control group or no random assignment (Box 4–J).

Sometimes researchers use subjects as their own control. There is no second group of subjects who are without treatment; rather, the subjects in the experimental group double as the control group. They receive the treatment, but they also experience a period of no treatment, which is considered the control period. In research notation, the design looks like this:

$$O \quad X_1 \quad O \qquad O \quad X_2 \quad O \qquad O \quad X_3 \quad O$$

It can be seen that an observation pre-test occurs, and then the first treatment is given, followed by a post-test. Then an amount of time similar to the treatment period elapses when no treatment is given, followed by a second post-test. This test becomes the pre-test for the second period of treatment, which then follows, and so on, until the desired number of treatment and nontreatment periods have occurred. During the nontreatment period, one would not expect to see any change in the dependent variable if in fact the treatment is the influence causing change, just as one would not expect to see change in the dependent variable in a control group. A graph of the expected results of this research design would look something like the drawing in Figure 4–1.

If the results did look similar to this, it would be fairly certain that the improvement in the dependent variable was due to the treatment procedure, and that when the treatment was not occurring, subject improvement leveled off. Of course, in reality, improvements are unlikely to start and stop as abruptly as the graph would indicate; there would probably be some effect of the treatment spilling over into the control period.

Although quasi-experimental research generally demands manipulation while either control or randomization may be missing, it should be noted that there are some designs that have neither control or randomization, yet fall into the quasi-experimental category because an independent variable is manipulated. The classic case is the single-case experiment, that is, one subject (or group of subjects) who receives pre-test, treatment, and post-test. (Campbell and Stanley [1969] refer to this as a pre-experimental design.) There are no control subjects, and there obviously cannot be any random assignment. Research notation for this design looks like this:

$$O \quad X \quad O$$

This design is fraught with difficulties, and some feel it is of little value. The pros and cons of this design are discussed in more detail in Chapter 5, which describes quantitative research designs.

Nonexperimental Designs

Nonexperimental designs have no manipulation of an independent variable. Control and randomization are not possible or even relevant facets of this type of research. These are usually designs in which the researcher intends to investigate (a) a variable that cannot be manipulated or changed because it is fixed (e.g., age, weight, and height); or (b) a variable that cannot be changed because it has already happened (e.g., head injury, drug abuse, an event in history such as a medical discovery); or (c) a variable in which the investigator wants to measure and compare two or more existing variables to see if there is a relationship between them (e.g., height and weight, therapist style and patient attendance at treatment, head injury recovery and position in the family). Because the variables in all three cases are being studied after they have occurred, this type of

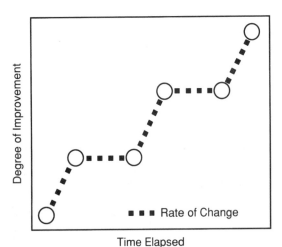

FIGURE 4–1 Representation of expected results when subject is used as his or her own control.

research is often referred to as *ex post facto* (roughly translated as "after the fact") research. Nonexperimental research is also called descriptive research because one is simply describing characteristics and events connected with a sample while not manipulating them in any way.

Included in the *ex post facto* category of designs are correlational studies, in which one looks for a relationship between two or more variables; survey research using structured interviews or questionnaires; the case study (sometimes called the single-case report), in which a single subject is observed and new interpretations and suggestions for treatment emerge; and methodological research, in which the reliability and validity of newly devised tests, tools, or instruments are tested. All of these will be discussed in the next chapter. There is another type of research, called evaluation research, that some people feel falls in a category of its own—partway between quantitative and qualitative types of research. However, in this book evaluation research will be included in the nonexperimental category of quantitative research.

Quantitative and Qualitative Research

People tend to have an intuitive leaning toward either quantitative or qualitative styles of methodology. There are those who feel great satisfaction from the tangible, countable nature of quantitative data. There is an obvious end point to the data analysis, and they like the certainty of knowing when they are done. They like the feeling of contributing to the knowledge base when they have answered a specific research question, knowing they have offered statistical proof that "this is so." Qualitative researchers, on the other hand, are comfortable studying amorphous phenomena; they love the challenge of the quest for meaning and the sense of discovery at the end of a long and complicated adventure with their data. They enjoy being totally immersed in their topic and generally have great positive emotional feeling for their data. They are often reluctant to end their study, a tendency compounded by the fact that there is usually no clear end point. These researchers feel comfortable

presenting their results in descriptive terms, knowing that often they have raised more questions than they have answered.

Comparison of Quantitative and Qualitative Research

To help you decide which type of research method to choose for your study, it might be helpful to summarize and compare the two types here. The following characteristics of the two styles of research draw heavily from the work of Bogdan and Biklen (1982).

Purpose

The purpose of quantitative research is theory-testing: to establish facts, show causal explanations and relationships between variables, allow prediction, and strive for generalizability. The purpose of qualitative research, on the other hand, is to develop concepts that will sensitize readers to cultures, describe multiple realities and interpretations, develop grounded theory, and develop an understanding of the perspectives of the actors and of that particular setting.

Designs

Quantitative research designs are predetermined and structured, and do not change during the course of the study; they are formal and specific according to a defined model and are used as a detailed plan of operation. Qualitative research designs fall at the other end of the spectrum. They are general in nature rather than confined, evolving throughout the study and remaining flexible to allow for change; they are used as a "hunch" as to how to proceed.

Data

The data gathered in quantitative research designs are quantifiable and statistical, using counts and measures. Variables are defined ahead of time, and data are managed according to the procedures outlined in the research proposal. Data gathered in qualitative designs are descriptive and deal with qualities. They may consist of field notes, artifacts, people's own words, personal documents, or official documents. Qualitative data are extensive and difficult to manage.

Their management requires specific techniques, just as numerical data do.

Subject Samples

In quantitative studies, the subject samples tend to be large, requiring random selection to yield precisely defined subjects who will be typical of those in the population. There is usually a control group to control for extraneous variables. In qualitative studies, the group of participants is small and may be nonrepresentative of the larger group. Sometimes researchers stratify their participant selection in order to sample people with different roles or statuses in the community.

Investigator's Relationship with Subjects

The quantitative researcher has circumscribed contact with the subjects on a short-term basis. He or she is detached and distant, keeping the roles of researcher and subject distinct. The researcher's role is to observe and measure, and care is taken to prevent the researcher from influencing the data through personal involvement with the research subjects. It is of utmost concern that the researcher be objective.

During a qualitative study, on the other hand, the investigator usually has intense contact with participants over a long period of time. There is an emphasis on trust. The informants are viewed as participants in an egalitarian relationship, and the investigator may empathize with the informants and their situations.

Techniques or Methods

The techniques or methods used in the two styles of research vary greatly. Those used in quantitative methods include experiments and quasi-experiments, structured surveys, structured interviewing, structured observation, data sets, manipulation, control, and statistical analysis of data. Techniques used in qualitative methods include observation, participant observation, reviewing documents and artifacts, open-ended interviewing, coding, searches for patterns, pattern matching, and narrative and displays for portrayal of data.

Instruments and Tools

The instruments and tools for data collection used in quantitative studies are varied and can be quite complicated. They may consist of scales and tests, inventories, questionnaires, or various types of hardware. In a qualitative study, the researcher is often the only "tool" for data collection. He or she may make use of guiding questions, as in an interview, as well as using mechanical tools such as audio or video tape recorders and a transcriber.

Data Analysis

Perhaps the greatest difference in the two styles of research is in how the data are analyzed. Data analysis occurs at the conclusion of data collection in a quantitative study. It tends to be deductive and tends to use statistical manipulation in accordance with the proposal guidelines. It is a straightforward operation that is often completed rather speedily. On the other hand, data analysis is ongoing throughout qualitative studies, using a constant comparison method. Data are analyzed as they are gathered, then reanalyzed in the light of new information, in a recursive manner. Qualitative data analysis is inductive in nature and addresses models, themes, and concepts. Techniques such as coding, memoing, event listing, pattern-matching, charting, matrices, and triangulation may be used.

A fundamental difference is that the quantitative researcher seeks evidence to prove or disprove hypotheses that were developed before the study, whereas in qualitative data analysis theory is built as the data are grouped and analyzed—theory emerges from the bottom up. "You are not putting together a puzzle, whose picture you already know. You are constructing a picture which takes shape as you collect and examine the parts" (Bogdan & Biklen, 1982, p. 29).

Outcome

As you can readily see, the outcomes of the two types of research will be quite different. Quantitative research studies will answer specific research questions by producing statistical evidence to prove a point. While the researcher certainly discusses the findings, there is a common saying that the data, meaning the statistical outcomes, speak for themselves. The outcome of qualitative research, more often than not, is a lengthy descriptive document, presenting the data in words rather than numbers. The write-up is rich, textural, anecdotal, and full of thick description in narrative form. The final analysis provides either verification of an existing theory or new grounded theory, together with well-formulated research questions that now need to be investigated.

Problems

Finally, let us consider some of the problems that may be encountered in conducting either form of research. In quantitative studies, (a) the researcher may have difficulty controlling variables that will affect the study; (b) the study's validity may be called into question, as some may feel that highly controlled experimental studies have little relevance to real life; (c) obtrusiveness of the investigator and data collection methods may affect the subjects or environment; and (d) the researcher (or readers) may be tempted to reify the topic variables—that is, to regard these abstractions as if they were material things. Problems of qualitative research include: (a) the nonstandardization of procedures; (b) the difficulty of managing large amounts of data and data reduction methods; (c) the extremely time-consuming nature of the whole process; and (d) the difficulty of using naturalistic methods to study large populations.

Summary

While reading this chapter, you may have decided that your project lends itself to a quantitative design, and you have some early ideas about which type of design would be preferable. You should first decide if your project falls into an experimental or nonexperimental mode. That is, do you intend to manipulate an independent variable, to actually offer some treatment, or will you be engaged in *ex post facto* research in which you will investigate a variable that is fixed or already has occurred? If you are planning to provide treatment or manipulation, can you meet the other two criteria for a true ex-

perimental design—control and randomization? If not, which of the quasi-experimental designs is appropriate for your study?

If you know you would prefer to conduct qualitative research, you will wish to read further about these designs before deciding which one is appropriate for you. The next chapter describes some of the actual designs used in experimental, quasi-experimental and nonexperimental quantitative studies, while Chapter 9 will describe naturalistic designs.

Stumbling Blocks

One of the difficulties in experimental research design is deciding which is the independent and which is the dependent variable. If the study calls for a treatment approach, the decision is relatively easy. The treatment is the independent variable. It is also obvious that the variable you hope to change is the dependent variable, the one that will be measured to look for the change.

The independent variable is one whose boundaries are defined in advance by the researcher. It is selected because it is seen as being causative or very important to the logical purpose of the research project. In cause-and-effect or experimental research, the independent variable is always the one assumed to cause something to happen, and the dependent variable is always the one being changed.

In *ex post facto* research, in which the independent variable cannot be manipulated because it is fixed or has already happened, it is still feasible to use the term "independent variable" and to assume that it is causative in nature. One usually makes this assumption based on experience and reading. However, the independent variable may not be easy to identify because it is not being manipulated by the researcher and is not easily identified as treatment.

A common mistake regarding the independent variable in nonexperimental research is thinking that one can still claim a cause-and-effect relationship between independent and dependent variables. In *ex post facto* research, as stated earlier, the independent variable cannot be manipulated by the researcher because it is fixed or has already happened. In this case, a variable (e.g., depression) is studied after the fact to see if it is likely to have affected another variable (e.g., productivity). Because this is not being tested in a true experimental manner, it is not possible to claim a cause-and-effect relationship but only an associative relationship. This puts the study in the realm of correlational (nonexperimental) research. Because we are not now manipulating the independent variable (depression), the results should be expressed in terms of association or relationship between variables and not in terms of cause and effect.

The true meaning of the term "random" often escapes people. In everyday usage, "random selection" means picking haphazardly, with no apparent pattern. But, as was noted earlier, "random" has a specific meaning for selection and assignment of subjects in a research study. If the researcher does not apply correct randomization procedures, results of the study cannot be generalized to similar populations.

Perhaps the most common stumbling block to completing a qualitative study is "drowning in the data." Because of the nature of these designs and data collection techniques, and indeed because it is desirable for a meaningful study, the data or words soon mount up, and the novice researcher may despair of ever being able to make sense of it all. As you will see later, certain techniques can be used to reduce data to meaningful chunks and to make it all manageable, but these must be learned systematically, just as one learns statistical procedures. It helps to have a plan, before data collection begins, about how you will organize the collection format and the storage of tapes, transcripts, and artifacts.

Many researchers feel tempted to end the data analysis before it is truly completed. Time marches on, and the investigator begins to feel that the study will never be done. Graduation may be fast approaching, and the pressure is on to get finished. I can only say that the quality of the study will be greatly compromised if data analysis ends too soon, before theoretical constructs have been verified or generated and before meaningful hypotheses have been produced. Before you give up in dismay, ask for help and support in getting finished.

WORKSHEETS

Does your project lend itself to quantitative or to qualitative methods? For example:

You will probably use a quantitative method if:

- You hope to prove a hypothesis
- You wish to look for the effect of one variable upon another
- You wish to look for a relationship between two or more variables
- You wish to find out some specific facts about a large group of people
- You have access to a large group of people who meet your criteria

You will probably use a qualitative method if:

- You wish to generate new theory
- You wish to generate new hypotheses to be tested later
- You wish to use a phenomenological approach to find out how a few individuals feel
- You wish to gather the data in a naturalistic setting
- You have access to a natural setting in which you can spend a lot of time and will be allowed to gather data from staff, patients, and records

A. If you think you may use a quantitative design:

Do you intend to offer treatment to a group of patients?

If not, go on to Section B.

If so, name the treatment.

What is the independent variable that you will manipulate?

What dependent variable do you expect to change as a result?

RANDOMIZATION

Think about your subject selection criteria. What attributes have a bearing on your study (e.g., age, gender, type of disability, degree of disability, location of residence)?

Is it possible for you to obtain a list of all the individuals who meet your criteria:

_____ In your facility?

_____ In a group of similar facilities in your area?

_____ Nationwide?

If so, do you know how to go about random selection and random assignment?

What method of random selection and random assignment to groups will you use?

CONTROL

Is it possible for you to have a control group of subjects? Describe how:

METHODOLOGY

Based on the answers to the foregoing questions, do you have a:

True experimental design? _____

Quasi-experimental design: _____

Lacking randomization? _____

Lacking control? _____

Use research notation to map out your design.

B. You are doing nonexperimental research.

Are you interested in studying a:

_____ Variable that is fixed?

_____ Variable that has already occurred?

_____ Comparison of one or more variables that have occurred?

Name the variable(s):

C. You are doing qualitative research.

What is the topic you wish to know more about?

List some research questions that would get you started:

In what settings would you look for participants?

Name some possible participants by title or position:

Describe some of the ways you would collect data:

Observation

Participant observation

Interviews

Examining records

Keep in mind the flexibility of the qualitative research process. Many of your initial ideas may change as the project progresses. Answering the preceding questions will give you a beginning focus that will probably be revised while you are collecting the data.

References

Bogdan, R.C., & Biklen, S.K. (1982). *Qualitative research for education: An introduction to theory and methods*. Boston: Allyn and Bacon.

Campbell, D.T., & Stanley, J.C. (1969). *Experimental and quasi-experimental designs for research*. Skokie, IL: Rand McNally.

Carpenter, C. (1994). The experience of spinal cord injury: The individual's perspective—implications for rehabilitation practice. *Physical Therapy, 74*(7), 614–629.

Crepeau, E.B. (1994). Three images of interdisciplinary team meetings. *American Journal of Occupational Therapy, 48*(8), 717–722.

Depoy, E., & Gitlin, L.N. (1994). *Introduction to research: Multiple strategies for health and human services*. St. Louis, Mosby–Year Book.

Geertz, C. (1973). Thick description: Toward an interpretative theory of culture. In *The interpretation of cultures*. New York: Basic Books.

Glesne, C., & Peshkin, A. (1992). *Becoming qualitative researchers: An introduction*. NY: Longman.

Helfrich, C., Kielhofner, G., & Mattingly, C. (1994). Volition as narrative: Understanding motivation in chronic illness. *American Journal of Occupational Therapy, 48*(4), 311–317.

Hofmann, R. (1995). *Some general pedagogical comparisons of qualitative and quantitative research*. Paper presented at 1995 Conference on Qualitative Research in Education, University of Georgia, Athens, GA.

Jongbloed, L. (1994). Adaptation to a stroke: The experience of one couple. *American Journal of Occupational Therapy, 48*(11), 1006–1013.

Jongbloed, L., Stacey, S., & Brighton, C. (1989). Stroke rehabilitation: Sensorimotor integrative treatment versus functional treatment. *American Journal of Occupational Therapy, 43*(6), 391–397.

Kielhofner, G. (1979). The temporal dimension in the lives of retarded adults: A problem of interaction and intervention. *American Journal of Occupational Therapy, 33*(3), 161–168.

King, L.J. (1974). A sensory-integrative approach to schizophrenia. *American Journal of Occupational Therapy, 28*(9), 529–536.

Mattingly, C., & Fleming, M.H. (1994). *Clinical reasoning: Forms of inquiry in a therapeutic practice*. Philadelphia: F.A. Davis.

McCuaig, M. & Frank, G. (1991). The able self: Adaptive patterns and choices in independent living for a person with cerebral palsy. *American Journal of Occupational Therapy, 45*(3), 224–234.

McDermott, R. (1976). *Kids make sense: An ethnographic account of the interactional management of success and failure in one first grade classroom*. Unpublished doctoral dissertation, Stanford University.

Miles, M.B., & Huberman, A.M. (1994). *Qualitative data analysis: An expanded sourcebook*. Thousand Oaks, CA: Sage.

Moore, D.A. (1989). *Guided visual imagery as an occupational therapy modality*. Unpublished master's thesis, Tufts University, Medford, MA.

Sachs, D., & Labovitz, D. (1994). The caring occupational therapist: Scope of professional roles and boundaries. *American Journal of Occupational Therapy, 48*(11), 997–1005.

Schultz, C.H. (1994). Helping factors in a peer-developed support group for persons with head injury. Part II: Survivor interview perspective. *American Journal of Occupational Therapy, 48*(4), 305–309.

Schwartzberg, S.L. (1994). Helping factors in a peer-developed support group for persons with head injury. Part I: Participant observer perspective. *American Journal of Occupational Therapy, 48*(4), 297–304.

Spencer, J., Young, M., Rintala, D., & Bates, S. (1995). Socialization to the culture of a rehabilitation hospital: An ethnographic study. *American Journal of Occupational Therapy, 49*(1), 53–62.

Spradley, J.P. (1980). *Participant observation*. New York: Holt, Rinehart & Winston.

Yerxa, E.J. (1991). Seeking a relevant, ethical, and realistic way of knowing for occupational therapy. *American Journal of Occupational Therapy, 45*(3), 199–204.

Additional Reading

Cox, R.C., & West, W.L. (1986). Selecting a research design. In *fundamentals of research for health professionals*. Laurel, MD: RAMSCO Publishing.

Goetz, J.P., & LeCompte, M.D. (1984). *Ethnography and qualitative design in educational research*. San Diego. Academic Press.

Lehmkuhl, D. (1970). Let's reduce the understanding gap: 3. Experimental design: What and why? *Physical Therapy, 50*(12), 1716–1720.

Morse, A. (Ed.) (1985). *New dimensions in research for health professionals* [Cassette recordings and workbook]. Laurel, MD: American Occupational Therapy Foundation and RAMSCO Publishing.

Oyster, C., Hanten, W., & Llorens, L. (1987). *Introduction to research: A guide for the health science professional*. Philadelphia: J.B. Lippincott.

Partridge, C.J., & Barnitt, R.E. (1986). Research design. In *research guidelines: A handbook for therapists*. Rockville, MD: Aspen Publishers.

Payton, O. (1994). *Research: The validation of clinical practice* (3rd ed.). Philadelphia: F.A. Davis.

Stein, F., & Cutler, S.K. (1996). *Clinical research in allied health and special education* (3rd ed.). San Diego: Singular Publishing Group.

Taylor, S.J., & Bogdan, R. (1984). *Introduction to qualitative research methods: The search for meanings*. New York: John Wiley & Sons.

Wolcott, H.F. (1992). Posturing in qualitative inquiry. In LeCompte, M.D., Millroy, W.L., & Preissle, J. (Eds.), *The handbook of qualitative research in education* (pp. 3–52). New York: Academic Press.

5

Quantitative Research Designs

In this chapter, some of the major quantitative research designs will be described and their advantages and disadvantages discussed. There are, of course, many more designs than are presented here, but beginning researchers should be able to find a design to fit their needs in getting started in the research process. This chapter is divided into experimental designs, quasi-experimental designs, and nonexperimental designs.

Experimental Designs

The Classic Design

The classic design with experimental and control groups, random selection, pre-testing, and post-testing has already been presented in Chapter 4. Using research notation, the design is represented thus:

$$R \quad O \quad X \quad O$$
$$R \quad O \qquad O$$

You will remember that this design provides for the three essential components of experimental research: randomization, control, and manipulation of the independent variable. Using this design, subjects are randomly selected and randomly assigned to either an experimental or a control group. Pre-tests and post-tests are administered to both groups. The resulting data from the pre-tests will enable the researcher to see whether or not the two groups are truly alike. Post-test scores can be compared to see which group shows the greatest change in the dependent variable. Finally, the pre-test and post-test of each group can be compared to see how much change occurred for the experimental versus the control group.

If circumstances dictate, the random assignment to groups could be performed after the pre-test; however, the assignment should be in no way influenced by the results of the pre-test. Following random assignment, equivalency between the two groups may be assumed; yet performing a pre-test provides a further check on equivalency. This double check is particularly useful in dealing with small samples. Nevertheless, mortality (loss of participants), particularly that which differs between experimental and control groups, should be a continuing concern.

Follow-up

If you wish to know if the effect of the intervention is long-lasting, the design may be further improved by adding a follow-up observation or post-test (O_2 and O_4), thus:

$$R \quad O \quad X \quad O_1 \quad O_2$$
$$R \quad O \qquad O_3 \quad O_4$$

This will enable you to see if any improvement following the treatment has been

---

Box 5–A

A 1989 study compared "the effectiveness of excitatory and inhibitory multisensory stimulation for reducing instances of stereotypic behavior (STB) in a severely multiply disabled population. Thirty-six subjects were randomly assigned to three groups (excitatory, inhibitory stimulation, and control groups) and the two experimental groups received a treatment intervention for 30 days. . . . STB was measured before, after, and 2 months after the intervention period."

The design would have been notated thus:

$$R \quad O \quad X_1 \quad O \quad O$$
$$R \quad O \quad X_2 \quad O \quad O$$
$$R \quad O \qquad \ \ O \quad O$$

(Iwasaki & Holm, 1989, p. 170)

---

maintained over time. Box 5–A illustrates the point with a follow-up observation occurring 2 months after the post-test.

Omitted Pre-test

Sometimes, the results of the treatment may be influenced by the fact that a pre-test has been administered. For example, subjects may benefit from practicing a task used in the pre-test, thus diminishing the effect of the intervention. In this case, the pre-test may be omitted as long as there have been random selection and random assignment to groups. The resulting design looks like this:

$$R \quad X \quad O$$
$$R \qquad \ \ O$$

However, if the investigator is not sure whether or not the pre-test has an effect, or knows that it has an effect but feels that it provides crucial information, the Solomon four-group design can be employed.

Solomon Four-Group Design

The Solomon four-group design is a powerful research design, but requires many subjects and a great deal of researcher time. It is constructed thus:

$$R \quad O \quad X \quad O_1$$
$$R \quad O \qquad \ \ O_2$$
$$R \qquad \ \ X \quad O_3$$
$$R \qquad \qquad O_4$$

There is random assignment to four groups, two experimental and two control groups:

- One group receives the pre-test and the experimental treatment followed by a post-test.
- A second group is given a pre-test and a post-test but no treatment.
- The third group is not given a pre-test but receives the experimental treatment and a post-test.
- The fourth group receives only the post-test.

In comparing the post-test results, the researcher is able to test not only for differences between experimental and control groups but for any interaction between pre-test and experimental treatment by comparing groups 1 and 3 (on O_1 and O_3) and groups 2 and 4 (on O_2 and O_4).

Factorial Designs

The experimental designs mentioned so far are designed to cope with one independent variable only, whereas researchers are typically concerned with more than one variable in the same study. Factorial designs may be used to investigate two or more independent variables and their interaction with the dependent variable. These designs allow the researcher to use the same subjects to study the effects of the independent variables on the dependent variable as well as any joint effect or interaction effect. In factorial designs, each independent variable is called a factor.

For example, in Henry, Nelson, and Duncombe's study (1984) regarding choice-making in group and individual activities, the investigators wished to assess subjects' responses to having or not having a choice in

	Individual activity	Group activity
Choice	Group 1	Group 3
No Choice	Group 2	Group 4

FIGURE 5–1 Chart depicting the Henry, Nelson, and Duncombe study (1984).

	Individual	Group	Combination
Choice	1	2	3
No Choice	4	5	6

FIGURE 5–2   Representation of a 3 × 2 design.

completing an activity. Forty subjects were divided into four groups:

1. Individual activity with a choice
2. Individual activity with no choice
3. Group activity with a choice
4. Group activity with no choice

The two independent variables were the type of activity (individual or group) and the factor of choice (choice or no choice). Therefore, the study was concerned with the effects of these variables on the dependent variable—affective response. The study is charted in Figure 5–1. There are two levels for each independent variable or factor: individual and group levels for the activity factor and choice and no choice levels for the choice factor. Thus, this is called a 2 × 2 design.

If one of these factors had contained three levels, by adding a group who received a combination of group and individual activities, for instance, it would be a 3 × 2 design and would be represented as shown in the chart in Figure 5–2. In a different variation, a third variable or factor, such as age, could be added to the original design with two levels for each factor, making it a 2 × 2 × 2 design as depicted in Figure 5–3. Age is actually a pseudoindependent variable because it is not being manipulated by the researcher; it is an already occurring attribute of the subjects. However, in factorial designs, pseudoindependent variables are often treated in the same manner as true independent variables.

As more variables are added, both the complexity of the design and the number of subjects required increases. Specific statistical procedures are used to analyze these designs, and usually the services of a statistician are required.

Quasi-experimental Designs

Lack of Randomization

In studying the effect of depression on self-care activities in hospitalized patients, Clark (1964) selected depressed patients from two wards and treated them as two separate groups. The design looked like this:

$$O \quad X_1 \quad O$$
$$O \quad X_2 \quad O$$

Although subjects in the two groups cannot be assumed to be equivalent because they were not randomly assigned, the researcher will have information about their pretreatment status based on the data from the pre-tests. If they are found to be substantially different at the pre-test stage, the researcher can either abandon the groups and start the study over or use statistical techniques to take into account the differences.

Convenience Samples

Major differences are likely to occur when the two groups are convenience samples (i.e., groups that are already formed by some event preceding the research study). They may be groups of patients in two different wards of the same hospital, or two different nursing homes, or two day-care centers, for example. Box 5–B illustrates the use of convenience samples.

It is quite common for clinical researchers to use ready-formed groups because this is so practical. Some critics look askance at the practice, saying it is impossible to make reasonable comparisons between such groups. Others point out that using convenience

Individual Activity				Group Activity			
Choice		No Choice		Choice		No Choice	
Over 50	Under 50	Over 50	Under 50	Over 50	Under 50	Over 50	Under 50
1	2	3	4	5	6	7	8

FIGURE 5–3   Representation of a 2 × 2 × 2 design.

Box 5–B

Hardison and Llorens (1988) studied the effects of a crafts group for teenage delinquent girls with suspected vestibular processing difficulties. Subjects were selected from two different group homes. Subjects from one group home became the experimental group and subjects from the other the control group.

samples is such a practical solution to a very real problem that we should impose whatever controls we can and be alert to the variables that can have an impact on such research. The crucial question to ask is whether the two groups truly come from the same population. The researcher may take the trouble to match subjects in the two groups so that there are commonalities in such items as socioeconomic status, gender mix, age, diagnosis, or other attributes considered important to the study. Cox and West (1986) offer a helpful description of the matching process and when it should be used. An example of matching is shown in Box 5–C.

The problem of nonrepresentation is less likely to occur if the subjects have been randomly assigned to the research groups, even though they were not randomly selected from the target population. This obviously cannot be achieved if convenience samples are taken from different locations, but can be achieved with a convenience sample taken entirely from one facility. Random assignment may ensure that the two groups are similar in characteristics, even though they may not be representative of the population.

Cohort Designs

When using cohort designs, a control group is again used to assess the changes made in the experimental group, but this time the groups are not observed at the same time. The groups follow each other through a setting such as classes of students moving through a therapist training program or groups of trainees entering a sheltered workshop for a training period. One group is selected as the experimental group and subjected to a unique experience, while another group acts as the control group and experiences the usual events of the setting.

The subjects in these groups are obviously not randomly chosen, because the groups are naturally occurring. Nonetheless, the two groups may be considered somewhat similar in that they both meet the admission requirements of the setting. The design may be depicted thus:

$$O \quad X \quad O$$
$$O \qquad O$$

There are internal validity problems with this design because of the difference in the time of the observations. History (i.e., some sort of global event that has an effect on all subjects in the sample) may play a part in accounting for the differences in data from the post-tests (Box 5–D).

The cohort design can be improved by employing recurrent institutional cycles, using three different cohorts. The design is as follows:

$$X \quad O_1$$
$$O_2 \quad X \quad O_3$$
$$O_4$$

The first group receives the experimental treatment followed by a post-test; the second group receives the traditional pre-test, treat-

Box 5–C

Bohannon (1987) used matched controls in his study to determine whether the relative muscular endurance of patients with paresis secondary to neuromuscular disorders was different from that of comparable healthy persons. The subjects were five persons with neuromuscular disorders: cauda equina lesions (2); nerve root compression (1); muscular dystrophy (1); and Guillain-Barré syndrome (1). Bohannon matched the five control subjects by sex, age, weight, height, and peak knee extension torque of the lower extremity.

Box 5–D

In studying the impact of depression on self-care management in a group of hospitalized depressed patients, a therapist reported that the death of President John F. Kennedy, which occurred partway into the study, had a profound impact on the patients (Clark, 1964). She surmised that this historically tragic event compounded the results of her study.

ment, and post-test; and the third group receives only a pre-test. The ideal pattern of results from this design would be similarity of responses on pre-tests O_2 and O_4 and on post-tests O_1 and O_2. The effect of the treatment would be evident by comparing scores on pre-test O_2 and post-test O_3.

Lack of Control

Time-series designs have no control group, and the subjects in the experimental group act as their own control.

Single-Group Time-Series Design

In the single-group time-series design, subjects are given a pre-test, followed by experimental treatment and a post-test. A period of time is allowed to elapse, equivalent to the amount of the experimental treatment time, and then another post-test follows. Periods of treatment and nontreatment are alternated with tests. During the treatment periods, the subjects in the group compose an experimental group, and during the nontreatment periods they act as a control group. Thus, we have the commonly used expression "acting as their own control," which was mentioned in Chapter 4. The design is notated as follows:

$$O \ X \ O \quad O \ X \ O \quad O \ X \ O$$

The group may be randomly selected to increase the likelihood of its being representative of the population under study. Of course, the issue of random assignment to groups is a moot point because there is only one group. This design provides a high degree of internal validity, meaning that one can be fairly sure that any changes that occur in the dependent variable at post-tests are due to the experimental treatment.

Follow-up

In a variation of the time-series design, a researcher may wish to assess the permanence of change in the dependent variable and may do so by administering several post-tests after the intervention; thus:

$$O \ X \ O_1 \ O_2 \ O_3 \ O_4$$

However, this design does have a flaw, in that it is difficult to know if improvement at the first post-test (O_1) was due to the intervention or to something else, including: (a) some other event that occurred concurrently; (b) something special that occurred with the procedure, instrument, or therapist; or (c) an inherent characteristic in the subject such as a seasonal improvement. There is no subsequent treatment period to use as a test for these possibilities.

Multiple Pre-tests

A third possible design of the time-series type will control for some of these flaws:

$$O \ O \ O \ O \ X \ O \ O \ O \ O$$

The multiple pre-tests will give a more accurate picture of how subjects score on the dependent variable before the experimental treatment, will control for seasonal or cyclical changes in abilities, and will eliminate the effect of history. An even more preferable design would be:

$$O \ O \ O \ X \ O_1 \ X \ O_2 \ X \ O_3 \ O_4 \ O_5$$

Here history is controlled for, the effects of experimental treatment can be viewed on more than one occasion (at O_1, O_2, and O_3), and the permanence of the effect can be measured (O_3 through O_5). The disadvantages of this design are that it is often impractical to wait long enough to administer several pre-tests before treating the patient and that the entire study becomes lengthy (Box 5–E).

Box 5–E

Ottenbacher (1982) uses a variation of the time-series analysis in his study of the effects of a sensory stimulation program and resultant duration of postrotary nystagmus on three learning-disabled children. He used a period of 5 weeks to gather baseline data on their postrotary nystagmus, then alternately treated and tested the children over 20 weeks. They received treatment three times per week and were tested twice per week, so the resulting design looks approximately like this:

$$O \ O \ O \ O \ O \quad X \ O \ X \ O \ X \quad X \ O \ X \ O \ X \quad \ldots \ldots \quad X \ O \ X \ O \ X$$

Despite the fact that these are quasi-experimental designs, they are effective and can be quite practical for the clinical researcher. It is sometimes easier to gain permission to include patients in quasi-experimental studies than it is to include them in experimental studies; for example, it is difficult to deny treatment to patients in control groups. Finally, the fact that these designs are carried out in clinical settings, with all the concomitant interferences and lack of control inherent in such settings, makes them more likely to be generalizable to other clinical settings. It is, after all, in day-to-day clinical practice that we wish to put the results of research into effect.

Nonexperimental Designs

The nature of problems in the health sciences usually prevents investigators from proving causal effects; that is, they cannot often state definitively that the changes they see at the end of their studies are caused solely by the treatment intervention. One reason for this is that various forms of disability and illness are frequently the target of study, and the rehabilitation professional has access to people only *after* they have acquired the disability or illness. Therefore, *ex post facto* ("after the fact") designs must be employed when the dependent variable has already occurred. Nonexperimental designs are many and varied. A representative sampling will be reviewed here.

Correlational Research

Most nonexperimental studies in rehabilitative health care fall in the correlational category. Correlational research is similar to experimental research in that a hypothesis is being tested; however, it is different in that there is no manipulation of independent variables, and a cause-effect relationship is not being simulated. Instead, in correlational research, the investigator is looking for a relationship between variables. Rather than hypothesizing, for instance, that being blind will cause an individual to have heightened tactile sensitivity, one might conjecture that there is simply a relationship between the variables "blindness" and "heightened tactile sensitivity." Blindness has already occurred by the time the researcher is studying it, making this *ex post facto,* or nonexperimental research.

The researcher tests a hypothesis, comparing two or more variables by measuring differences and looking for a relationship. The procedure for the correlational research design is similar to that for experimental designs; that is, reviewing the literature, formulating research questions or hypotheses, deciding whether the hypotheses should be directional or null hypotheses, defining and operationalizing terms, selecting a sample from a population, and selecting data collection and interpretation methods.

In correlational research, however, specific statistical tests are used for data analysis that look for an association between the two variables. This association is known as a correlation coefficient and yields a value between -1 and $+1$, where 0 indicates no relationship and the two extremes indicate a perfect negative (or inverse) relationship (-1) or a perfect positive (or direct) relationship ($+1$) (Box 5–F).

Because this is nonexperimental research and, therefore, is not subjected to the stringent rules of experimental research, similar results need to be found in many studies before therapists can claim relationships between variables concerning their patients.

Survey Research

Surveys are used frequently to gather information about a large population in order to answer a set of hypotheses. They are cross-

---

Box 5–F

A correlational study was conducted by Short-DeGraff, Slansky, and Diamond (1989) to see if there was a relationship between preschoolers' self-drawings and results on the Goodenough-Harris Draw-a-Person Test (DAPT) and the General Information subtest of the Wechsler Preschool and Primary Scale of Intelligence (WPPSI). High correlations were obtained between the man, woman, and man/woman converted scores of the DAPT and the self-drawings ($r = 0.93$ and $r = 0.91$). Low correlations were found between all of the figure drawing and WPPSI scores (average $r = 0.3$).

sectional in the sense that they generally describe the group at one point in time, and they are used to measure the "what is" about a group rather than providing information on "why" (Cox & West, 1986). Information collected in survey research covers a vast array of topics and may include items ranging from attitudes, values, opinions, motives, and levels of information to concrete information on such things as the respondents' work situation, environment, living situation, behaviors, and so on.

To qualify as research, the survey must be carefully crafted to answer a well-defined set of questions that have been grounded in a literature review and have significance and relevance. The manner of analysis and interpretation of the data also make this a research design rather than solely a status survey to elicit some facts about a particular group. The method of analysis needs to be chosen and applied judiciously; interpretations and application to the population must be made with care.

Information may be collected either directly through a face-to-face interview or telephone interview, or indirectly through the mail or private completion of a questionnaire. These forms of data gathering are discussed in a later chapter on the collection of data.

It is crucial that the relevant population be defined clearly and that its characteristics and limits be described. Sample selection methods must ensure representation because the method generally used in conducting survey research is the drawing of conclusions about a large group from a smaller sample of persons (Box 5–G). If you are not confident that the sample is representative of the population, the resulting discussion will be invalid for the larger group about whom you are generalizing.

Methods of selection, or sampling, are crucially important in survey research. Random selection is described in Chapter 4 of this book. Also, Kalton's *Introduction to Survey Sampling* (1983) offers an excellent overview of methods to use when sampling for a survey.

Quantitative Case Study Research

There is little agreement among researchers as to what exactly constitutes a case study. There are those who consider it useful only as a pilot study and a prelude to a "full" experimental study, those who feel it can stand on its own as a quantitative study (Yin, 1994), and those who feel it has great merit as a form of qualitative inquiry (Merriam, 1988). In this book, I have chosen to describe two types of case study research designs, the quantitative case study and the qualitative case method. The qualitative case method will be discussed in Chapter 9.

That which is referred to as quantitative case study research in this book is often referred to as single-subject, single-case, small-N, or idiographic research in other publications. In this type of case study, an individual, unit, or event is studied in great depth over time—anywhere from a few weeks to several years. Thus, it is a longitudinal study rather than the cross-sectional study of the survey type. In quantitative case studies, the case being studied is usually an individual person or event.

Data are generally gathered by one researcher at various points throughout the life of the case and may occur in a natural setting such as the home or, more often, in a clinical setting such as a hospital.

Case studies often fall into the category of exploratory studies, those which have as their goal the generation of hypotheses for further study under experimental conditions. They can be generalized to theoretical propositions, rather than to populations in the way that experiments are and, in this sense, the case does not represent a "sample." The investigator's goal is to expand and generalize theories rather than to enumerate frequencies. Case studies have been used very effectively in the rehabilitation litera-

---

Box 5–G

In Bailey's study (1990) on reasons for attrition from occupational therapy, she defined her population as female certified occupational therapists who were no longer working as occupational therapists. She selected her sample randomly from (a) female occupational therapists who had completed the 1986 AOTA Member Data Survey saying that they were not currently working, (b) those who had let their AOTA membership lapse, and (c) those whose names had been provided by colleagues because they were working in non-occupational therapy jobs.

ture and have provided accounts of treatment techniques and procedures that have been helpful to therapists in their practice. The regular case reports section of the *American Journal of Occupational Therapy* has been especially helpful in this regard.

Ottenbacher and York (1984) found that single-case studies tend to be practice-based and practitioner-oriented, and they have listed reasons why clinicians find case studies particularly doable and useful forms of research in their clinics. Single-case studies are often easier to manage for therapists who have difficulty gathering groups of homogeneous patients to form experimental groups. Furthermore, group studies are usually concerned with comparing the average change between two groups and clinicians may not be as interested in the average changes of a group as they are in changes in individuals. They are interested not only in the patient's overall change by the end of the study, but also in the course of that clinical change over time. Single-subject studies allow the clinician an opportunity for continuous assessment of a client's progress at various points during treatment. The clinician not only can monitor changes throughout treatment, but also can alter the intervention based on the study data, should this be indicated. This is not usually possible with group study designs. Data can be collected during the intervention period and compared with data collected when intervention is not being provided (the process of using subjects as their own control that was described earlier). For these reasons, clinicians tend to find single-case studies manageable and desirable in the clinical setting, while readers find them valid and relevant to their own practice.

When trying to decide whether to use a case study rather than another type of exploratory study such as a survey, it is useful to bear in mind that "how" and "why" questions are best answered by case studies. For example, Stein and Nikolic (1989) asked, "How could a stress management training program be used to assist a young man with schizophrenia control his anxiety?" Therapists often ask how and why a particular adaptive aid or treatment procedure worked with a particular patient. For instance, Rogers, Marcus, and Snow (1987) asked, "Why did their sensory training program work with a severely regressed elderly patient?" This case illustrates the essential points of the case study approach so well that it is in-

cluded as a lengthy example (Box 5–H). The authors wanted to generate ideas about the role of sensory training in putting severely regressed elderly patients in touch with their

---

Box 5–H

In a case report in the *American Journal of Occupational Therapy* (1987), Rogers, Marcus, and Snow recount the story of Maude, a 90-year-old woman diagnosed with senile dementia and many other ailments such as gout, hypertension, head injury, depression, and possible cancer. Maude was nonambulatory, incontinent, and dependent for all her self-care needs, and she spent most of her day nonresponsive, sitting with her eyes closed. She had been a facility resident for many years and represented the severely regressed, sensorily deprived elderly patients with whom the authors were concerned.

Maude received an intensive sensory training program, 4 days a week for 5 weeks. The daily greeting procedure and 10 core activities of the program are described in detail, together with supplementary stimulation activities and concluding procedures. Maude made dramatic gains as a result of the program. She showed a consistent increase in independent functioning during the sessions, in all 10 core activities. Her initial belligerence and hostility toward the leader subsided and were replaced by open affection. She became meaningfully talkative, initiated conversations with the leader, and made comments about other participants. At the end of the program, she had become oriented to person and place, was able to look at the examiner when addressed, could respond to questions with short appropriate phrases, and showed appropriate facial expressions. Similar improvements were noted by other staff members at the facility, and her gains lasted for the year during which there was follow-up.

In the discussion, the authors provide several hypotheses, conjecturing that Maude's increase in interaction may have promoted additional stimulation from the staff because they found her easier to communicate with and more rewarding to be with; they hypothesize about sensory training being based on the concept that deficiencies in physical and mental stimulation contribute to cognitive impairment; and about the common characteristics of sensory deprivation seen in normal individuals. Finally, the investigators give information about the specific activities that appeared most helpful in the treatment sessions.

environment rather than enumerating the times or the degree to which "Maude" was able to respond to the activities. Their hope was that other therapists would try these ideas with similar patients, testing the hypotheses and elaborating on the theory.

Investigators sometimes wonder when to use a single-case study rather than a multi-case study. Use a single-case study if:

1. You can identify *the* critical case that illustrates all the propositions of the study

2. One case is the extreme or unique case and there are no others easily available

3. You have a revelatory case that was previously unavailable to researchers

4. It is being used as a pilot study case for the multicase study approach (Yin, 1994)

Use a multicase study approach if:

1. You wish to build theoretical constructs across cases, thus presenting a stronger outcome.

2. You want "to build a general explanation that fits each of the individual cases, even though the cases will vary in their details."

3. You have the opportunity of more than one similar case. Then you should adopt replication logic (i.e., all cases should be as similar as possible and you should expect to obtain similar outcomes). If you get very different findings, you need to rethink the original theory for the study (Yin, 1994).

If you chose the multicase study approach, how many cases should you use? If there are not too many variables under study, use two or three cases; if there are many variables, increase to five or six cases. It is appropriate to use a pilot study case for a multicase study and use it to revise such things as choice of subject, method of data collection, and type of data collected. It is not appropriate to change the original purpose or intent of the study.

The criterion for a successful case study is that theoretical propositions or hypotheses have resulted that can be tested in an experimental manner. Ultimately, the hope is that the hypotheses will be supported and give indications that will allow therapists to pre-scribe specific treatments for appropriate patients.

In quantitative case study research, the investigator is often designing and testing a specific treatment protocol for a client with a particular disability, such as Stein and Nikolic's (1989) stress management program, or designing and testing a device such as a splint or a piece of adaptive equipment, specific to an individual. In these types of studies, the researcher gathers baseline data on the client's condition in order to test whether the program or device has had the desired effect. It can be seen that this is similar to the classic experimental design with a pretest, intervention, and post-test, but is conducted on an individual rather than a group.

Data for the quantitative case study are likely to be gathered in several ways: observing and counting such things as behaviors that are targeted for change, using hardware to measure such things as joint flexion and extension or muscle strength, or using a formal index to evaluate some portion of self-care activities. These data will provide the baseline information that will be measured against data from later collection periods, usually conducted at various points throughout the study. Baseline data are often supplemented by documentary evidence such as information in patients' charts, reports of case conferences, previous assessments or progress reports, or administrative memoranda. While providing the researcher with a rich source of data for comparison, these data also "flesh out" a picture of the subject for the reader.

It may be appropriate to use statistical data analyses for a quantitative case study if you have sufficient data. For instance, if you have collected data after various phases of treatment, and perhaps at several follow-up points after treatment has ended, this could yield a dozen or more groups of data that could be tallied and otherwise statistically manipulated in order to show change over time. A pictorial presentation, such as a graph, is often an informative way to indicate changes that occur.

Case studies are a useful and fascinating way for therapists to learn the investigation process. Most of us have at least one client whose progress and style of learning could benefit others, while the case study process itself requires discipline and is thought-provoking.

Methodological Research

For many years, therapists have been interested in developing and fabricating their own adaptive aids, equipment, tests, and other instruments for use in the evaluation and treatment of their patients. They wish to test and improve the validity and reliability of such materials (Box 5–I), and methodological research methods may be used to achieve these goals. Methodological research develops, validates, evaluates, and produces standardized measures. If the instruments used in clinical research are reliable and valid, the researcher can have more confidence in the results of the research, and results can be compared across studies.

The precise set of procedures used in standardizing measures is described by Benson and Clark (1982) in their article, "A Guide for Instrument Development and Validation." The stages include:

1. Deciding on the purpose of the measure and the population of concern (such conditions as age, gender, diagnosis, symptomatology, place of residence, vocational goals, and psychological attributes)

2. Elucidating the content of the measure by using personal experience, review of relevant literature, and opinions of experts in the field

3. Organizing and compiling the content into a logical and meaningful sequence

4. Testing the resulting measure on a large sample of the chosen population

5. Subjecting the results to statistical tests for reliability and validity

6. Improving the design and content of the measure based on the findings

7. Retesting the measure

8. Repeating the last four steps several times until you are satisfied with the results

9. Writing an accompanying manual outlining the research process used, the population for whom the measure is intended, the results of the tests for reliability and validity, and exact procedures for using the measure

As you can readily see from this list, "methodological research develops, validates, and evaluates standardized measures. Such research establishes the validity and reliability of research instruments, which improves the quality of research" (Oyster, Hanten, & Llorens, 1987, p. 97). We often use self-made instruments in research studies without showing sufficient concern or caution in interpreting data produced by such nonstandardized measures. As Oyster and colleagues (1987) point out, ". . . it is important to recognize that [methodological research] may be one of the most significant contributors to the evolution of health science research as an exact science" (p. 98).

Evaluation Research

Evaluation research is designed to determine, first, how a new program should be developed and designed and, second, how well an existing program is doing and what should be done, if anything, to improve it. Thus, the results of evaluation research will provide answers to the questions "What should we do?" and "How well are we doing?" The first part is formative research, in that it represents a collection of data or opinion that can be used to form a policy upon which to design a program. Data and opinions are collected from both the users and the providers of the program.

The second part is summative research, in which an existing program and its policies are evaluated. It is usual to write the program goals and objectives in behavioral terms and then collect evidence in the form of data to determine whether the goals and objectives are being met. It is quite difficult to write goals and objectives in behavioral and measurable terms while keeping them meaningful for the program's mission, but

---

Box 5–I

A group of physical therapy investigators conducted a methodological study to determine the "reliability of lumbar flexion and extension range-of-motion measurements obtained with the modified-modified Schober and the double inclinometer methods on subjects with low back pain." They found that the modified-modified Schober method was a reliable method of measurement for these subjects, and thus expanded the range of patients on which this tool could be used.

(Williams, Binkley, Bloch, et al., 1993, p. 26)

Box 5–J

A study was conducted to assess the effectiveness of an occupational therapy program in the treatment of alcohol and drug dependency (Stensrud & Lushbough, 1988). The program was viewed as a demonstration project. If it was deemed successful, occupational therapy would be incorporated into the Alcohol and Drug Dependency Treatment Center.

this is essential if the data are to be used to evaluate the effectiveness of the program.

Data are gathered from many sources, including past and present consumers of the program, representatives of all levels of providers in the program, written policies and procedures, client records, and the physical plant and its equipment. Often large quantities of data need to be organized and applied to each of the program's stated goals and objectives. The evaluator then must make judgments as to whether or not the goals and objectives are being met (Box 5–J).

A program evaluator from outside the program is often employed, the advantages being that the evaluator is more likely to be objective about the program's good and bad points and is free of the burden of implementing recommended changes. If evaluators knew that they would have to make the required changes at the end of an evaluation, they might be biased in the type of changes being recommended. The negative side of having an outside evaluator is that it takes time for the outsider to be accepted by program staff. Also, staff have been known to sabotage evaluations by not cooperating or by being dishonest with the outside evaluator.

Validity and Reliability of Quantitative Research

In order to feel that their studies are of value, researchers engaged in any of the foregoing research methods will wish to address the credibility of their studies. In order to do so, the principles of study validity and reliability need to be understood. Whereas reliability is concerned with the replicability of scientific findings, validity is concerned with the accuracy of scientific findings.

Validity

A study is valid only if investigators are truly addressing the constructs they set out to study and measure. Validity needs to be addressed from two points of view. First, internal validity—are investigators actually observing and measuring what they think they are observing or measuring? And, second, external validity—to what extent are the ideas generated or tested by the investigators applicable to other groups?

Internal Validity

The effects of history (the events that have happened throughout the study), maturation of the subjects during the study, testing of the subjects, instrumentation used in the study, subject selection, and subject mortality (how and how many subjects were lost before completion of the study), can all have an impact on the internal validity of a study. These will be dealt with in some detail.

1. **History.** In a study in which measurement of an independent variable (the variable being examined for change) is occurring before and after some sort of manipulation or treatment, internal validity may be compromised. This can happen if something happens to the subjects or the environment that was not planned in the study design, such as a subject having an injury or losing interest in the study and not making an effort during the treatment sessions. This will affect the final measurement scores. Historical contamination can be prevented by careful sampling and by controlling subjects' activities during the study.

2. **Maturation.** This is also related to the passage of time during the study; in fact, it is directly related to time rather than to events that happen between pre-test and post-test. Maturation refers to the subjects' growth, development, or changes that occur naturally over time. Studies in which the subjects are children are particularly vulnerable to maturation problems. For example, it might be difficult to determine if a year-long remedial writing program has resulted in improvement in a child's handwriting, or if that improve-

ment would have occurred anyway with the passage of time.

3. **Testing.** If the same test is being used several times throughout the study, it is possible that subjects [illegible]

4. **Subject Selection.** [illegible] subjects to the groups.

5. **Subject Mortality or Attrition.** However well a study is prepared, it is difficult to prevent subject attrition due to such things as illness, a geographic move, or death. Extra subjects should be recruited into the study to account for these losses. This is particularly important in a case study.

6. **Instrumentation.** The condition of the instruments themselves may influence measurements. For example, an instrument may not be calibrated accurately or it may be old, worn out, or in bad condition and not give accurate readings. Mailed surveys or attitude surveys may include cultural, racial, intelligence, or language bias that would influence the results.

External Validity

Controlling influences on external validity is a tougher proposition. As researchers take pains to add control subjects to their experiments to produce sound research designs, they make their experiments less likely to generalize to situations outside the research setting. The reader is left to decide if the studies are valid or relevant to "real-life" situations, often one of the biggest criticisms of experimental research. If researchers wish their studies to be useful in clinical situations, they must often compromise on the control subjects incorporated in the study design. Some of the most common threats to external validity are mentioned here.

1. **Hawthorne Effect.** If subjects are exhibiting the Hawthorne effect, they are performing better on the study task simply because they are getting special attention, and not necessarily because of the treatment they are receiving.
2. **Replication.** When researchers report on their studies, they must describe their methods in sufficient detail that others may replicate the studies. If you cannot be assured that the same methods have been followed in replicated studies, then findings cannot be generalized confidently, thereby threatening external validity.
3. **Generalizability.** Generalizability refers to the extent that the results found in the study sample will also be found in the population. Does the sample being studied truly represent those in the defined population? Random selection of the sample from the population is the only sound way to hope for generalizability.
4. **Multitreatments.** In a study in which subjects are given more than one treatment as the independent variable, the results cannot be generalized to other settings in which only one of those treatments is used. Effects of more than one treatment must be viewed as cumulative and intermingled. Studies that use a single treatment as the independent variable and a single measure for the dependent variable are more likely to achieve external validity.
5. **Researcher Effect.** Sometimes subjects react to the study in a certain way because of their relationship with the researcher, whether it be positive or negative. This is a particularly important consideration if the dependent variable has to do with interpersonal relationships or emotion-laden topics.

Reliability

A study is considered reliable if, when it is repeated, similar findings are produced. The closeness of outcome measures following repetitions of the same study, indicate the dependability of the procedures. Whenever close agreement occurs among several measures of the same phenomenon, the reliability of the procedure, instrument, or research will be high and consumers may have confidence in that portion of the study. Reliability might also refer to the extent to which an instrument agrees with itself, and three types of reliability pertaining to test instruments will be described in a later chapter: test-retest reliability, split-half reliability, and interrater reliability.

Some problems confounding the reliability of the study itself, rather than instruments used, need to be discussed. In the following cases, the study instrument might be reliable but the study itself will not be if these items are not considered.

1. **Subject Fatigue.** This can be a problem when subjects are expected to perform physical or mental tasks repeatedly, and are tired toward the end of the testing procedures. As a consequence, they do not perform to the best of their ability and results are affected. Physiological abilities can change in response to diurnal or circadian rhythms, which may result in different results at different times for the same person.

2. **Subject Motivation.** Subjects are not always interested in the study and may not perform at their best because of lack of motivation. They may even dislike participating in the study, which would certainly influence the effort they put into the testing process. Sometimes they are not in their best mood. In these cases, test results will be varied and will not be reliable indicators of the subjects' abilities.

3. **Subject Learning.** If there are repeated tests on the same instrument within the study, subjects are likely to achieve some learning. They may perform better on later tests simply because they have learned the material on the test rather than because of an experimental intervention.

4. **Subject Ability.** Subjects' ability to respond to certain questions or tasks will vary according to skill level or knowledge of the topic. Responses may vary for the same subject, if he or she chooses to create a response to appease the examiner or to make himself or herself look better.

5. **Tester Skill.** If a tester does not administer certain tests in exactly the same manner each time, responses could vary for the same subject.

6. **Different Testers.** People administering the test differ in such things as their degree of enthusiasm, delivery of instructions, voice, personality, and ability to handle the situation. The same subject may achieve different results depending on the tester.

7. **Test Environment.** Changes in the environment from test to test can influence a subject's responses. Distractions such as noise or interruptions are particularly intrusive on test results.

Once you have decided on the research method you will employ in your study, you will want to make an effort to control for as many of these threats to validity and reliability as possible. Go through the threats listed here one at a time, checking them against the steps you propose to follow in your study method.

Summary

Some examples have been provided of designs that may be employed in the three categories of research: experimental, quasi-experimental, and nonexperimental. Naturally, there are many more types of quantitative research designs than have been mentioned here. Some further designs can be found in the Additional Reading list at the end of this chapter. In particular, there are many variations on the basic themes presented in the experimental and quasi-experimental categories. Careful reading of such texts as Campbell and Stanley's *Experimental and Quasi-Experimental Designs for Research* (1969) and Kerlinger's *Foundations of Behavioral Research* (1979) will guide investigators toward the best design for their particular sets of circumstances.

WORKSHEETS

If you are doing experimental or quasi-experimental research and you did not find a suitable research design in Chapter 4, look through the designs presented in this chapter and choose the most appropriate for your project.

EXPERIMENTAL RESEARCH

1. The classic:

   R   O X O
   R   O   O

2. With follow-up:

   R O X O_1 O_2
   R O O_3 O_4

3. Omitted pre-test:

   R X O
   R   O

4. Solomon four-group:

   R O X_1 O_1
   R O O_2
   R X_2 O_3
   R O_4

5. Factorial designs:

   _____ How many factors?   _____ How many levels for each factor?

Plot out the independent variables in a table so that you can see what your design will look like:

QUASI-EXPERIMENTAL RESEARCH

1. Lack of random assignment:
$$O \quad X_1 \quad O \quad or \quad O \quad X \quad O$$
$$O \quad X_2 \quad O \qquad \quad O \qquad O$$

2. Cohort designs:
$$O \quad X \quad O$$
$$\qquad \qquad O \qquad O$$

3. Recurrent institutional cycles:
$$X \quad O_1$$
$$\qquad \quad O_2 \quad X \quad O_3$$
$$\qquad \qquad \qquad \quad O_4$$

4. Lack of control:
$$O \quad X \quad O \qquad O \quad X \quad O \qquad O \quad X \quad O$$

5. With follow-up:
$$O \quad X \quad O_1 \quad O_2 \quad O_3 \quad O_4$$

6. Multiple pre-tests:
$$O \quad O \quad O \quad O \quad X \quad O \quad O \quad O \quad O$$

or:
$$O \quad O \quad O \quad O \quad X \quad O_1 \quad X \quad O_2 \quad X \quad O_3 \quad O_4 \quad O_5$$

NONEXPERIMENTAL RESEARCH

If you decide that your project is best suited for a nonexperimental design, review the methods offered and choose the most appropriate:

1. Correlational Research

2. Survey Research

3. Quantitative Case Study Research

4. Methodological Research

5. Evaluation Research

WRITING THE RESEARCH PROTOCOL

Now it is time to put into operation the design you have chosen by writing a research protocol. In other words, you need to insert your specific variables, subjects, and procedures into the research design, creating a personalized "road map" for carrying out the project.

Let us say you have chosen the classic experimental design to test your hypothesis, you must now insert the method of random selection and assignment you plan to use, the criteria you will use to select subjects, your definition of dependent and independent variables, exact procedures you will use for the experimental treatment, and the exact procedures you will use to observe or pre-test and post-test the dependent variable(s).

The following is a sample of a research protocol used for a study of verbalization in patients with chronic schizophrenia (Bailey, 1978):

Subject Selection Criteria. Adult (18 years or older), men and women, chronic (diagnosed as schizophrenic for 5 years or more), nonparanoid (chart diagnosis) schizophrenic (chart diagnosis) patients (residents of an institution).

Method of Selection. Subjects will be randomly selected from two subpopulations of nursing home residents who meet the selection criteria. One group will form the experimental group and the other the control group.

Hypothesis. That sensory stimulation, with emphasis on vestibular input, will increase the quantity, quality, and speed of response of verbalization in adults with chronic, nonparanoid schizophrenia.

Dependent Variable. The quantity, quality, and speed of response of verbalization.

Independent Variable. Sensory stimulation program with emphasis on vestibular input.

Procedures for Treatment. Administer a planned, graded program of sensory stimulation, with emphasis on vestibular stimulation, to all subjects in the experimental group for:

> half an hour per day
>
> 5 days per week
>
> for 12 weeks

The program will be provided in the same room of the nursing homes (the day room) each day, using a variety of sensory equipment. The group will be led by the same therapist each day, assisted by occupational therapy students.*

The control group will attend a sedentary crafts program (with as little vestibular input as possible), for the same amount of time, in the same room, led by the same staff as the experimental group.*

PROCEDURES FOR OBSERVATION

Pre-test: Individual subjects in experimental and control groups will be asked 17 questions, and their responses will be recorded on audio tapes. The tester will be a person unknown to all subjects and not involved in the activity groups.

The following items will be measured using the tape recordings:

1. Number of words used in response to all questions

2. Quality of speech (as specified on attached sheet)†

3. Length of time from end of question to beginning of response (measured in seconds by stop watch)

Post-test: Individual subjects in experimental and control groups will be asked the same 17 questions as in the pre-test, and their responses will be recorded on audio tapes. The tester will be the same person as was used for the pre-test. The same measurements for quantity, quality, and speed of response will be used. Figure 5–4 illustrates the data collection sheet used in this project.

---

* The actual program for the sensory stimulation group and the craft group were written in detail for each session.
† A specific checklist for "grading" quality of speech was provided to the tester.

Name: _____   Experimental #: _____

Control #: _____

Date of birth: _____   Sex: M   F

Residence: _____

Physician: _____

Diagnosis: _____

Length of time with this diagnosis: _____

Medications: Initial _____

At termination _____

Any special precautions: _____

Informed consent obtained: _____

Physician's permission to participate obtained: _____

Pre-test date: _____   Tester: _____

Post-test date: _____   Tester: _____

Treatment group attendance: X if in experimental group

C if in control group

Comments

Jan. 24 - Jan. 28   ____ ____ ____ ____ ____   _____

Jan. 31 - Feb. 4   ____ ____ ____ ____ ____   _____

Feb. 7 - Feb. 11   ____ ____ ____ ____ ____   _____

Feb. 14 - Feb. 18   ____ ____ ____ ____ ____   _____

Feb. 21 - Feb. 25   ____ ____ ____ ____ ____   _____

Feb. 28 - Mar. 4   ____ ____ ____ ____ ____   _____

Mar. 7 - Mar. 11   ____ ____ ____ ____ ____   _____

Mar. 21 - Mar. 25   ____ ____ ____ ____ ____   _____

Mar. 28 - Apr. 1   ____ ____ ____ ____ ____   _____

Apr. 4 - Apr. 8   ____ ____ ____ ____ ____   _____

Apr. 11 - Apr. 15   ____ ____ ____ ____ ____   _____

Apr. 18 - Apr. 22   ____ ____ ____ ____ ____   _____

Investigator: _____

FIGURE 5–4   Data collection sheet used for sensory stimulation research project.

References

Bailey, D.M. (1978). The effects of vestibular stimulation on verbalization in chronic schizophrenics. *American Journal of Occupational Therapy, 32,* 445–450.

Bailey, D.M. (1990). Reasons for attrition from occupational therapy. *American Journal of Occupational Therapy, 44*(1), 23–29.

Benson, J., & Clark, F. (1982). A guide for instrument development and validation. *American Journal of Occupational Therapy, 36*(12), 789–800.

Bohannon, R.W. (1987). Relative dynamic muscular endurance of patients with neuromuscular disorders and of healthy matched control subjects. *Physical Therapy, 67*(1), 18–20.

Campbell, D.T., & Stanley, J.C. (1969). *Experimental and quasi-experimental designs for research.* Chicago, IL: Rand McNally.

Clark, M. (1964). *The effect of depression on self-care management* (unpublished paper).

Cox, R., & West, W. (1986). *Fundamentals of research for health professionals.* Laurel, MD: RAMSCO Publishing.

Hardison, J., & Llorens, L.A. (1988). Structured craft group activities for adolescent delinquent girls. *Occupational Therapy in Mental Health, 8*(3), 101–117.

Henry, A., Nelson, D., & Duncombe, L. (1984). Choice making in group and individual activity. *American Journal of Occupational Therapy, 38*(4), 245–251.

Iwasaki, K., & Holm, M.B. (1989). Sensory treatment for the reduction of stereotypic behaviors in persons with severe multiple disabilities. *Occupational Therapy Journal of Research, 9*(3), 170–183.

Kalton, G. (1983). *Introduction to survey sampling.* No. 35 of Quantitative Applications in Social Sciences Series. Newbury Park, CA: Sage Publications.

Kerlinger, F. (1979). *Foundations of behavioral research.* New York: Holt, Rinehart & Winston.

Merriam, S.B. (1988). *Case study research in education: A qualitative approach.* San Francisco: Jossey-Bass.

Ottenbacher, K. (1982). Patterns of postrotary nystagmus in three learning disabled children. *American Journal of Occupational Therapy, 36*(10), 657–663.

Ottenbacher, K., & York, J. (1984). Strategies for evaluating clinical change: Implications for practice and research. *American Journal of Occupational Therapy, 38*(10), 647–659.

Oyster, C.K., Hanten, W.P., & Llorens, L.A. (1987). *Introduction to research: A guide for the health science professional.* Philadelphia: J.B. Lippincott.

Rogers, J.C., Marcus, C.L., & Snow, T.L. (1987). Maude: A case of sensory deprivation. *American Journal of Occupational Therapy, 41*(10), 673–676.

Short-DeGraff, M.A., Slansky, L., & Diamond, K.E. (1989). Validity of preschoolers' self-drawings as an index of human figure drawing performance. *Occupational Therapy Journal of Research, 9*(5), 305–315.

Stein, F., & Nikolic, S. (1989). Teaching stress management techniques to a schizophrenic patient. *American Journal of Occupational Therapy, 43*(3), 162–169.

Stensrud, M.K., & Lushbough, R.S. (1988). The implementation of an occupational therapy program in an alcohol and drug dependency treatment center. *Occupational Therapy in Mental Health, 8*(2), 1–15.

Williams, R., Binkley, J., Bloch, R., Goldsmith, C., & Minuk, T. (1993). Reliability of the modified-modified Schober and double inclinometer methods for measuring lumbar flexion and extension. *Physical Therapy, 73*(1), 26–37.

Yin, R.K. (1994). *Case study research: Design and methods.* No. 5 of Applied Social Research Methods Series. Thousand Oaks, CA: Sage Publications.

Additional Reading

Cook, T.D., & Campbell, D.J. (1979). *Quasi-experimentation design and analysis issues for field settings.* Boston: Houghton-Mifflin.

Creswell, J.W. (1994). *Research Design: Qualitative and quantitative approaches.* Thousand Oaks, CA: Sage Publications.

Fink, A. (1995). *How to report on surveys.* Thousand Oaks, CA: Sage Publications.

Fink, A., & Kosecoff, J. (1985). *How to conduct surveys.* Newbury Park, CA: Sage Publications.

Fowler, F.J. (1995). *Improving survey questions: Design and evaluation.* Thousand Oaks, CA: Sage Publications.

Frey, J.H., & Oishi, S.M. (1995). *How to conduct interviews by telephone and in person.* Thousand Oaks, CA: Sage Publications.

Hacker, B. (1980). Part I Single subject research strategies in occupational therapy. *American Journal of Occupational Therapy, 34*(2), 103–108.

Hacker, B. (1980). Part II Single subject research strategies in occupational therapy. *American Journal of Occupational Therapy, 34*(3), 169–175.

Kazdin, A.E. (1982). *Single-case research designs: Methods for clinical and applied settings.* New York: Oxford University Press.

Kraemer, H., & Thiemann, S. (1987). *How many subjects? Statistical power analysis in research.* Newbury Park, CA: Sage Publications.

Kratochwill, T.R. (1978). *Single subject research: Strategies for evaluation change.* New York: Academic.

Mangione, T.W. (1995). *Mail surveys: Improving the quality.* No. 40 in Applied Social Research Methods. Thousand Oaks, CA: Sage Publications.

Schuman, H., & Presser, S. (1996). *Questions and answers in attitude surveys: Experiments on question form, wording, and context.* Thousand Oaks, CA: Sage Publications.

6

Establishing Boundaries for the Quantitative Research Study

A research study needs to be given boundaries and to be put into a suitable context for readers. Readers should be able to understand quickly where a study fits into the scheme of professional literature, should be made aware of any of the author's assumptions about the underlying principles of the study, should know if there are any overriding problems that are likely to influence the results or interpretation of the results, and should be able to find the meanings of all terms used if they are not obvious. This information will enable readers to understand the researcher's general intentions and to follow the researcher's train of thought. Your report should include sections on the study's definition of terms, assumptions, scope, limitations, and subject criteria and selection.

Defining and Operationalizing Terms

Some of the terms in the study need to be defined; others need to be operationalized. In both cases, the specific meanings of the terms in your study need to be made clear to the reader. First, let's consider the simple definitions.

People who read your study may come from a variety of professional backgrounds and may not be familiar with terms idiosyncratic to your discipline or specialty. Defining your terms will help the reader know their precise meaning in the context of the study. Some terms that need definition are those that are specific to your field or that have everyday language counterparts with which they might be confused, such as the word "grounded," which has a meaning in ethnography that is quite different from its nautical or electrical meanings.

It is especially important to define terms that occur in the problem statement, the purpose of the study, and the research questions or hypotheses, because a misunderstanding here could threaten the reader's grasp of the entire study. Definitions may come from sources such as dictionaries, medical textbooks, lists of synonyms, and glossaries, and may range from the simple substitution of words to elaborate explanations several paragraphs long (Boxes 6–A and 6–B). Some researchers (see Ritter in Box 6–A) use existing definitions from authorities and cite the authors, which is a useful and acceptable procedure.

In experimental research, some terms need to be operationalized. Operationalizing terms goes one step further than simply sub-

---

Box 6–A

For a study whose hypothesis was that regular aerobic exercise will improve the cardiovascular fitness of adults with developmental disabilities, simple definitions were used for two relevant terms:

Aerobic exercise—Exercise during which the energy needed is supplied by the aerobic metabolism. Slow, rhythmic movement of large body muscles. Aerobic exercise is required for sustained periods of physical work and vigorous athletic exercise. (Cooper, 1968).

Developmental disabilities—Conditions due to congenital abnormality, trauma, deprivation, or diseases occurring up to the age of 22 years that interrupt or delay the sequence and rate of normal growth, development, and maturation (Massachusetts Developmental Disabilities Council, 1985).

(Ritter, 1989, p. 15)

Box 6–B

Willoughby and Polatajko reviewed the literature concerning the debate over the nature of motor problems in children with developmental coordination disorder (DCD): do these problems have a physiological basis or are they the result of a developmental delay? They felt it was essential to sort out the terminology used in the literature:

A number of terms have been used to identify children with DCD. Ayres (1972) used the term *developmental dyspraxia* to apply to a particular group of children because she believed that these children possessed a motor planning problem. Gubbay (1975) and Henderson and Hall (1982) used the term *clumsy,* but Johnston, Short, and Crawford (1987) have suggested that the term *clumsy* is not ideal, as it has unfavorable connotations. Many other terms have also been used and continue to be used such as *physically awkward, poorly coordinated* (Cratty, 1994), *perceptuomotor dysfunction,* and *motor delay* (Henderson, 1994). Because no one term has won universal acceptance, in this article, the term *DCD* has been chosen to describe children with motor coordination problems who otherwise appear to be without disabilities.

(Willoughby & Polatajko, 1995, pp. 787–788)

---

stituting one term for another. The purpose is to remove words that do not describe observable phenomena from the definition so that their meaning for a particular study cannot be misinterpreted. The purpose is to achieve clear scientific communication so that studies can be accurately replicated. To achieve clarity, concepts are defined in terms of the operations by which they are measured. For example, time is measured in commonly identifiable quantities; thus, the treatment protocol in a study might be measured by total number of treatment sessions, number of sessions per week, and length of each treatment session in minutes. The goal is to provide readers with information that will allow them to know what to do in order to experience that which is being defined.

Operational definitions may apply not only to measurable items, such as degrees of flexion, but also to concepts, such as independence or self-esteem. Operational definitions should always point to a specific example or referent. Chase (1966) listed four possible referents that could serve as the basis of operational definitions:

1. Material objects at given places and dates: this splint here; this patient with carpal tunnel syndrome; this rehabilitation hospital.

2. Collections of objects at given places and dates: the patients with cardiac conditions in Sunnyview Nursing Home on August 4, 1996.

3. Happenings at given places and dates: the passage of the Health Maintenance Organization legislation in Washington, DC, on July 29, 1986.

4. Processes verified scientifically: normal body temperature is approximately 98.6°F.

Francis, Bork, and Carstens (1984) add a fifth referent:

5. The personal experience of a given individual as reported by that individual: Freud's Oedipus Complex as his way of experiencing and explaining certain behavior patterns. Descriptions of personal experience are valid representations of individual thought even if there is no corresponding external referent. Even Thomas Szasz's notion of "the

---

Box 6–C

In Middlebrook's study entitled *The effect of functional movement patterns on hemodynamic response in older individuals,* the definition of heart rate reads:

> Heart Rate (HR): "The number of ventricular beats per minute" (Astrand & Rodahl, 1970; p. 122) resulting from contraction of the ventricles. This measurement was taken by counting the number of QRS complexes detected by the ARS beeper on the ECG monitor in a 15-second period, then multiplying by 4. It was recorded in beats per minute (bpm).

(Middlebrook, 1988, p. 25)

---

myth of mental illness" can be operationally defined in terms of what Szasz thinks a person must know to understand that myth.

The first sentence in Box 6–C would have been sufficient for a simple definition. However, Middlebrook wanted to operationalize the term *heart rate* in order to make it specific to her study, so she added the last two sentences to make an operational definition. Boxes 6–D and 6–E contain examples of simple definitions and operational definitions from two theses. It is worth taking time to define terms accurately and completely to prevent confusion later on.

Assumptions

The next step in establishing your study's boundaries is to think about your own assumptions regarding the study and the premises upon which it is formulated. Researchers customarily examine their assumptions carefully and state them to the reader near the beginning of the study. Readers need not agree with your assumptions but are able to follow the logic of your propositions and to understand why you approached the study as you did.

Assumptions are underlying principles that the researcher believes or accepts but that are difficult to prove in any concrete way. They are frequently untested and untestable hypotheses, basic values, or views about the world. They include such values as

---

Box 6–D

The purpose of a 1986 study by Ball was to determine the nature of the relationship between grip strength and hand function and between pinch strength and hand function, and the correlation between strength and function in dominant and nondominant hands. Thus, it was necessary for Ball to define and operationalize grip strength, pinch strength, hand function, and dominant hand.

Grip Strength: Measure of force registered by a Jamar dynamometer when an individual exerted maximal effort while holding the dynamometer handle between partly flexed fingers and the palm, and counterpressure was applied by the thumb which was wrapped over the dorsum of the fingers.

Pinch Strength: Measure of force registered by a B&L Pinch Gauge when an individual exerted maximal effort while holding the pinch gauge:
  a) between the pad of the thumb and the radial side of the middle phalanx of the index finger (lateral pinch),
  b) between the tips of thumb and index finger; all joints of these fingers were flexed and thumb was abducted (2-point tip pinch),
  c) between the tips of thumb, index and long fingers; all joints of these fingers were flexed and thumb was abducted (3-point tip pinch),
  d) between the pads of thumb and index finger; DIP joints were extended or only slightly flexed. Thumb was abducted (2-point pad pinch),
  e) between the pads of thumb, index, and long fingers; DIP joints were extended or only slightly flexed. Thumb was abducted (3-point pad pinch). (Mathiowetz, Weber, Volland, & Kashman, 1984; Sherik, Weiss, & Flatt, 1971; Smith & Benge, 1985).

Hand Function: Measured by performance on the Jebsen Hand Function Test (HFT). Low scores on time indicated a high degree of proficient hand function; high scores on time indicated a low degree of proficient hand function. (Jebsen, Taylor, Trieschmann, Trotter, & Howard, 1969).

Dominant Hand: The dominant hand was the hand which the subject preferred most often in Annett's Hand Preference Questionnaire (Annett, 1970a).

(Ball, 1986; pp. 6–7)

Box 6–E

The purpose of a 1989 study by Moore was to evaluate the effectiveness of an individualized guided visual imagery program for patients with psychosomatic, psychogenic, or chronic somatic disorders. He defined terms in the following manner:

Psychogenic Illnesses: somatic illnesses created by the mind or mental state.

Psychosomatic Illnesses: somatic illnesses exacerbated by the mind or mental state.

Somatic Illnesses: states of illness that originate in the body secondary to trauma, disease process, or malfunction of one or more body systems.

Responses: monitored physiological states including electromyograph, galvanic skin response, heart rate, respiration rate, peripheral thermal reading, amount of medication.

Individualized, guided visual imagery: images created by the therapist or the patient that use one or more of the five senses to create a temporarily believable illusion, that is specifically designed to meet the needs of the patient as dictated by their individual personality, preferences, and language format.

(Moore, 1989; pp. 7–8)

---

the notion that people are basically good or that people want to function independently in their day-to-day activities. These ideas would be very difficult to prove with the population at large or even with a small research group.

Two kinds of assumptions need to be examined: first, assumptions about the ideological principles upon which the study is based, and second, assumptions that are made concerning the procedures used in the study. We all adhere to certain ingrained principles that will affect the way we approach situations and therefore the way we design research studies.

For example, in following their ideological principles, a client-centered researcher and a financially oriented researcher might approach Ritter's (1989) study about the use of aerobic exercise with adults who have developmental delays from quite different viewpoints. The client-centered researcher might hold the assumption that adults with developmental delays deserve the fun and sense of well-being often promoted by aerobic exercise and would investigate ways of bringing such exercise to those residing in sheltered living situations with this in mind. The money-conscious administrative researcher might feel that aerobic exercise contributes to physical health and that regular participation may reduce the cost of medical care for adults with developmental delays who are financially supported by the state.

The two researchers are likely to adopt different study methods when addressing the benefits of aerobic exercise for developmentally delayed adults who receive state support. The first researcher would probably investigate the results of the exercise on the well-being and enjoyment level of subjects, while the second might investigate the results of the exercise on the health status and resulting health care costs of the subjects.

The second type of assumption relates to the procedures used during the research study. Usually these pertain to the instruments used and the willingness of subjects to participate in the study. For instance, researchers are often obliged to assume that the measuring instrument being used is valid and reliable because, at least in human subject research, it is often difficult to prove validity and reliability conclusively. The most notoriously unreliable instruments (in experimental research when replication is desirable) are interviews and questionnaires, yet it is sometimes impossible to conduct a quantitative study without them. Box 6–F illustrates how one author clearly stated an important assumption in her study.

There are other basic assumptions associated with the use of measuring instruments, such as assuming that the subjects will answer questions honestly and respond to tests of skill to the best of their ability. In making

---

Box 6–F

Kircher points out an ideological principle that readers must be aware of if they are to look at her study from her viewpoint:

It is assumed that an activity must have meaning to the performer to be purposeful.

(Kircher, 1984, p. 166)

...dural assumptions, the researcher ...hink in advance of events that may ...ring the study and must try to con-...; for those events to avoid having to make procedural assumptions about them. For example, in some studies in which performance of a test of skill is being measured, it is imperative for the study that subjects try as hard as they can on the test. To ensure this, some researchers have devised reward systems to compensate subjects according to their motivation level. When these types of strategies are used, assumptions need to be made less frequently and only for items beyond the researcher's control and ingenuity.

Making your assumptions known in the early stages of describing a study is most important so that readers know where you stand on issues related to the research and where they should keep a critical eye on procedures.

Scope of the Study

In completing the worksheet on the significance of your study following Chapter 3, you showed why your study, among all possible studies that the problem might generate, was worth undertaking. Any problem can be approached from different angles; however, you have selected a specific approach, and it is necessary to explain that approach to the reader. This is known as defining the study's scope. It is insufficient to state merely which approach you are taking. You must provide a rationale, a set of constructs and principles that will guide the reader to a clear and focused understanding of your frame of reference. This set of guiding constructs and principles, called the conceptual framework of the study, serves as a structure for the scope.

For example, in King's work (1974) with chronic schizophrenic patients, she made it clear to readers that she was taking the guiding constructs and principles of A. Jean Ayres's theories on sensory integration and adapting them for use with a new client population. She explained the portion of Ayres's theory she was using, defined her research population precisely, and stated why she thought the particular frame of reference described was an appropriate approach to use. King's article is an excellent example of documentation for a research project's scope.

The scope section may not always be as elaborately and meticulously presented as King's, however. She chose to spend so much time on this point because she was presenting a new treatment choice for a particular client population. Her study encompassed the crucial underlying constructs and principles that the reader needed to understand and accept in order for the ensuing research to be logical and meaningful. In studies in which the point of the study is not contingent on the scope or conceptual framework chosen, it is customary to merely set the stage for the reader with a paragraph on the subject (Box 6–G).

The conceptual framework focuses the study and narrows it to just one of a myriad possibilities. It tells the reader what the focus is, what will be covered in the project, and what will not be included. For instance, if a sensory integrative approach is to be taken in a study, it would be unreasonable to expect the researcher to cover the possibilities of what might happen to subjects if a behavioral approach had been used.

Informing the reader of the conceptual framework and therefore the scope of the project puts the study in context within the work that was previously accomplished using that framework. In this way, it is immediately apparent to readers that King's

---

Box 6–G

Middlebrook's study of the effect of functional movement patterns on hemodynamic responses in older individuals contains a good example of a brief description of the conceptual framework of her study, which in this case was a previously documented frame of reference.

> This investigation was based on the biomechanical frame of reference, which, according to Trombley (1983), "deals with increasing strength, endurance, and range of joint motion in patients who have an intact central nervous system but who have dysfunction in the peripheral nervous system or the musculoskeletal, integumentary, or cardio-pulmonary systems" (pp. 1–2). In the present investigation, the endurance of subjects performing an upper extremity activity was studied through monitoring. . . .

(Middlebrook, 1988; pp. 27–28)

work adds to the body of knowledge about sensory integrative techniques as a form of treatment. Knowledgeable readers on that topic know that a new group of patients is being added to those who currently benefit from sensory integrative treatment.

Besides setting the study in a context for the reader, defining the scope of the study often helps investigators put limits on their own work. In this way, the scope acts as a delimiting factor, marking the boundaries of material that should be covered.

Limitations of the Study

In setting forth the limitations of your study, you should include conceptual and methodological shortcomings that cannot be overcome in the study design. Limitations in experimental research may include such things as inability to randomly select the subjects, or to include a control group, or lack of a standardized instrument to measure variables. Nonexperimental research may have insurmountable methodological problems, such as lack of an appropriate mailing list of the people you want to poll in an attitude survey, which could force you to make do with an overinclusive or underinclusive list (Box 6–H). Conceptual limitations could include such problems as an underlying prin-

---

Box 6–H

In Nelson's study of self-esteem and professionalism in female occupational therapists, limitations are identified as follows:

Since the sample size was not large, and the cross-section of respondents not wide, it was impossible to make generalizations about the entire population of occupational therapists. Because this was a case study of occupational therapists in Massachusetts, it was difficult to draw conclusions about occupational therapists at large. Another limitation was that the variables chosen for study (self-esteem and professionalism) are only contributing factors to some of the larger problems of the profession outlined here. That is, they comprise a small piece of the larger puzzle.

(Nelson, 1989; pp. 5–6)

---

ciple of the study not being widely accepted outside your professional specialty.

Naturally, listing the limitations of a study does not excuse you from making all possible attempts to overcome the problems. But after all possible improvements have been made, pointing out the remaining limitations shows that you are aware of them and will consider them when discussing the results.

Subject Criteria and Selection

At this point, a word about the subjects in your quantitative research project is in order. Although most experimental studies, particularly those investigating the efficacy of treatment, use individuals to supply the evidence, some may rely on documents, records, and verbal reports as evidence. Thus, research subjects may be people or written materials. It is important that your readers know from which population the sample you studied came and how they were selected.

First let's review the distinction between a **population** and a **sample**. A population is the total group or set of events to which your hypotheses apply. The population shares a specific set of characteristics or criteria that have been established by the researcher. For example, you may be studying all occupational therapists working in the United States who are from 40 to 60 years old and who are working with children in a classroom setting. A sample is a smaller subset of the population that has been selected to participate in the project (e.g., 100 therapists randomly selected from the above population).

The criteria of a study population are determined from a literature review and the goals for the study (Box 6–I). Selection criteria are established gradually, as the assumptions and theoretical base of the study unfold. In experimental studies, the criteria are dictated by the theory behind why a researcher feels the intervention being studied will be helpful. For example, King's theory (1974), based on many years of observation, was that among patients with schizophrenia, only those of the nonparanoid type can be expected to benefit from sensory-integrative treatment; therefore, her population criteria included patients with nonparanoid schizo-

---

Box 6–I

In designing an alternative splint for clients with carpal tunnel syndrome (CTS), Mawn (1990) wanted to test the splint on subjects who had not used a splint previously and had not been operated on for CTS before the study. This was to allow a controlled study, comparing subjects using the new splint to a control group using other methods of treatment. Additionally, Mawn wanted subjects of both sexes who were employed and taking sick leave because of CTS symptoms to determine if they could return to work using the new splint sooner than those in the control group. Thus, the population criteria were: Men and women with CTS, who had not received a splint or had an operation, and who were on sick leave from their jobs.

Box 6–J

Clifford and Bundy administered the Preschool Play Scale and Preschool Play Materials Preference Inventory to 66 preschool-age boys in order to examine whether or not play preference and play performance of boys with sensory-integrative (SI) dysfunction were different from the preferences of normal boys in this age group. The *population* under study were all preschool-age boys in Massachusetts participating in day-care centers or day camps. The *subjects,* who were not randomly selected, consisted of 66 4-, 5-, and 6-year-old boys, divided into two groups matched in age, verbal intelligence (single-word receptive vocabulary), and socioeconomic status. Group 1 consisted of 35 normal boys recruited from day-care centers and a day camp in the Boston area. Group 2 consisted of 31 boys diagnosed by an experienced occupational therapist with training in SI theory and evaluation as having SI dysfunction. Group 2 subjects were recruited from three occupational therapy private practices, an occupational therapy teaching clinic, and two children's hospitals, all in Massachusetts.

(Clifford & Bundy, 1989, pp. 205–206)

---

phrenia. Examples of populations, samples and selection criteria from actual studies may be found in Boxes 6–J, 6–K, and 6–L.

Whereas the population criteria are established *before* subject selection, detailed information about the subjects in the sample is given *later,* after they have been recruited into the study. For example, in the Mawn study (1990) testing a new splint on patients with carpal tunnel syndrome (see Box 6–I), this might include such information as the subjects' type of employment, how long they have been absent from their jobs, and any previous treatment they had received for carpal tunnel syndrome.

Once the subject selection criteria are decided, you will use one of the probability sampling methods to select your subjects from the larger population. Random selection (described in Chapter 4) is one of the most popular types of probability sampling. Probability sampling allows the researcher to specify for each characteristic of the population the probability that it will be included in the sample. You might, for example, set the criteria of a study population as all adults in a specific rehabilitation system who have left hemiplegia and who are dependent in dressing, and then randomly select a specific number of those people to be in your sample. When the study is completed, you will be able to generalize the study findings from the sample to the original population of adults with left hemiplegia. Random

sampling increases the likelihood that the study results will be similar to results that would have been found if the entire population had been studied. In general, keep in mind that your sample should represent the population as closely as possible.

Box 6–K

In Moore's study (1989) investigating whether guided visual imagery was a viable modality for occupational therapists, a retrospective chart review was used as the research method. In this instance, the *population* consisted of all the charts of patients seen at a hospital in Massachusetts during a specific 2-year period. The *subjects* were the charts of those patients seen by one occupational therapist who were diagnosed with psychogenic, psychosomatic, or chronic somatic disorders, and who had received guided visual imagery as a treatment modality.

Box 6–L

In her 1988 study Middlebrook used all the men and women in Massachusetts between the ages of 60 and 79 as her *population*. The subjects in her *sample* were the 23 women and 7 men who volunteered to participate and who were "without a history of cardiovascular disease, systemic hypertension (blood pressure greater than 150/90 mm/Hg), chronic obstructive pulmonary disease . . ., or cerebrovascular accident. The medical histories of the subjects were determined by self-report."

(Middlebrook, 1988; p. 27)

As we saw in Chapter 4, random selection is quite difficult to achieve. Many researchers, in fact, find they can conduct their studies only if they use as subjects the patients they have on their caseload, what is known as a convenience sample. Though convenience samples pose difficulties from an experimental researcher's viewpoint, they do provide a way for novice investigators to get started with the research process.

Stumbling Blocks

Assumptions

People often make the mistake of including in their assumptions those notions they hold about the study that can be proved; in other words, ideas that are referenced in scientific literature. If an idea can be proved scientifically, it need not be presented as an assumption but rather should be presented in the literature review as part of the reason for conducting the study in a certain manner. Only beliefs that are difficult to prove concretely, beliefs that are untested or untestable hypotheses, basic values, or views about the world, should be included in the assumptions section.

Scope

The distinction between the assumptions underlying a research project and the scope of the project is sometimes blurred. Remember that assumptions are individual and often unrelated beliefs about the nature of the topic. The scope, on the other hand, presents an encompassing conceptual framework in which to place the whole study. This frame of reference will color all aspects of the research and will provide a backdrop against which the reader may view the entire study.

Limitations

I advise students not to give litanies of limitations for their studies. It may begin to look as if the study never should have been attempted, when in fact the study may have proved quite useful in advancing an area of knowledge. There is a middle ground to be achieved between listing every conceivable problem and quirk in a study and being fair with the reader and presenting those things that could truly bias the results. Knowledgeable readers will pick up obvious limitations but will respect an author who acknowledges problems and considers them in the interpretation of the findings.

Convenience Samples

Although there might be compelling financial or temporal reasons for using a convenience sample, this is perhaps the least desirable sampling method. You can never be sure that the qualities of convenience-sample members will compare with those of other members in the population and will consequently lose the ability to generalize the results of the study.

WORKSHEETS

DEFINITION OF TERMS

Have someone outside your discipline review the problem statement, purpose of the study, and research questions or hypotheses. Have the person point out words or phrases he or she does not understand.

List here words you feel need either a simple definition or an operational definition:

Problem statement words:
Definition   Operational definition

Words from the purpose of the study:
Definition   Operational definition

Hypothesis words:
Definition   Operational definition

Go through the list and decide for each word if the definition should come from a dictionary, glossary, textbook, professional authority or group, and so forth.

Write a definition for each word in the:

Problem statement:

Purpose:

Hypothesis:

ASSUMPTIONS

Read through the problem statement, the background, the purpose, and the significance of the study. As you read, see if you have made any assumptions about your population, the environment in which they function, or the intervention being proposed that need to be presented to the reader.

Assumption 1:

Assumption 2:

Assumption 3:

SCOPE OF THE STUDY

What is the underlying framework or scope for your study? Are you following an accepted theoretical frame of reference, such as a behavioral or developmental approach or a biomechanical model? State your conceptual framework here:

Write two or three paragraphs describing why you are approaching the study from this perspective and how the chosen conceptual framework will shape the study.

LIMITATIONS

Reread the early sections of your study looking for conceptual limitations. List them here:

Reread the methodology section of your study looking for procedural limitations. List them here:

SUBJECT CRITERIA

Will the subjects for your study be clients, patients, written records, tape recordings, verbal reports, observations, or other?

Define the selection criteria for the population (from whom your sample will be chosen):

Examples:

- All the written records, photographs, and tape-recorded interviews relating to the founding of the American Physical Therapy Association.
- All occupational therapists working in psychiatric hospitals in Massachusetts.

Add relevant criteria to the description of the population based on the literature review and the design of the study.

Example:

- Occupational therapists currently working in Massachusetts state-supported psychiatric hospitals who are working with patients with schizophrenia.

SUBJECT SELECTION AND ASSIGNMENT

Do you know the approximate number in the population?

How will the sample be selected from the population?

_____ Random selection _____ Other

Describe the procedure:

How many will the sample comprise?

Will the sample be divided into experimental and control groups?

How will group assignment be made?

_____ Random assignment _____ Other

Describe the procedure:

References

Ball, J.H. (1986). *Pinch and grip strength related to performance on the Jebsen Hand Function Test.* Unpublished master's thesis, Tufts University, Medford, MA.

Chase, S. (1966). *The tyranny of words.* New York: Harcourt, Brace & World.

Clifford, J., & Bundy, A. (1989). Play preference and play performance in normal boys and boys with sensory integrative dysfunction. *Occupational Therapy Journal of Research, 9*(4), 202–217.

Francis, J., Bork, C., & Carstens, S. (1984). *The proposal cookbook: A step by step guide to dissertation and thesis proposal writing.* Naples, FL: Action Research Associates.

King, L.J. (1974). A sensory-integrative approach to schizophrenia. *American Journal of Occupational Therapy, 28*(9), 529–536.

Kircher, M.A. (1984). Motivation as a factor of perceived exertion in purposeful versus nonpurposeful activity. *American Journal of Occupational Therapy, 38*(3), 165–170.

Mawn, M. (1990). *The dorsal-ulnar splint as a treatment for carpal tunnel syndrome: A case study.* Unpublished master's thesis, Tufts University, Medford, MA.

Middlebrook, J.A. (1988). *The effect of functional movement patterns on hemodynamic responses in older individuals.* Unpublished master's thesis, Tufts University, Medford, MA.

Moore, D.A. (1989). *Guided visual imagery as an occupational therapy modality.* Unpublished master's thesis, Tufts University, Medford, MA.

Nelson, B.J. (1989). *Self-esteem and professionalism in female occupational therapists.* Unpublished master's thesis, Tufts University, Medford, MA.

Ritter, J. (1989). *Aerobic exercise with adults with developmental disabilities.* Unpublished master's thesis, Tufts University, Medford, MA.

Willoughby, C., & Polatajko, H.J. (1995). Motor problems in children with developmental coordination disorder: Review of the literature. *American Journal of Occupational Therapy, 49*(8), 787–794.

Additional Reading

Berger, R.M., & Patchner, M.A. (1988). *Planning for research: A guide for the helping professions.* No. 50 in the Sage Human Services Guides Series. Newbury Park, CA: Sage Publications.

Stein, F. Research Design. In Stein, F., & Cutler, S.K. (1996). *Clinical research in allied health and special education* (3rd ed.). San Diego: Singular Publishing Group.

7

Data Collection Techniques

Sometimes the research method dictates data collection techniques. For example, an ethnographic research method implies the use of field data collection techniques such as observation and tape-recorded interviews, whereas survey research always involves either structured interviews (by telephone or in person) or written questionnaires. However, when using other research methods, it may be less clear which data collection technique to use, and the investigator often has a wide array of choices.

To illuminate the choices, let us categorize data collection possibilities and discuss each of them. Techniques may be conveniently grouped as follows:

1. Observation
2. Interview
3. Written questionnaire
4. Record and artifact review
5. Hardware instrumentation
6. Tests, measures, and inventories

Observation

This data collection technique may be used in any of the quantitative or qualitative research designs and is commonly used in conjunction with other techniques. Observations may be made of human subjects, videotape recordings of subjects or events, or nonhuman items such as pieces of equipment. Observation is structured differently depending on the type of research approach being used; that is, it is formalized in advance in quantitative methods and ever-changing according to the context in qualitative methods.

Observation in Quantitative Research

When observing the frequency or type of events occurring in a quantitative study, a method for recording observations needs to be carefully prepared and the observers should be well trained. Rather than being asked to observe and record subjective items such as "dependence" or "enjoyment," it is preferable for observers to be given objective criteria believed to represent those subjective items. For example, "dependence" may be represented by the number of times a subject asks for assistance, and "enjoyment" may be represented by the number of smiles, laughs, or verbal statements that would indicate happiness. Observers should be provided with a protocol defining the items to be observed and a method for recording those items, such as noting any occurrence, frequency of occurrence, or length of time between occurrences, on a previously designed form.

Videotapes can be useful for training purposes. The observer rates the tapes and the researcher checks the ratings until he or she is satisfied that the observer is making correct and reliable ratings. If there is more than one observer or rater, the researcher will probably want to use a technique called interrater reliability, which means that the raters are checked not only individually but also against one another. This reliability check is carried out until all raters score similarly and the researcher has confidence, borne out by statistics, that they will rate consistently well.

The importance of raters' impartiality to protection of the internal validity of the study cannot be emphasized enough. This issue is addressed more fully in the Stumbling Blocks section at the end of this chapter.

Observation in Qualitative Research

The term "participant observation" is used to refer to the ethnographer who spends large amounts of time in the setting under study (the field), gathering data from a wide variety of sources (Spradley, 1980). The researcher keeps field notes of everything observed that might be remotely useful to the study, such as the environment, the participants' appearance and manner, routines, unusual events, human groupings at specific times, and so on. The participant observer works hard to be accepted in the setting—not to be treated as special—to be able to see what normally occurs. Therefore, clipboards, cameras, and other obvious observation tools are frequently kept to a minimum at the site. Although observers take copious field notes to get the fullest picture of events, they usually return home to flesh out the field notes that same day while information is still fresh in their minds. Participant observers will probably be conducting loosely structured interviews, or simply asking occasional questions for clarification as well as observing.

Miles and Huberman (1994) recommend that, as the raw field notes are being processed later the same day, any reflections that come to mind be included immediately to make the transcript a more useful later resource. Some examples of items that might be remembered and added to the notes include:

- What the relationship with informants feels like, now that the observer is off the site

- Second thoughts on the meaning of what a key informant was *really* saying during an exchange that seemed somehow important

- Doubts about the quality of some of the data; second thoughts about some of the interview questions and observation protocols

- A new hypothesis that might explain some puzzling observations

- A mental note to pursue an issue further in the next contact

- Cross-allusions to material in another part of the data set

- Personal reactions to some informants' remarks or actions

- Elaboration or clarification of a prior incident or event that now seems of possible significance (Miles & Huberman, 1994, p. 66)

Styles of observation used in qualitative research fall on a continuum from nonparticipant observation to active participant observation. As the name implies, nonparticipant observers do not engage in any of the subjects' activities at the site, devoting their energies to viewing, noting, and remembering events in as much detail as possible. Participant observers, on the other hand, may be deeply involved in the site activities and may be indistinguishable from some of the informants. There is a range between these two extremes, and observers can choose the degree to which they participate, depending on their goals and purposes.

Establishing just the right amount and type of participation at the site can be difficult, with different considerations arising at different sites. Observing and being accepted by children presents its own challenge. Should you try to behave as a peer and engage in their activities, or retain an obviously adult role on the fringe of activities and risk appearing aloof or as if you are spying?

Participant observation in small groups where group members attempt to be open and honest with one another presents another challenge. Observers feel pressure to become group members, to share their own thoughts and feelings, and in so doing are likely to become so involved as to lose the opportunity to observe. Alternatively, if observers resist the expectation to participate, they may risk being seen as hostile or as awkward appendages, and they may thus impede the real work of the group. If therapist field workers are trying to observe treatment sessions, there are patient sensitivity issues to consider. Will the therapist and patients reach the point of feeling comfortable with a third person present so that the observer can gain a true understanding of what is going on? Or will this always be a contrived situation, in which therapist and patients are acting in the manner they feel is expected of them? Is there an appropriate place for participation here, or will the role always be that of total observer?

Questions concerning how much, with whom, and how you participate in the various settings tend to work out as the research focus develops and as your personal style and comfort level become apparent to you. Exactly how much and the type of your participation and observation will probably vary during the course of the study. You may start out being somewhat detached while waiting to be accepted, increase your participation as you and the informants get to know one another, and perhaps pull back a little as you prepare to leave the field site. Bogden and Biklen (1982) suggest that, no matter what your level of participation at any given time, you carry with you an imaginary sign saying:

> "My primary purpose in being here is to collect data. How does what I am doing [now] relate to that goal?" (p. 130)

How long should observation sessions be? Probably, for the first few sessions, an hour or less is plenty of time to get started at a site. This will allow you to get a feel for the site and for the informants to begin to get used to your presence. As you decide on the key events you will be observing for your project, the length of observations will become more prescribed. The key to this decision is not to stay any longer than your memory can serve you or than is practical to give you time to write up your notes immediately after the observation. It is crucial that note writing be done immediately, while the events are fresh in your memory. Most of us find it more fun to be at the site observing than at home writing up field notes, so the natural temptation is to stay on at the site "just in case something important happens that I ought to see." The veteran field worker does not give in to this temptation.

It can be seen that the unstructured, free-flowing observation style of qualitative research is the antithesis of the type of observation that occurs during quantitative studies. The goal here is to gather as much data as possible that reflect on the research questions under study; whereas in quantitative studies, only data that have been previously elucidated and clearly defined are collected, in a prescribed manner.

Interview

Interviewing is one of the techniques used to gather data in survey and ethnographic research. In ethnographic research, interviews are always conducted face-to-face, but they may be conducted either face-to-face or by telephone in survey research. Interviews conducted face-to-face are more intimate, allowing the interviewer to interact directly and develop rapport with the interviewee. This may be important if sensitive issues are being explored; the interviewee can be put at ease, reassured, and encouraged to give candid answers. Additionally, the interviewer has a chance to "read" the nonverbal cues given by the interviewee, which may indicate confusion or lack of understanding, so that a question can be rephrased. Nonverbal information may also be an important part of understanding the full response to the question.

The disadvantage of face-to-face interviews is the amount of effort required to set up the interview—contacting subjects, arranging mutually convenient times and places, traveling, and setting up rooms. Telephone interviewing cuts down on travel time and arrangements are easier to make, but the personal contact and the chance to observe nonverbal cues are lost. Also, it is easier for a subject to refuse an interview on the telephone.

In survey research, the interview format may be structured or unstructured, sometimes referred to as formal or informal. In structured interviews, the same questions are always asked, and they are asked in the same order. Although this format may appear stilted and formal, the answers will be easier to compare from one subject to another and the information from all subjects will be consistent.

In unstructured interviews, the interviewer must be trained to know what information is essential for the research, and must be entirely familiar with the questions before starting the interview. Although informal interviewing is often more comfortable for the interviewee and is useful in obtaining a great deal of detailed information, the volume of material can be difficult to organize and analyze, and often is not comparable from one subject to the next. Accordingly, one cannot compare across subjects easily or compile frequencies and percentages easily. If the researcher is carrying out survey research, the implication is that he or she will discover something about a whole group of people and will want similar information from each person to compare and contrast.

Unstructured interviews are often used in a pilot study, to set the parameters of the study. Once the issues have been clarified, a structured interview can be used for the formal study. In using unstructured interviews, the researcher is often "fishing," not wanting to be boxed in by specific formal questions. However, there is the danger of getting too far off track and of losing the original sense of purpose for the study. Results from the procedure can be amorphous because the material differs from subject to subject, and it can be difficult to know what to do with it all. Nevertheless, one can get an in-depth feel for that individual subject or topic, and in this way the unstructured interview can be useful as a tool in pilot studies.

Unstructured interviews may also be beneficial when questioning subjects about sensitive or awkward topics. The skillful interviewer can reword or reorder questions and introduce additional questions to put the subject at ease and to move at each subject's own pace. Unstructured interviewing can be used in this manner as an important method for gaining an interviewee's perspective in qualitative research. It is discussed later, from this aspect, in the chapter on qualitative research designs.

Structured or formal interviews, on the other hand, are probably best used by inexperienced interviewers and by beginning researchers. The data will be more easily tabulated and analyzed, and interpretations are more likely to be accurate and meaningful.

In deciding on the wording of questions, prime consideration should be given to the language style and idiom used by subjects, which may well be different from that used by the researcher. Try to use words and language similar to those used by the subjects. It is especially important not to use words foreign to respondents, such as medical terms (e.g., use "stroke" rather than "cerebrovascular accident"). Remove highly charged words from the interview and substitute more moderate words with the same meaning (Box 7–A).

One of the problems with data obtained from interviews is that it is difficult to know if subjects are telling the truth or trying to impress the interviewer by saying what they think the interviewer wants to hear. They may also be embarrassed or ashamed to tell the truth on sensitive issues. Experienced interviewers can gain skill in reading nonverbal cues to determine the degree of truthfulness in answers.

There is a great deal to be learned about the construction of individual questions and the interview as a whole. Because most of this information pertains to questionnaires as well as interviews, it will be discussed in the following section on written questionnaires.

Written Questionnaires

There are three ways to distribute written questionnaires. They may be mailed to respondents, or given to respondents person-

---

Box 7–A

Converse and Presser state:

"Forbid" and "allow" . . . are logical opposites, and thus substituting one for the other in the question "Do you think the United States should [allow/forbid] public speeches against democracy?" might easily be assumed to have no effect. Yet it turns out that many more people are willing to "not allow" such speeches than are willing to "forbid" them.

(Converse & Presser, 1986, p. 41)

ally with instructions to mail them back to the researcher, or respondents may be asked to complete questionnaires in the presence of the researcher. If questionnaires have been mailed or left for subjects to complete and return, there are special considerations. First, the questions must be very clear and unambiguous because the researcher will not be present to answer inquiries. This is of particular concern because if a question has been misinterpreted and answered incorrectly, the whole questionnaire must be discarded unless special statistical procedures are followed in analyzing results.

Another big concern researchers have regarding mailed questionnaires is whether there will be sufficient responses to justify the study. A reasonable response rate to expect if you are mailing to a group known to have an interest in the topic under study is about 30 percent. But there are ways to improve a response rate. The survey must be attractive and pleasing so that recipients will not discard it without reading the cover letter and initial instructions. The cover letter must be written to catch and hold the recipients' attention, and the topic must interest them sufficiently that they will want to answer the questions.

Questionnaires must be short enough that respondents will finish them but long enough to obtain the required information. There is a great deal written on the topic of how long questionnaires should be (Fink & Kosecoff, 1985). Self-administered questionnaires are generally limited to 30 minutes, whereas face-to-face interviews can continue for about an hour (Boxes 7–B and 7–C). One good rule of thumb is to view your questionnaire as objectively as you can and to ask

---

Box 7–B

A local health clinic is concerned about continuing to meet the needs of a changing community. In recent years, many more of its patients are older than 65 years of age, and a substantial percentage speak English as a second language. A bilingual volunteer will be devoting two mornings a week for 8 weeks to a 45-minute face-to-face interview with users of the clinic. A 50-item survey form has been designed for the purpose.

Box 7–C

The neighborhood clinic is also concerned that its services be appropriate for a population that is getting older and includes many people who prefer not to speak English. The city has decided to sponsor a survey of its clinic patients' needs. To minimize the amount of time that staff and patients will have to spend on the survey, a 10-minute, six-item self-administered questionnaire is prepared. To facilitate the survey's efficiency, questionnaires are left at the receptionist's desk.

---

yourself if you would stick with it and answer all the questions if it came to you in the mail.

Make sure that the cover letter tells the recipients why they should be interested in the study and what benefits they can expect from participating (even if the sole benefit is that they will be assisting a therapy student to complete her or his thesis and will thereby be indirectly helping to add one more person to the pool of working therapists). Capture their interest in the project by telling what you hope to achieve as a result of the study.

Always give a deadline for returning the questionnaire—approximately 2 weeks after it has been received. Research shows that recipients rarely return questionnaires after 2 weeks. Unless returns are confidential, keep a master list of those to whom you have mailed questionnaires and check off their returns. If you have not heard from them in 2 weeks, send them a reminder postcard.

Always enclose a stamped, addressed envelope. This will greatly increase the response rate. Recipients will generally not make the required effort to find an envelope and your address on the cover letter (which has often been destroyed), and may resent having to pay postage for your research project.

Question Construction

When constructing questions for questionnaires and interviews, two types of questions—closed-ended and open-ended—may be used. Closed-ended questions are those that require only a simple answer, usually "yes" or "no" or a check mark against a series of options, whereas open-ended questions are those that respondents can answer in as many words as they please.

Open-ended questions are most useful in dealing with complicated information when slight differences of opinion are important to know. Second, they provide a good way to elaborate on a closed-ended question, such as:

Do you teach clinical reasoning skills to your therapy students?   Yes _____ No _____

If yes, please explain how and at what point in the curriculum:

Third, open-ended questions may be used as a way of finding out which issue in a series of closed-ended questions is the most important or most relevant to the respondent. For example, a series of specific questions about specialty certification may be followed by the question "What is your opinion of specialty certification?" This technique is useful in that it often makes respondents feel better after having been "boxed in" for possible answers—they can now say what they want to say. You might not use the open-ended piece of information in tabulating results, but it keeps the respondents interested and involved, and increases their chances of completing the survey.

Open-ended questions are useful in allowing respondents to answer in any style and manner they wish without giving them suggestions. This reduces the chance of their giving what they perceive as socially acceptable answers. Similarly, questions that may be viewed as sensitive or threatening are usually best handled as open-ended questions and may be more honestly answered on an anonymous questionnaire than in a personal interview.

Respondents are often more willing to go quickly through a questionnaire composed of closed-ended questions rather than writing several sentences that they have to think about and compose. However, the closed-ended responses may not satisfy the investigator who would prefer more detailed and personal responses. There is a trade-off here, and the choice must be made by the researcher (Box 7–D).

In closed-ended questions, response formats should be mutually exclusive and, when ratings are required, there should be a wide array of choices. In the "yes/no" answer, there are differing opinions about whether to

---

Box 7–D

"In an open versus closed question experiment, people were asked what they thought was the most important problem facing the nation (Schuman & Presser, 1981). As the survey began, the U.S. was hit with an unexpected natural-gas shortage. This was reflected on the open version, where 22% said the 'energy shortage' was the most important problem. On the closed version, designed without knowledge of the energy problem, there was hardly a trace of concern about the shortage, with over 99% choosing one of the five offered alternatives. . . . Thus, when not enough is known to write appropriate response categories, open ended questions are to be preferred."

(Converse & Presser, 1986, p. 34)

---

include the "don't know" option. Some people feel it gives respondents an easy way out and would rather force them into a positive or negative answer, while others feel it is only fair and that respondents deserve that option (Box 7–E).

There are several ways in which respondents may be asked to respond to items. As well as the simple "yes/no" response, they may be asked to fill in the blank or to choose a relevant response from a list. Yet other questions rely on some sort of rating scale, the best known being the semantic differential and the Likert rating scales. The semantic differential, developed by Charles Osgood (Osgood, Suci, & Tannenbaum, 1957), is used as a measure of affective meaning. Respon-

---

Box 7–E

"The problem [addressed in the question] is intensified by the standard survey practice of not including 'don't know' or 'no opinion' as a response option mentioned in the question. Experimental research shows that many more people will say 'don't know' when that alternative is explicitly offered than when it is not. Such filtering for no opinion generally affects from about an eighth to a third of those interviewed."

(Converse & Presser, 1986, p. 35)

dents are given a domain of concern and are asked to rate their affective responses about that domain on a list of bipolar scales. These are seven-point scales with opposing adjectives at the two extremes. Generally, three dimensions exist into which these adjective pairs can be categorized—the evaluative dimension (good/bad), the potency dimension (strong/weak), and the activity dimension (fast/slow). Box 7–F shows one use of the semantic differential.

In the Likert scale (Likert, 1932), a statement is given to respondents to indicate the domain of concern, and the respondents are asked to indicate their level of agreement with that statement on a five-point or seven-point scale. The five-point scale is typically worded as follows: "Strongly agree, Agree, Neutral, Disagree, Strongly disagree." The seven-point scale would add "Very strongly agree" and "Very strongly disagree" at either end.

Incomplete sentences are sometimes used to find out such things as opinions, attitudes, knowledge, styles of behavior, or personality traits. A phrase is provided to indicate the domain of concern, and the respondent is asked to complete the sentence. For example,

"My opinion about placing adults who are mentally retarded in group homes is. . . ."

Multiple-choice items can be used to elicit opinions or attitudes from respondents. A statement is provided, sometimes in question form, and respondents are asked to select from the list the item that most reflects their opinion, attitude, or even a likely action, as shown in Box 7–G.

In rank-ordering items, a list of items is provided and respondents are asked to place a number beside each, indicating their order of importance. Sometimes only the first two or three items of importance are asked for, and sometimes the whole list must be prioritized. It should be remembered that for most people it is difficult to prioritize more than about 10 items.

Questionnaire Construction

The survey questions should be sequenced so that they follow one another in a logical order. First, draw subjects into the interview and gain their interest with broad, general questions. Avoid sensitive questions until the respondent is comfortable and, in the case of a face-to-face interview, until rapport has been established.

It is a good idea not to give too many questions that require a simple "yes" or "no" or too many requiring a rating at different levels (such as "Rate on a scale of 1 to 5") in a sequence, because respondents lose interest and concentration after a while and answer without giving the questions much thought.

Box 7–F

Henry, Nelson, and Duncombe (1984) used the semantic differential to elicit subjects' responses on how they felt about themselves following a choice/no choice situation in an activity group, on three affective factors: evaluation, power, and activity. They used Osgood's short-form semantic differential where subjects were asked to assign a rating on a 7-point scale for each of 12 scales, 4 scales being identified with each factor. The actual scale looked like this:

nice	awful
fast	slow
quiet	noisy
sour	sweet
powerless	powerful
young	old
bad	good
weak	strong
alive	dead
deep	shallow
big	little
unhelpful	helpful

Box 7–G

Stein and Cutler give the example of a researcher surveying some postmyocardial-infarction patients on their attitudes toward their disability. This multiple-choice question might be found on the survey:

"If I had a severe pain in my chest I would first do the following:
1. Call my private physician.
2. Call an ambulance.
3. Call the emergency rescue unit of the police.
4. Lie down and rest.
5. Other, please specify:_____."

(Stein & Cutler, 1996, p. 120)

Break up these questions with others written in a different format.

Often researchers add a general open-ended question at the end of a questionnaire, designed to give respondents an opportunity to add any information they did not have a chance to include during the process. On mailed questionnaires, it is quite common for respondents to write notes to the investigator, explaining things they think are unclear or adding items they feel are relevant. The final general question gives respondents a legitimate place to do this.

If you are planning to use a survey to collect data for your research project, you are strongly advised to read one of the excellent books written about this specialized topic. Several such books are listed in the Additional Reading list at the end of this chapter.

Record and Artifact Review

Review of written records may be a means of data gathering in many types of research, including experimental, ethnographic, historical, and case study designs. In some types of research, such as the historical type, reviewing records and archival material may be the sole means of gathering data, whereas in others it is only one technique.

> Documents provide both historical and contextual dimensions to your observations and interviews. They enrich what you see and hear by supporting, expanding, and challenging your portrayals and perceptions. Your understanding of the phenomenon in question grows as you make use of the documents and artifacts that are a part of people's lives. (Glesne & Peshkin, 1992, p. 54)

Written documents may include patients' medical records, minutes of meetings and case conferences, letters, speeches, articles, books, diaries, graffiti, notes, membership lists, newsletters, newspapers, and illustrations. Artifacts may include physical materials such as adaptive equipment, adapted clothing, photographs, audio and video recordings, and films. One way to obtain written materials is to ask informants to keep diaries, journals, or other kinds of records. You might be able to collaborate with therapists so that clinical notes can simultaneously meet the needs of the institution and the research study. If you are interested in clients' satisfaction with their rehabilitation, you might be able to play a role in the design of a client satisfaction form that would assist the institution as well as your study.

Traditionally, records used as research data are divided into primary and secondary sources. **Primary sources** are first-hand accounts about the topic under review, such as autobiographies or eyewitness accounts, and **secondary sources** are accounts written about the topic by others that are not based on personal experience, such as medical records (which are written by clinicians and not by the patients having the experience). Investigators should try to verify both the truth about the writing of the documents (did this person actually write it?), as well as the truth about the content of the documents (did this actually happen?). (For more on this topic, see the section in Chapter 9 on the historical research design.)

Conversely, written materials may be used to corroborate investigators' observations or what interviewers tell them. Also, they may raise useful questions about the study and shape new directions for observations and interviews. They can provide historical, demographic, and sometimes personal information that is unavailable from other sources.

In summarizing and interpreting the data gathered, the researcher must use logical analysis and try to be as objective as possible. In a historical study, when examination of records is often the only form of data gathering possible, the researcher usually cannot confirm that one event in the past caused another to occur. In this case, the investigator must make assumptions or draw inferences that assign causality. The more information is uncovered about an event, the more likely is the cause of the event to become known. Investigators must be careful to restrict interpretations about causes and generalizability to the evidence gathered.

Hardware Instrumentation

Many studies performed by therapists employ physical measures of such functions as joint range, muscle strength, or galvanic skin response. Physical or mechanical instruments that provide a valid and reliable measurement are usually more desirable in experimental research than the subjective ack given by subjects. Before relying on e of equipment as a measuring instru- n a research study, however, the ther- hould make sure that it is reliable and .. The use of equipment for measuring is also desirable in research because it provides a simple method for operationally defining independent variables (Box 7–H).

In these days of sophisticated equipment, many choices are available for measuring independent variables. Therapists use instruments, commonly known as hardware, such as cable tensiometers, spirometers, electroencephalographs, and goniometers. In his book *Elements of Research in Physical Therapy,* Currier (1984) describes the use of scientific hardware, considerations of instrumentation such as manufacturers and specifications, and areas of research interests and the associated hardware used to measure relevant physiological responses. A list of publications that will assist the researcher in identifying and locating hardware is included in Appendix C.

Unfortunately, many variables cannot be measured with hardware, and other means must be found to define and quantify them. These other means are generally written tests and measures, which will be discussed in the next section.

Tests, Measures, and Inventories

A great deal of research data used by health professionals are gathered on written tests, measures, and inventories. Variables that can be measured by these written means include psychological factors, cognitive abilities, perceptual motor skills, child development stages, prevocational skills, vocational

---

Box 7–H

For example, in a study measuring the range of motion in the affected elbow joints of patients with hemiplegia following a certain treatment technique, range of motion at the elbow could be operationally defined as the number of degrees registered on a goniometer placed on the joint angle while in extension and in flexion.

---

interests, personality factors, attitudes, and values. A list of the major suppliers of tests is given in Appendix D.

Some of the better-known tests have been gathered and critiqued in such bibliographic texts as Asher's book (1996) on tests used in the practice of occupational therapy in mental health, and two collections of tests and measures used for psychological assessment (Chun, Cobb, & French, 1985) and personality and social psychological attitudes (Robinson, 1991). Perhaps the best-known and most comprehensive books on the subject are the Buros Institute's *Tests in Print IV: An Index to Tests, Test Reviews, and the Literature on Specific Tests* (Murphy, Conoley, & Impara, 1994), which lists tests of intelligence, development, attitudes, and vocational interests, and *The Eleventh Mental Measurements Yearbook* (Kramer & Conoley, 1992), which contains reviews of the tests and references regarding their use. Other sources for tests are the catalogs from the major test publishers. A list of bibliographic sources for tests is given in Appendix E.

Should you find that there is no existing test to gather exactly the type of information you are interested in, you will probably be designing your own test. In order for your test to be valid and useful, you must be sure to follow accepted test construction techniques. You are referred to Benson and Clark's (1982) article "A Guide for Instrument Development and Validation" for a step-by-step description of the procedure for test construction.

Validity and Reliability of Test Instruments

Tests, measures, and inventories can be standardized or nonstandardized. Standardized tests have been subjected to a process called normalizing, which establishes a level of validity and reliability in relation to the "normal" population.

Validity

A test that is valid is one that measures what it claims to measure; for example, an intelligence test truly measures a child's intelligence rather than his or her school performance or concentration and motivation.

Reliability

A test that is reliable is one that will measure in the same manner and result in the same answers when measuring the same characteristic, time after time. For example, a reliable intelligence test will give the same intelligence quotient (IQ) score for the same individual time after time, all else being equal.

Three types of reliability pertaining to test instruments are important to understand:

1. *Test-retest reliability* is concerned with the reliability of scores over time. Subjects are measured regarding some characteristic; a period of time is allowed to elapse; and the same subjects are remeasured on the same characteristic. The scores of the two administrations are then examined and, assuming that the conditions and the characteristic being measured are stable, the scores should be similar.

2. *Split-half reliability* concerns the extent to which different parts of an instrument are measuring the same thing. For instance, are two different items on a test for self-esteem both actually measuring components of self-esteem? If not, the whole test may be suspect, and the compiled score may not truly represent the subject's self-esteem score. To assess this type of reliability, the test is divided into two parts and subjects' scores on the two groups of items are compared. The two scores should be similar in order for the test to be considered reliable.

3. *Interrater reliability* is the extent to which different raters or observers perceive the same person or characteristic similarly. There are two parts to this concept: first, are observers consistent in their ratings within themselves, and second, are observers consistent in their rating with other observers? Here again, ratings should be similar if observers are to be considered reliable.

The manual that accompanies a standardized test should include information about the process by which norms were established, details of the population used as normative groups, and the actual degree of validity and reliability achieved for the test. You should review this information to see if the test is rigorous enough for the purpose of your study. It is important that you use the test only on the type of subjects described in the manual. The researcher must learn the test administration procedures, and the test should be given exactly in the manner described in the manual. The reliability and validity of a test can be ensured only if the test is administered to the prescribed population, under the prescribed conditions, and in the prescribed manner. Once any of these items has been changed, the investigator cannot claim for his or her particular study the degree of reliability and validity listed in the manual.

Moving on to the Next Step

Now that you have decided on the methods you will use to collect data, you must decide on techniques to analyze those data. Your data collection may have generated either quantitative or qualitative data. Quantitative data result from variables that can be enumerated in some way so as to be tabulated and subjected to statistical procedures. The analysis of quantitative data will be discussed in Chapter 8. Qualitative data, on the other hand, are non-numerical and cannot be measured directly (e.g., attitudes, values, degree of participation, degree of pain experienced, and adjectives describing feelings). When numbers or units are assigned to components of such variables (known as attributes), statistical analysis can be made using appropriate, nonparametric statistical procedures. These are also discussed in Chapter 8. When no such assignment of a numerical value is given to the attribute, other methods of data analysis must be used. These methods are addressed in Chapter 10.

Stumbling Blocks

Observation in Quantitative Research

A common problem in making observations for quantitative research is the inability to be impartial or objective, especially if the observer is also the main investigator, the one whose study is being observed. We all tend to see what we want to see, and this is often true of the researcher who wishes to see positive results in his or her research study. For this reason, it is a good idea to have more than one observer watching and recording the same event. If possible, the person responsible for designing the study should not make the observations. It is also desirable for the observers to be ignorant of the hypothesis of the study and to know as little as possible about the premises behind the study, so that this information will not bias what they see. They also should not know whether subjects are in the experimental or control group while they are making observations. Observer bias is one of the major problems affecting the internal validity of an experimental study, and the researcher should do everything possible to eliminate that bias. Oyster, Hanten, and Llorens (1987) offer an excellent segment on observer bias in *Introduction to Research: A Guide for the Health Science Professional.*

Interviews

In conducting a formal interview, the issue of pacing is important. There is the danger of moving too quickly because the interviewer is familiar with the material and does not need as much time as the subject to think about the questions. If the interview is rushed, subjects may feel unimportant, as if there is insufficient time for them. Subjects also need time to understand the questions fully and to think about their answers.

Questionnaires

When designing a questionnaire, often the temptation is to adopt the attitude that "as long as I'm at it, why don't I ask . . ." and to add on a few more questions just because the questioner is curious. The temptation to ask for material that will not serve any useful purpose to the study should be overcome. Not only is it a waste of respondents' time, but also it may irritate them or cause them to run out of patience. A golden rule in survey construction is "Do not ask for information

unless you can act on it" (Fink & Kosecoff, 1985, p. 25). This rule also applies to asking questions that will raise hopes you cannot fulfill (Box 7–I).

Do not be too personal. A respondent may find the following questions insulting: "Are you divorced, married, or single?" "How much money do you make in a year?" "How do you feel about your therapist?" If respondents find these questions too personal, they will either not answer them at all or not answer them honestly. When personal information is essential to a survey, there are ways to phrase the questions to make them more tolerable, such as:

In which category was your salary last year?

1. Below $10,000
2. Between $10,000 and $20,000
3. Between $20,000 and $30,000
4. Between $30,000 and $40,000
5. Between $40,000 and $50,000
6. Over $50,000

Be careful not to lead respondents into giving you the answer they think you want. This may be done by adding positive or negative inferences to topics. For example, if you ask a subject about "working hard on his or her job," it implies that the job is taxing when the subject may not view it that way. In this case, you would be imposing your own attitude about the job onto the subject.

Box 7–I

"In a survey of a community's needs for health services, it would be unfair to have people rate their preference for a 24-hour emergency room staffed continuously by physicians if the community were unable to support such a service. Remember that the content of a survey can affect respondents' views and expectations."

(Fink & Kosecoff, 1985, p. 25)

WORKSHEETS

Review the techniques for data collection presented in this chapter and decide which techniques you will be using:

_____ Observation

_____ Interview

_____ Questionnaire

_____ Record and artifact review

_____ Hardware

_____ Tests, measures, and inventories

Remember that you may need to use more than one technique to collect the necessary data for your study.

Observation. If you are using this technique:

Which hypothesis do you plan to address with the observation?

What events, items, and behaviors need to be observed?

Write an observable definition for each item:

What method will be used to record the observations? Sketch out a data collection chart or protocol.

Who will actually do the observing and recording?

Will they need training?

_____ Yes   _____ No

If so, who will do the training?

Design a training procedure:

If there is more than one observer, will you test for interrater reliability?

_____ Yes   _____ No

Describe the procedure you will use:

Interview or questionnaire. If you plan to use an interview or questionnaire to gather data:

Which hypothesis do you plan to address with the interview or questionnaire?

What specific information will you need in order to address this hypothesis?

What demographic data will you need in order to determine if the sample is representative of the population?

_____ Will you conduct the interview in person?

_____ Will you conduct the interview over the telephone?

_____ Will you use a written questionnaire to be left with subjects?

_____ Will you mail out a questionnaire?

Will the interview be:

_____ Structured?

_____ Unstructured?

If you are mailing out a questionnaire, compose the cover letter. Remember to include:

- Why the survey will be of interest and benefit to respondents
- The main goal for the survey
- A deadline for returning the questionnaire
- A stamped, self-addressed envelope

Make the cover letter and survey attractive.

You are now ready to compose the questions. First, decide on the exact pieces of data you need to know. Then, decide which format would best suit the question (e.g., yes/no or multiple-choice format). Spend time on this until you feel you have the wording exactly right.

Conduct a small pilot study to see if your questions elicit the type of information you expected and if they are clear and unambiguous to respondents. (Read the section on pilot studies before doing this.)

Rewrite the questions based on the feedback from the pilot study.

Record and Artifact Review. If you plan to use a record or artifact review to gather data:

Which hypothesis will the record review address?

What data will you need to address this hypothesis?

Where will you find this information (specify for each):

Written material?

Physical material?

Mechanical material?

Which are primary sources?

Written:

Physical:

Mechanical:

Secondary sources?

Written:

Physical:

Mechanical:

Do you have sufficient primary sources to make this a viable method of data collection?

_____ Yes   _____ No

Hardware. If you plan to use this technique to gather data:

Which hypothesis will you address with the hardware?

What data do you need to gather in order to address this hypothesis?

Is there existing hardware to provide these data?

_____ Yes   _____ No

Or will you have to develop your own?

_____ Yes   _____ No

For existing hardware, is it standardized?

_____ Yes   _____ No

If so, what is the level of reliability? _____

validity? _____

If you are developing your own hardware, can you standardize it?

_____ Yes   _____ No

If yes, describe the procedure:

Tests, Measures, Inventories. If you plan to use tests, measures, or inventories to collect data:

Which hypothesis will be addressed by a test/measure/inventory?

What data do you need in order to address this hypothesis?

Is there an existing test that will elicit these data?

_____ Yes   _____ No

If yes, is it standardized?

_____ Yes   _____ No

If yes, what is the level of reliability? _____

validity? _____

What is the scoring procedure?

Contact the publisher to find out if the test is available.

If you are constructing your own test, will you be able to standardize it?

_____ Yes   _____ No

Construct the test, using the Benson and Clark (1982) article as a reference.

Conduct a pilot study and rework the test items based on the feedback. (Read section on pilot studies.)

What is the scoring procedure?

References

Asher, I.E. (1996). *Occupational therapy assessment tools: An annotated index* (2nd ed.). Bethesda, MD: AOTA.

Benson, J., & Clark, F. (1982). A guide for instrument development and validation. *American Journal of Occupational Therapy, 36*(12), 789–800.

Bogdan, R.C., & Biklen, S.K. (1982). *Qualitative research for education: An introduction to theory and methods.* Boston: Allyn and Bacon.

Chun, K.T., Cobb, S., & French, J.R. (1985). *Measures for psychological assessment.* Ann Arbor, MI: Institute for Social Research, University of Michigan.

Converse, J.M., & Presser, S. (1986). *Survey questions: Handcrafting the standardized questionnaire.* No. 63 in Quantitative Applications in the Social Sciences Series. Newbury Park, CA: Sage Publications.

Currier, D.P. (1984). *Elements of research in physical therapy.* Baltimore: Williams & Wilkins.

Fink, A., & Kosecoff, J. (1985). *How to conduct surveys: A step-by-step guide.* Beverly Hills, CA: Sage Publications.

Glesne, C., & Peshkin, A. (1992). *Becoming qualitative researchers: An introduction.* New York: Longman.

Henry, A.D., Nelson, D.L., & Duncombe, L.W. (1984). Choice making in group and individual activity. *American Journal of Occupational Therapy, 38*(4), 245–251.

Kramer, J. & Conoley, J. (Eds.). (1992). *The eleventh mental measurements yearbook.* Lincoln, NE: Buros Institute of Mental Measurements.

Likert, R. (1932). A technique for the measurement of attitudes. *Archives of Psychology, 52*, 140–145.

Miles, M.B., & Huberman, A.M. (1994). *Qualitative data analysis: An expanded sourcebook.* Thousand Oaks, CA: Sage Publications.

Murphy, L., Conoley, J., & Impara, J. (Eds.). (1994). *Tests in print IV: An index to tests, test reviews, and the literature on specific tests.* Lincoln, NE: Buros Institute of Mental Measurements.

Osgood, C., Suci, G., & Tannenbaum, P. (1957). *The measurement of meaning.* Urbana, IL: University of Illinois Press.

Oyster, C., Hanten, W., & Llorens, L. (1987). *Introduction to research: A guide for the health science professional.* Philadelphia: J.B. Lippincott.

Robinson, J.P. (1991). *Measures of personality and sociopsychological attitudes.* San Diego, CA: Academic Press.

Spradley, J.P. (1980). *Participant observation.* New York: Holt, Rinehart & Winston.

Stein, F., & Cutler, S.K. (1996). *Clinical research in allied health and special education* (3rd ed.). San Diego: Singular Publishing Group, Inc.

Additional Reading

Converse, J.M., & Presser, S. (1986). *Survey questions: Handcrafting the standardized questionnaire.* No. 63 in Quantitative Applications in the Social Sciences Series. Newbury Park, CA: Sage Publications.

Fink, A., & Kosecoff, J. (1985). *How to conduct surveys: A step-by-step guide.* Beverly Hills, CA: Sage Publications.

Rubin, H.J., & Rubin, I.S. (1995). *Qualitative interviewing: The art of hearing data.* Thousand Oaks, CA: Sage Publications.

Schuman, H., & Presser, S. (1981). *Questions and answers in attitude surveys: Experiments on question form, wording, and context.* New York: Academic Press.

8

Analyzing Quantitative Data

Next is the part that many people hate! What to do with this mass of numbers that has been collected? What statistical manipulations to apply? Some people have such a fear of this part of the research process that they never get beyond it. The fear and/or lack of knowledge may be real or imagined but should not be allowed to stand in the way of the therapist as a researcher. If you feel at all uncertain about quantitative data analysis, get help from a statistician.

Consulting a Statistician

Consulting a statistician has a price, but most people I know who have hired someone feel it is worth the cost. You may be fortunate enough to be connected to a university or other facility that employs a statistician who is willing to help free of charge or for a nominal fee. Otherwise, you may have to contact a statistician (call your local college or university for suggestions) and inquire about charges; hourly rates may be quite high, so it would pay to shop around.

The question of when to seek statistical assistance during the research process is worthy of discussion. A statistician should be consulted in the design stage of the project, while you are still deciding on the instruments or measures you will use to collect

data. You will be the one to decide on the actual measures used and whether these measures will collect the type of data you want as reliably as you wish; however, the statistician understands how the data will be analyzed and may have some advice concerning the format in which the data are to be collected.

For example, in knowing that you wish to compare two groups' performances on pretests and post-tests in order to determine which group made the most progress, the statistician may advise that data resulting from a certain measure are not in a format suitable for such comparisons. An unclear response from subjects such as, "I feel somewhat better," does not lend itself to objective comparisons, either for that one subject or among subjects.

More often, some crucial piece of information concerning subjects has been omitted from a questionnaire (e.g., their ages). If you wish to group people by age for comparisons, this information will of course be important. Although the therapist obviously has the ability to spot this type of error, it sometimes takes an objective reader who is accustomed to studying data to notice it.

Helping the therapist design formats for the collection of data is another way the statistician can be helpful. Knowing how the data will be entered on a computer, for instance, allows the statistician to understand that this will be more easily accomplished if numbers are arranged linearly with a separate line for each subject.

Finally, a statistician may determine that a certain statistical test will be best suited to achieve the analysis you wish to make and can advise on how many subjects are needed in order to use that test. You would want this information early in the planning stages of your project. Thus, it can be seen that seeking assistance from a statistician early in the research design process is helpful in ensuring that data will be collected in such a way that they can be manipulated effectively.

Anything but basic statistics is beyond the scope of this text. However, it is hoped that a simple explanation of some of the processes involved in organizing and manipulating data will enable the reader with a fear of statistics to cope with the material and to know when to get help.

Descriptive Versus Inferential Statistics

Statistics may conveniently be divided into two categories: descriptive and inferential statistics. Descriptive statistics are those that describe, organize, and summarize data. They include such things as frequencies, percentages, descriptions of central tendency (mean, median, mode) and descriptions of relative position (range, standard deviation).

These procedures allow for the description of all the individual scores in a sample on one variable by using one or two numbers, such as the mean and standard deviations. They can be used to describe each dependent variable, such as the percentage and mean of each item physical therapists checked off on a list of reasons for moving into supervisory positions and their ages when they moved. Descriptive statistics can also be used to give the variation or spread of scores within each group studied, such as the mean and range of scores for experimental and control groups in a study on a new treatment technique for carpal tunnel syndrome.

Inferential statistics, on the other hand, allow one to make inferences from the sample to the population in order to speculate, reason, and generalize about the population

from the sample findings. Sufficient subjects are needed in the sample to be able to do this; in addition, random selection should be used. The types of statistical tests used in inferential statistics include t tests, F tests, and tests for r. These tests result in probability statements that help one draw conclusions about differences or relationships between groups. For example, if a difference is found between the mean scores of two groups at the end of a study, the researcher must decide whether a similar difference is likely to be found between the same mean scores in the whole population. The t, F, and r tests would allow the researcher to make this decision.

Both descriptive and inferential statistics are often used in the same research study. Descriptive statistical methods are the same regardless of the type of data being used; however, inferential statistical methods do vary according to the type of data used.

Types of Data

The data that have been collected in your study may be characterized in four different ways: nominal, ordinal, interval, and ratio.

Nominal Data

Nominal data are the numbers applied to nonnumerical variables (e.g., a group of people's disabilities could be coded as follows: right hemiplegia = 1, left hemiplegia = 2, paraplegia = 3, and so on). Each category of data must be mutually exclusive, meaning that no individual or variable could be assigned to more than one group. There is no ordered relationship between categories, meaning that one category could not be considered to come before or after another category. This type of data is sometimes referred to as "discrete" as opposed to "continuous." There is no limit to the number of categories that can be included in a nominal scale. Because there is no numerical value to categories, they cannot be meaningfully added, subtracted, or multiplied, and so forth. One cannot calculate an average (mean) disability, for example.

Examples of categories are male and female; inpatient, outpatient, and day treatment settings; and patients with schizophrenia, bipolar disease, or depression. A nominal scale may also be used to code such responses on a survey as "yes/no" or "never/sometimes/always."

Ordinal Data

Ordinal data are numbers that still are discrete but are ordered; however, the intervals between the categories are not known and cannot be assumed to be equal. Numbers can be assigned to groups, and the numbers can be put into a meaningful sequence. For instance, a review committee may rank-order a series of program proposals and assign first, second, and third place; but the top-ranked proposal may be considerably better than the ones ranked second and third, whereas the ones ranked fourth, fifth, and sixth may be similar to each other in quality. These differences among intervals would not be reflected in the numerical assignment. Other examples would be ratings on a Likert scale such as "Strongly agree," "Agree," "Neutral," "Disagree," "Strongly disagree;" or classifications for client ability such as "Needs full assistance," "Needs partial assistance," "Independent." An ordinal data scale indicates a greater or lesser degree of something, or it may reflect a "precedes" or "superior" concept.

Interval Data

Interval data also are ordered in a logical sequence. However, this time the intervals between the numbers are considered equal and represent actual amounts. These are continuous data. Examples are intelligence scores, degrees of muscle strength, and degrees of perceptual motor skills. Items are ordered on a continuum; however, there is no actual zero point. For instance, the zero reading on a dynamometer does not reflect a total absence of muscle strength; it is not a measure of anything.

Ratio Data

Ratio data are numbers that are also continuous with equal intervals between numbers. Additionally, ratio data have a meaningful zero point. In other words, the zero point indicates a total absence of whatever ability or property is being measured. For instance, there can legitimately be zero range of motion or visual acuity. "Ratio data can be multiplied and divided, enabling one to say that

a range of motion of 40 d[...] of a 20-degree range" (H[...] 1976, p. 431).

Parametric and Nonparametric Data

Nominal and ordinal data ar[...] **nonparametric data**, whereas i[...] ratio data are **parametric data**. [...] tance of making this distinction i[...] one will know what kind of statistics can be used to manipulate these data. Although most of the descriptive statistics can be used on both parametric and nonparametric data (the exception being that mean and standard deviations cannot be used on nominal data), different inferential statistics must be used on the two types of data. This is because of the properties of the data, such as the data being ordered or the intervals between numbers being equal. Some tests are not powerful enough to cope with unordered, unequal data, whereas others are. Nominal data need such nonparametric tests as the chi-square or Mann-Whitney tests; interval data can be manipulated using t tests and analyses of variance. Table 8–1 may be helpful in summarizing categories of data with their corresponding parametric and nonparametric classifications and types of statistical tests.

Some rules need to be applied to the distribution of data in order for one to be able to use parametric tests:

1. The sample must be representative of the target population so that the variables being measured fall within the normal distribution for that population (e.g., random selection has occurred).

2. Variables must have been measured in a manner that generates interval or ratio data.

3. Initial differences between subjects in the two groups under study must have the opportunity to be similar (i.e., random assignment to groups or matching must have occurred).

When any of these conditions has not been met, nonparametric statistics should be used; that is, when:

1. Random selection has not occurred, so that the sample is not considered representative of the population and vari-

...E 8–1   Categories of Data with Corresponding Classifications and Inferential Tests

Categories of Data	Classification	Examples of Inferential Tests
Nominal data: named categories, unordered	Nonparametric	Pearson's chi-square Fisher's exact Goodman and Kruskal's tau b
Ordinal data: ordered categories, unequal intervals	Nonparametric	Pearson's chi-square Spearman rho Wilcoxon rank sum Mann-Whitney Kruskal-Wallis Kendall's tau
Interval data: ordered data with equal intervals between categories	Parametric	t tests Analysis of variance (ANOVA) Analysis of covariance (ANCOVA)
Ratio data: equal intervals with zero point	Parametric	t tests Analysis of variance (ANOVA) Pearson product moment correlation

ables are probably not normally distributed.

2. Variables have been measured in a manner that generates nominal or ordinal data.

3. The numbers of subjects in the sample are small.

Because nonparametric data do not meet strict statistical criteria, substantial differences must be found between sets of scores before those differences are considered meaningful.

Frequently nonparametric statistics should be used in health science research because pathological human conditions are being studied. The variables of illness or pathology often are not distributed normally in the target population. Also, it is often difficult to locate many subjects with the requisite pathology, so sample groups tend to be small.

Descriptive Statistics

A great deal of quantitative data can be effectively analyzed using descriptive statistics. In fact, if a nonexperimental research design is used, almost all of the data will be appropriately analyzed descriptively because random selection may not have been used for the sample and there may not be a control group. It is difficult to make inferences from a sample to a population (the purpose of inferential statistics) if random sampling and control criteria have not been met.

The initial description and compilation of data can be achieved using descriptive statistics; that is, providing the frequencies, percentages, and means for all the characteristics under study so that the reader has a thorough understanding of the subjects and variables. It is customary to present percentages alongside the frequencies, both in the text and in illustrative tables.

It is often useful to give the reader the group's average score—that is, their **central tendency.** The mean, median, or mode can be used to describe central tendency. The mean is computed by adding all the scores and dividing the total by the number in the group. The median is the midpoint among all the scores. Each score must be listed before finding the midpoint, which incidentally may end up not being a whole number. The mode is the most commonly occurring score. There may be more than one mode; for instance, in a list of IQ scores, four people may score 110 and four may score 115. In this instance, the total group of scores would be referred to as bimodal. Oyster, Hanten, and Llorens (1987) provide a useful description of when to use which of the measures of central tendency.

The reader also may wish to know the **relative position** of subjects and their scores. For instance, a range will explain the section of the continuum in which the subjects scored, perhaps IQ scores from 90 to 120, resulting in a range of 31. Another way to describe relative position is to use the standard deviation, referred to as s or SD. The standard deviation indicates how the scores are grouped around the midpoint. To continue using the IQ example, a group of 7-year-olds with a mean IQ of 100 whose scores ranged from 90 to 110 would be quite different from a group of 7-year-olds with a mean IQ of 100 whose scores ranged from 80 to 120.

There are many useful ways to illustrate descriptive data, such as tables, pie charts, and graphs. These formats are described in Chapter 12.

Inferential Statistics

Inferential statistics are those that allow us to take the results from a research project and decide whether they are likely to occur in the target population. They also help us decide the chances of that occurring. If there is a statistically significant result, we may decide that the probability is great that we have in fact found a result that can be generalized to the target population.

Tests for inferential statistics can be divided into three groups:

1. Those that try to find if the differences observed between two sets of scores are significantly different

2. Those that examine two sets of scores to find the strength of association between them

3. Those that compare more than two sets of scores to find the extent to which they vary among each other

Significant Differences

In this group, the tests assist the researcher in deciding whether the changes in the mean pre-test and post-test scores of the experimental group are, in fact, a result of the experimental treatment rather than chance. They allow comparison of results from the sample with that which was hypothesized as normally occurring in the target population. The tests can be used with a directional hypothesis or with a two-sided hypothesis.

Use the classic experimental research design as an example:

$$R \quad O_1 \quad X \quad O_2$$
$$R \quad O_3 \quad \quad O_4$$

Statistical difference tests would be applied to the scores from the pre-test and post-test results of the experimental group (O_1 and

O_2), and to the pre-test and post-test scores of the control group (O_3 and O_4), and finally to the post-test scores of the two groups (O_2 and O_4). The first result would indicate the degree of change following the experimental treatment; the second, changes following no treatment; and the third, the difference between end conditions of the experimental and control groups. If the difference between the scores on the third test (between O_2 and O_4) were statistically significant, it would indicate that changes could be attributed to the treatment rather than to chance (Box 8–A).

Significance testing is based on the laws of probability. It answers the question: What is the probability that this change occurred because of events in the research study, and what is the probability that this change would have occurred anyway, by chance? The tests that are used to make this determination result in a level of probability, and it is the researcher who decides whether or not this level is significant. In the social sciences, the usual convention is that 5 occurrences in 100 of the change being caused by chance is a reasonable number to accept, and that any result better than that is statistically significant. This result would imply that it is 95 percent certain that the improvement in post-test scores was caused by the treatment. This probability level is expressed as $p < .05$. Some scientific endeavors require more stringent proof, and a standard of $p < .01$, or 1 chance in 100 that the change

---

Box 8–A

An example of the classic experimental design can be found in Mitchell, Daines, and Thomas's (1987) study of the effects of ingestion of amino acids on burning pain threshold. One experimental group received L-tryptophan, a second experimental group received phenylalanine, and a control group received a placebo. At pre-testing, the three groups showed a wide difference in "normal" pain threshold, so a statistical test was used at the end of the study. The test, called analysis of covariance (ANCOVA), could adjust the post-test scores based on the pre-test differences. In measuring the results of the three groups on the post-test, the ANCOVA showed no significant difference between the groups.

occurred by chance, is set for those studies, otherwise known as a 99 percent success rate. Clinicians must decide on the significance level to be used, deciding how acceptable it would be for the dependent variable to be changed by the independent variable at various levels of certainty (Box 8–B).

The tests most commonly used to determine significance levels are Pearson's chi-square test on nonparametric (nominal and ordinal) data and the student's t test on parametric (interval and ratio) data. The chi-square and t tests can be used to compare two groups on only one variable at a time.

Pearson's Chi-square Test

In the Pearson's chi-square test, the data used for analysis are counts of category membership (e.g., "How many subjects are men and how many are women?" or "How many have right hemiplegia and how many have left hemiplegia?"). Pearson's chi-square test may be used when you wish to know if there are significant differences between pre-test and post-test scores for a given group, or if you wish to know if two groups are similar when you intend to use one as an experimental group and one as a control group. It can be used to compare groups on a single variable or on groups of variables, one at a time. This test is useful when the researcher is interested in similarities be-

tween groups of subjects (Box 8–C). If the researcher can determine the numbers of characteristics such as gender, age, or diagnosis, a chi-square test on the respondents will test whether the sample matches the population. The calculated value for the chi-square formula is evaluated using standardized tables that list critical values. When the chi-square exceeds the table value, the hypothesis is supported.

t Tests

There are three different t tests, each of which is used with a different research design, but all compare the mean scores of two groups. The single sample t test compares the mean for a sample against a known population mean for a particular variable. This test is rarely used because the mean score for a population is rarely available. The paired groups t test is used when subjects have been used as their own control group and when groups consist of individuals who have been matched on some characteristic. In this case, the pre-test and post-test scores are compared for the first group and the two scores from the matched pairs are compared for the second group. In the independent groups t test, the pre-test and post-test means are compared for the experimental and control

---

Box 8–B

A decision concerning significance level was made by therapists when they were studying the relationship between infant neuromotor assessment and preschool motor measures. In the research design section of their article, the authors state:

> Because we used multiple comparisons, the alpha level was set at .01. This level also was thought to be advisable because, with a sample size of 77, correlation coefficients could be large enough to be significant at the .05 level but not large enough to be clinically significant. (Deitz, Crowe, & Harris, 1987, p. 15)

Here, the clinicians are making a decision about the level of significance based on the idiosyncrasies of a specific test (Spearman's rank correlation coefficients).

Box 8–C

Coren and colleagues (1987) investigated the factors related to physical therapy students' decisions to work with elderly patients. They used chi-square tests to determine relationships between students' intentions to work with the elderly and their answers to questions concerned with such things as biographical information (students' age, whether they had ever lived with their grandparents, whether they had friends over the age of 65 years), experiential influences (courses in problems of the elderly, weekly home visits with the well elderly, clinical rotations in a geriatric setting), and attitudinal perceptions (concern that salaries might be lower in geriatric settings, lack of prestige in working with the elderly). Answers to the questions were of the nominal and ordinal type, so that chi-square tests were appropriate for data analyses.

Box 8–D

Shinabarger (1987) used an independent group *t* test to compare the range-of-motion scores for each of eight motions between subjects with diabetes mellitus in experimental and control groups.

Box 8–F

The Wilcoxon signed rank test was used in a study of the effects of a maternal preparation program on mother-infant pairs. Tests were performed separately on the experimental and control groups' prenatal and postnatal questionnaire scores.

(Hamilton-Dodd et al., 1989)

---

groups, and the two post-test scores are compared. This is the most commonly used *t* test (Box 8–D).

If you have decided on a direction for your hypothesis, a one-tailed *t* test should be used to determine significance of results. If a nondirectional hypothesis has been used, a two-tailed *t* test should be employed to determine the direction of the significance, if any (Box 8–E). The *t* test is quite powerful and can be used on groups of subjects smaller than 30.

Wilcoxon Signed Rank Test

The Wilcoxon signed rank test is used on nonparametric data and is equivalent to the correlated groups *t* test. It is performed on paired scores and will determine the significance of the difference between either pretest and post-test scores for individuals (Box 8–F) or scores on matched pairs of subjects.

Wilcoxon Rank Sum Test

The Wilcoxon rank sum test is the equivalent to the *t* test for independent groups, but is used on nonparametric data. For this test, ranks are assigned to scores for all subjects

in the study, and the ranks for all subjects in each group are summed. The test determines the degree of differences between group total scores (Box 8–G).

Mann-Whitney Test

The Mann-Whitney test is yet a third alternative to the *t* test for use on nonparametric data. It tests for differences between means on two independent groups and is equivalent to the independent groups *t* test (Box 8–H).

Tests for Correlation

These tests are used to examine two sets of scores to find the extent of their relationship to one another. The two sets of scores might be from one set of individuals or from two different groups of individuals. Once it is seen that one score moves up or down, the intent is to find out if the other score moves in a corresponding fashion. The objective is to find out how closely the scores covary; that is, whether they change together in a particular pattern, in a positive or negative way. If both scores increase together, they are said to be positively correlated; for example, height and weight scores for a group of subjects would probably increase together. If, on

---

Box 8–E

Liu, Currier, and Threlkeld (1987) investigated the effects of electrical stimulation on the blood circulation of an unexercised part of the body. They used an independent, two-tailed *t* test to determine equality between the experimental and control groups and to analyze the prestimulated heart rate, blood pressure, and pulsatility index. They found that the groups were similar on these variables before experimental intervention and thus did not need to make adjustments later via statistical analyses.

Box 8–G

Case-Smith, Cooper, and Scala (1989) used the Wilcoxon rank sum test "to estimate whether or not the differences between the summed scores were significant" (p. 247). The researchers compared efficient and nonefficient neonate feeders on neonatal oral motor assessment scores.

Box 8–H

In studying changes in students' perceptions of the professional role, Corb and colleagues (1987) employed a Mann-Whitney *U* test to investigate differences between students' and faculty members' perceptions of various concepts. Concepts related to professional role were investigated using a semantic differential technique with a seven-point scale, so that data generated were of the ordinal type (i.e., numerical values 1 through 7 representing respondents' agreement with one or other of the adjectives).

Box 8–J

Gogia and colleagues (1987) investigated the intertester reliability of goniometric measurements at the knee and the validity of the clinical measurements by comparing the measurements taken from radiographs. They used the Pearson product-moment correlation coefficient to compare the measurements recorded by two therapists and to compare measurements obtained by each therapist with those derived from the radiographs.

the other hand, scores for age over 60 years and scores for muscle strength were computed, age scores might increase while strength scores decreased. These scores would be said to be negatively correlated. The two sets of scores that are being compared in correlation testing can be entered on a scattergram to show the degree of correlation graphically (Box 8–I).

Tests for correlation yield a statistic called a correlation coefficient, expressed as *r*. An *r* may range from -1 (indicating a perfect negative relationship) to $+1$ (indicating a perfect positive relationship). A zero would indicate that there is no relationship between the two variables. Decimal factors are used to indicate *r* scores (i.e., .87 or $-.66$). As with the previous tests, a level of significance can be computed for an *r* score.

Pearson Product Moment Correlation

The most common correlation test is the Pearson product moment method, often called the Pearson *r*, which is used on parametric data. This test can be used on group

scores or individual scores. It indicates only systematic disagreements between scores and does not show the odd or occasional disagreement. It is often used to estimate reliability between tests, as in a test-retest situation, or between two testers to indicate intertester reliability (Box 8–J).

Spearman Rho

The Spearman rho method is the equivalent to the Pearson *r*. It is used in descriptive research resulting in nonparametric data when items have been ranked and the investigator wishes to compare two sets of rankings to see if there is any type of relationship between them. Like the Pearson, it results in an *r* value falling between -1 and $+1$ (Box 8–K).

It is important to remember that a relationship between two sets of scores does not necessarily mean that this is a cause-and-effect relationship. The researcher can claim only that a positive or negative relationship between the variables has been found, and no more.

Box 8–I

Taylor and colleagues (1987) used the scattergram to good effect in their article on the effects of interferential current stimulation for treatment of subjects with recurrent jaw pain. The scattergram illustrates the intensity of mean jaw pain on the vertical axis and the subject groups on the horizontal axis.

Box 8–K

The authors of a study on the relationship between infant neuromotor assessment and preschool motor measures state clearly why they used the Spearman test:

Because the assumptions for the use of parametric statistics were not met, the relationships were examined using Spearman's rank correlation coefficients.

(Deitz, Crowe, & Harris, 1987, p. 15)

Regression Analysis

Regression analysis is a technique that can be used after the correlation coefficient has been established. When a relationship has been found between two variables, one can attempt to predict future scores for the dependent variable based on the scores on which the correlation coefficient was found.

Comparison of More Than Two Variables

The investigator often wishes to explore more than two variables in the same study. In this case, different statistical tests are needed.

Analysis of Variance

Analysis of variance (ANOVA) is a statistical technique that can compare the mean scores of three or more groups in one study. It deals with multigroup questions, such as the one in Box 8–L.

The ANOVA yields an *F* ratio, which is evaluated using a standardized table to see if there is a significant difference between the largest and smallest of the study group means. If you wish to see if there are significant differences between any of the other means, you must use another test, such as the Duncan range test, the Newman-Keuls test, or the Tukey test (Box 8–M).

In addition to informing the investigator of differences between the means of the study

---

Box 8–L

Is there a difference in bilateral motor coordination measured by jumping jacks, symmetrical stride jumps and reciprocal stride jumps, in 5- to 9-year-old children (Magalhaes, Koomar, & Cermak, 1989)? In this study there were five groups: 5-, 6-, 7-, 8-, and 9-year-olds, each divided into girls and boys. Each group of children was tested on the three activities (independent variables) to measure their abilities against existing tests for bilateral motor coordination. A one-way analysis of variance (ANOVA) was used to determine the effect of age and sex on the three activities. The tests were also capable of determining the interaction among age, sex, and task.

Box 8–M

Lohmann and colleagues (1987) found through an ANOVA that there were significant differences in mean measurements of tibia vara between limbs when the lower extremity was in different positions under different conditions and used a Newman-Keuls test to see exactly where the differences were—between which two of the three groups.

---

groups (e.g., differences between total means for the 5-, 6-, 7-, 8-, and 9-year-olds), the ANOVA can give information about differences between the individuals within each group. If each of the 5-year-olds, for instance, had 10 trials on each of the activities, a mean could be computed for each child and those means entered into the ANOVA equation. The test would then compute whether there were significant differences among the 5-year-olds. ANOVA is powerful enough to be able to pick out odd or occasional differences in an individual's scores.

Analysis of Covariance

A similar test is the analysis of covariance (ANCOVA). It controls for initial differences between groups. If pre-test scores show that the dependent variable is substantially different for the groups owing to extraneous variables such as age or sex, an ANCOVA can take into account the extraneous variables by treating them as covariates and by extracting their effect from the data. If the groups are made more equitable to begin with, the final results can be compared and judged more fairly (Box 8–N).

Box 8–N

While testing for the possible effect of amino acids on burning pain threshold in two experimental groups and one control group, investigators used an ANCOVA to control statistically for the wide individual variance found in pre-test pain measures.

(Mitchell, Daines, & Thomas, 1987)

Kruskal-Wallis Test

The Kruskal-Wallis test is equivalent to the one-way ANOVA and can be used on non-parametric data. Like other nonparametric tests, this test is based on rankings of scores on the dependent measure in which all subjects are put into one group during the ranking procedure, then put back into their original treatment groups for the remaining analysis (Box 8–O).

Multiple Regression

This test provides a way of making predictions about the study variable by understanding the effects of two or more independent variables on the study variable (i.e., how much do the independent variables correlate with the study variable?). It is possible to take the procedure a step further by untangling the relative contributions of each of the independent variables. One can then use stepwise regression to look at the independent variables in various combinations to see which combination is most useful in predicting the occurrence of the study variable.

Only some of the many possible tests for manipulating data are reviewed here. A statistician will be familiar with other possibilities and will be able to advise on the appropriate statistical tests based on your specific research design.

Computer Analysis

All of the aforementioned tests can be computed by hand, but this is a tedious and time-consuming process and most people use a computer for statistical processing. With the help of a statistician or a computer assistant, therapists can enter the raw data onto the computer. It is also possible for the relative novice to perform the statistical manipulations by learning the entry keys for the relevant statistical software package. There are manuals for each package, but they are often difficult to follow without computer literacy. Three commonly used statistical software packages designed for the health and social sciences are:

1. SAS/STAT—SAS/STAT User's Guide, Version 6, ed. 4. SAS Institute, Inc., Cary, NC (1990).
2. SPSS—Statistical Package for the Social Sciences, 444 North Michigan Avenue, Chicago, 60611 (1995).
3. BMDP—Biomedical Data Package, University of California, Berkeley, (1990).

A fourth package, Minitab, is an effective statistical analysis software package that was developed for use in introductory statistics courses. It has since been made available for use on personal computers as *The Student Edition of Minitab* (Schaefer & Anderson, 1989). This edition comes with a clearly written manual and is powerful enough to do most of the statistical procedures likely to be used in therapists' and students' research studies. Statistical features include basic statistics, regression analysis, analysis of variance, and nonparametric tests, with graphics to enhance the display of data.

If you need to analyze more than just a small amount of data, using a computer is highly recommended. It is well worth the researcher's time to take a basic computer course to learn to move around the keyboard, to understand basic computer concepts, and to enter data.

Box 8–O

When investigating the differences in perception among three groups of respondents who assessed the importance of 80 competencies for physical therapists treating patients with arthritis, Moncur (1987) used the Kruskal-Wallis ANOVA to make group comparisons. Levels of importance of a competency were compared among the different practitioner groups by the Kruskal-Wallis ANOVA test.

Stumbling Blocks

It may not be easy to find a statistician with whom one is compatible and with whom one can communicate easily, but it is definitely worth the search and the cost. If you are not sure where to go for help, ask colleagues who have participated in research, or faculty at the local therapy training program. There is usually someone on the faculty whose job it is to assist with statistics, and he or she may be willing to work with private clients. Alternatively, you might be fortunate enough to find a fellow therapist or a colleague knowledgeable about statistics who can help you. Too often I have seen therapists or students struggling to understand a statistician and feeling that the problem was all their own. They have been reluctant to ask questions or to change consultants. Of course, the problem is never one-sided. Often it is the statistician who does not understand the clinical process and who is unable to design data collection and analysis methods that are appropriate. Either way, it is best to leave that situation and find someone else. You may even have to try two or three people before finding the one who is right for you.

Be sure that it is clear in your own mind what it is you hope to find out as a result of the data analysis. For example, know whether you want to determine the difference between pre-test and post-test results for the same group of subjects, or whether you want to know the difference between two post-test results for two different groups of subjects. Sometimes therapists get talked into performing complex and elegant statistical manipulations on their data by statisticians who are more interested in proving that they can do such manipulations than they are in helping therapists achieve their goals. The analyses may look impressive but often do not make much sense in real-life terms in relation to the data. As Partridge and Barnitt (1986) state, "It is . . . important to distinguish 'real life' significance from 'statistical' significance—they may be different . . ." (p. 76). A useful example to illustrate the point is given in Box 8–P. Cohen (1988) offers a further example of the concepts "sig-

nificant" and "meaningful" not being synonymous, as presented in Box 8–Q.

Finally, I recommend again that you consult with a statistician *before* you begin to collect data, to ensure that all the necessary data are collected in a useful format.

Box 8–P

"In a study of the efficacy of chest physiotherapy and intermittent positive pressure breathing in the resolution of pneumonia by Graham and Bradley (1978), the conclusion was that chest physiotherapy and intermittent positive pressure breathing do not hasten resolution of pneumonia; however, most therapists would not consider physiotherapy had a place in the treatment of acute pneumonia. The lack of statistically significant differences between treated and untreated groups was not of real life 'significance' or importance."

(Partridge & Barnitt, 1986, p. 77)

Box 8–Q

"For example, in the pain study significantly more subjects might have preferred to read *Time* magazine than *Newsweek*. Although such a difference may be meaningful to the sales managers of these publications, this information probably has little relevance to the outcome of the pain experiment."

(Cohen, 1988, p. 599)

WORKSHEETS

Review the research design and data collection methods you have selected for your project.

Are you using:

_____ An experimental design?

_____ A quasi-experimental design?

_____ A nonexperimental design?

Are you collecting data using:

_____ Observation?

_____ Interview?

_____ Questionnaire?

_____ Record review?

_____ Equipment?

_____ Tests, measures, inventories?

Will you be confined to descriptive statistics or will you also be able to use inferential statistics?

_____ Descriptive?

_____ Inferential?

For the *descriptive statistics,* which ones do you think would help the reader to understand your results?

_____ Frequencies and percentages

_____ Central tendency: mean, median, mode

_____ Relative position: range, standard deviation

For *inferential statistics:*

Will the results of the data collection techniques yield:

_____ Nominal data?

_____ Ordinal data?

_____ Interval data?

_____ Ratio data?

Therefore, will you be using parametric or nonparametric statistics to analyze your data?

_____ Parametric

_____ Nonparametric

Do you wish to test for:

_____ Significant differences between groups?

_____ Correlation between variables?

_____ A comparison of more than two variables?

What test(s) does it seem likely that you could use to make these determinations?

_____ *t* test(s)

_____ Chi-square

_____ Wilcoxon signed rank test

_____ Wilcoxon rank sum test

_____ Mann-Whitney test

_____ Pearson product moment correlation

_____ Spearman rho

_____ Regression analysis

_____ ANOVA

_____ ANCOVA

_____ Kruskal-Wallis test

INFORMATION SHEET TO TAKE TO THE STATISTICIAN

To help the statistician understand what you wish to achieve in your study, take some basic information with you when you meet. The following information would give the statistician a clear idea of your project.

Hypotheses:

Subjects:

      How many?

      How selected?

      In how many groups?

      How assigned to groups?

Methods: Type of research design (e.g, pre-test/treatment/post-test; survey; comparison of experimental and control groups).

Specific data collection methods (e.g., self-designed questionnaire; IQ test; values inventory, goniometer readings).

Type of data that will be generated (nominal, ordinal, interval, ratio; more than one type). Give actual examples of data.

Your initial thoughts on data analysis:

      If using descriptive statistics:

      _____ Frequencies and percentages

      _____ Central tendency

      _____ Relative position

      If using inferential statistics:

      _____ Significance between groups

      _____ Correlation between groups

      _____ Comparison of more than one variable

Therefore, some thoughts on specific tests:

References

Case-Smith, J., Cooper, P., & Scala, V. (1989). Feeding efficiency of premature neonates. *American Journal of Occupational Therapy, 43*(4), 245–250.

Cohen, H. (1988). How to read a research paper. *American Journal of Occupational Therapy, 42*(9), 596–600.

Corb, D.F., Pinkston, D., Harden, R.S., O'Sullivan, P., & Fecteau, L. (1987). Changes in students' perceptions of the professional role. *Physical Therapy, 67*(2), 226–233.

Coren, A., Andreassi, M., Blood, H., & Kent, B. (1987). Factors relating to physical therapy students' decisions to work with elderly patients. *Physical Therapy, 67*(1), 60–65.

Deitz, J.C., Crowe, T.K., & Harris, S.R. (1987). Relationship between infant neuromotor assessment and preschool motor measures. *Physical Therapy, 67*(1), 14–17.

Gogia, P.P., Braatz, J.H., Rose, S.J., & Norton, B.J. (1987). Reliability and validity of goniometric measurements at the knee. *Physical Therapy, 67*(2), 192–195.

Graham, W.G., & Bradley, D.A. (1978). Efficacy of chest physiotherapy and intermittent positive pressure breathing in the resolution of pneumonia. *New England Journal of Medicine, 229,* 624–627.

Hamilton-Dodd, C., Kawamoto, T., Clark, F., Burke, J.P., & Fanchiang, S.P. (1989). The effects of a maternal preparation program on mother-infant pairs: A pilot study. *American Journal of Occupational Therapy, 43*(8), 513–521.

Hasselkus, B.R., & Safrit, M.J. (1976). Measurement in occupational therapy. *American Journal of Occupational Therapy, 30*(7), 429–436.

Liu, H., Currier, D.P., & Threlkeld, A.J. (1987). Circulatory response of digital arteries associated with electrical stimulation of calf muscle in healthy subjects. *Physical Therapy, 67*(3), 340–345.

Lohmann, K.N., Rayhel, H.E., Schneiderwind, W.P., & Danoff, J.V. (1987). Static measurement of tibia vara. *Physical Therapy, 67*(2), 196–199.

Magalhaes, L., Koomar, J., & Cermak, S. (1989). Bilateral motor coordination in 5- to 9-year-old children: A pilot study. *American Journal of Occupational Therapy, 43*(7), 437–443.

Mitchell, M.J., Daines, G.E., & Thomas, B.L. (1987). Effect of L-tryptophan and phenylalanine on burning pain threshold. *Physical Therapy, 67*(2), 203–205.

Moncur, C. (1987). Perceptions of physical therapy competencies in rheumatology. *Physical Therapy, 67*(3), 331–339.

Oyster, C.K., Hanten, W.P., & Llorens, L.S. (1987). *Introduction to research: A guide for the health science professional.* Philadelphia: J.B. Lippincott.

Partridge, C.J., & Barnitt, R.E. (1986). *Research guidelines: A handbook for therapists.* Rockville, MD: Aspen Publishers.

Schaefer, R.L., & Anderson, R.B. (1989). *The student edition of Minitab: Statistical software adapted for education.* Reading, MA: Addison-Wesley Publishing and Benjamin/Cummings Publishing.

Shinabarger, N.I. (1987). Limited joint mobility in adults with diabetes mellitus. *Physical Therapy, 67*(2), 215–218.

Taylor, K., Newton, R.A., Personius, W.J., & Bush, R.M. (1987). Effects of interferential current stimulation for treatment of subjects with recurrent jaw pain. *Physical Therapy, 67*(3), 346–350.

Additional Reading

Cliffs studyware for statistics. (1993). Lincoln, NE: 1993 Cliffs Notes.

Greenstein, L.R. (1980). Teaching research: An introduction to statistical concepts and research terminology. *American Journal of Occupational Therapy, 34*(5), 320–327.

Kerlinger, F.N. (1973). *Foundations of behavioral research.* New York: Holt, Rinehart & Winston.

Koosis, D. (1985). *Statistics: A self-teaching guide.* New York: John Wiley & Sons.

Lee, E.S., Forthofer, R.N., & Lorimer, R.J. (1989). *Analyzing complex survey data.* No. 71 in Quantitative Applications in the Social Sciences Series. Newbury Park, CA: Sage Publications.

Lodge, M. (1981). *Magnitude scaling: Quantitative measurement of opinions.* No. 25 in Quantitative Applications in the Social Sciences Series. Newbury Park, CA: Sage Publications.

Reynolds, H.T. (1984). *Analysis of nominal data.* No. 7 in Quantitative Applications in the Social Sciences Series. Newbury Park, CA: Sage Publications.

Rowntree, D. (1981). *Statistics without tears: A primer for non-mathematicians.* New York: Charles Scribner's Sons.

9

Qualitative Research Designs

The Purpose of Qualitative Research

Since the publication in 1967 of Glaser and Strauss's book, *The Discovery of Grounded Theory,* qualitative researchers have been debating whether the purpose of qualitative research should be to develop new theory, verify existing theory, or both. Glaser and Strauss believe that the role of qualitative investigators is to develop theory, and their grounded theory approach (described in Chapter 10) is designed toward that end. Other researchers believe that the purpose of qualitative research is to verify existing social theories through analytic induction, similar to the goals of quantitative methods that test hypothetical propositions. Many qualitative researchers, however, think both purposes are appropriate.

Let's explore the processes of grounded theory and analytic induction.

> The grounded theory approach is a method for discovering theories, concepts, hypotheses, and propositions directly from data, rather than from a priori assumptions, other research, or existing theoretical frameworks. (Taylor & Bogdan, 1984, p. 126)

When generating grounded theory, researchers do not seek to prove their theories but merely to demonstrate plausible support for them by seeing if they "fit" and "work." If a theory "fits" the generated categories (la-beled or coded groups of data), it will be readily applicable to the data; if it "works," the categories will be meaningful to the behavior under study.

Analytic induction, not to be confused with Patton's (1990) description of inductive analysis, explained in Chapter 10, is a procedure for verifying or modifying existing theories and propositions based on newly collected qualitative data. It is designed to identify universal propositions. The steps are (a) to develop a rough definition of a phenomenon to be explained; (b) to formulate a proposition or hypothesis to explain the phenomenon; and (c) to study one case to see if there is a fit between the case and the hypothesis. If the hypothesis does not explain the case, the researcher either (d) reformulates the hypothesis or redefines the phenomenon. Next, the researcher looks for negative cases within the study group to disprove the hypothesis and, if they are found, (e) reformulates the hypothesis or redefines the phenomenon until the hypothesis has been adequately tested. In this way, a universal proposition is formulated.

Preparing for a Qualitative Research Study

The preparatory work for a qualitative study is similar to that for a quantitative study.

You must identify the problem you wish to study and generate research questions concerning the problem. Review the literature to gain an understanding of the depth and parameters of your problem, as well as other people's views on the topic. (It should be noted that some qualitative researchers disagree with this, believing that it is better to read after data collection to minimize their preconceived ideas.) You will need to formulate background material and decide on a theoretical base within which to design the study. Finally, you will choose a research design encompassing data collection and analysis techniques. Even the format for the final write-up should be considered in the early stages of the project. The early chapters of this book, therefore, are just as relevant to qualitative research projects as to quantitative studies.

General Components of Qualitative Research

All qualitative researchers tend to use similar principles, techniques, and approaches. When using a qualitative approach, the investigator will interview relevant people, observe various interactions and events, examine written documents, make decisions about the resulting information, and write a narrative for professional colleagues. As stated earlier, before a naturalistic researcher begins to ask the first question in the field, a problem, a theory or model, a research design, specific data collection techniques, tools for analysis, and a specific writing style will have been formulated.

Although researchers begin with planned research designs, naturalistic work tends not to be orderly. The researcher must be ready to follow where the data and the informants lead, which means being open to serendipity, creativity, luck, and a lot of hard work. Unlike quantitative research, data collection and data analysis in qualitative research begin and continue simultaneously. Data collection typically yields an enormous amount of data, and a preformulated data analysis technique is needed to make sense of it all. Several techniques are described in Chapter 10.

The Problem

Qualitative research begins with a problem or issue of interest that guides the entire project. It will dictate the style of the research design, the data collection techniques, and even the presentation of the findings.

Theory

Similarly, no study, naturalistic or otherwise, can be conducted without an underlying theory or model. It may be a formal anthropological or psychosocial theory or a personal model about how things work, but theory is crucial in the definition of the problem and in deciding how to tackle it.

A typical model for naturalistic studies is based on phenomenology. Because qualitative researchers are interested in taking an emic approach, the phenomenological model allows them to adopt the view that all things are relevant only from the informants' perspective (Box 9–A). Phenomenologically driven studies are usually inductive; their results are generated from the study data, and few explicit assumptions are made ahead of time about study informants or events. Glaser and Strauss' (1967) grounded theory method of analysis is entirely based on such an approach.

Four other theories used to guide naturalistic studies include cognitive theory, which assumes that we can describe what people think by listening to what they say (using linguistically driven techniques); and cultural or personality theory, which encompasses psychoanalytic theory. Some qualitative researchers adopt materialist theories and view the world according to observable

---

Box 9–A

Carpenter (1994) pursued her study purely from her informants' point of view by conducting semistructured, in-depth interviews with people who had sustained spinal cord injuries. She wanted to uncover accounts of meaningful aspects of the informants' disability experience. Carpenter's analysis of their accounts revealed three categories of meaning for the informants: rediscovery of self, redefining disability, and establishing a new identity.

Box 9–B

In a study of a national intervention program for school dropouts, Fetterman used a structural functionalist approach to map out the structure and function of the schools and their relationship to various government institutions. He also used innovation theory to "pigeonhole observations about the innovative program, ranging from its introduction through the intricate maze to its acceptance, rejection, and/or modification."

(Fetterman, 1989, p. 17)

---

behavior patterns related to class consciousness, class conflict, social organization, and economic forces. Another theory is concerned with the structure and function of organizations (Box 9–B).

Theories need not be elaborate sets of constructs, assumptions, propositions, or generalizations. They can be personal theories about how the world, or some small part of it, works. Therapists engaging in qualitative research may choose similar theories to those chosen for quantitative studies, which are often psychologically, sociologically, or medically oriented. Therefore, the section in Chapter 6 entitled "Scope of the Study," which discusses conceptual frameworks, will be relevant reading for the theoretical portion of a qualitative study.

Research Questions

Although the qualitative researcher will have developed some research questions during the research design phase, many more questions will typically be generated during the initial survey phase of field work. Research questions are fluid in naturalistic research, unlike the fixed hypothesis mode of quantitative research. Some questions may be dropped as irrelevant; some may be modified as additional data are gathered; and new questions may be added as the study proceeds. In qualitative research, the final report may be written in the form of hypotheses with supporting material. In this case, researchers frequently request that others test their proposed hypotheses further, under different conditions, or they may do so themselves in later studies.

Participant Selection

Qualitative research can be characterized as an inquiry in which the investigator observes and questions participants in their own setting, to learn their perspective on things—a naturalistic inquiry. Therefore, researchers will use purposeful sampling to choose participants who can offer the fullest and most relevant information about the topic under study. In purposeful sampling, you must establish the criteria or conditions necessary to be included in the study, then purposefully, choose a case or cases that match these criteria. The participants who turn out to be the most reliable and informative become the key informants. Others may have useful information to add and will be seen as secondary informants.

There are several types of purposeful sampling, and they are chosen according to the researcher's needs for a particular study. Some of the most popular types are:

- **Typical:** A case is chosen because it is thought to be like the majority (i.e., typical). For example, a therapist might want to see how a typical person with hemiplegia proceeds through a particular rehabilitation program.

- **Extreme or deviant:** After the norm for a typical case is established, the researcher might want to explore extreme cases in order to make a comparison, for example, a person with hemiplegia who does not complete the rehabilitation program or a person who completes the program in an extremely short time.

- **Comprehensive:** A situation in which all the cases in a sample can be examined, for example, all the people with hemiplegia completing a rehabilitation program with a particular treatment regimen.

- **Unique-case selection:** Selection is based on unique or rare attributes, for example, a person with double lower-extremity amputations who becomes an athlete.

- **Reputational-case selection:** A case is chosen on the recommendation of experienced experts, based on its reputation, for example, a highly successful caregiver support program for persons caring for a spouse with Alzheimer's disease. The program is recommended by an expert in caregiver support programs because of its excellent reputation.

- **Comparable-case selection:** Selecting cases on the same relevant characteristics over a period of time in order to compare results for replication, for example, selecting one person with hemiplegia who successfully completes a rehabilitation program, for each month, over a 6-month program.

- **Critical case selection:** The one case that makes the point dramatically, for example, a program succeeding in a particularly difficult location, a successful program with especially low overhead costs, or a rehabilitation program showing an extremely high success rate with severely disabled clients.

- **Convenience sample:** The case or cases that can be studied most easily, cheaply, or quickly, for example, persons with hemiplegia participating in the rehabilitation program run by the researcher.

Data Collection

Often, the only data collection "instruments" used during qualitative research are the investigators themselves. Although some quantitative methods rely heavily on physical instruments such as paper and pencil tests or goniometry, qualitative researchers generally collect data via observation, interviewing, and tape recording in the field. Because they are the ones observing the events and asking the questions, they are considered the data collection "instrument." Some of the actual processes for collecting data include observation, interviewing, filming, photography, and record and artifact review.

Data Analysis

Qualitative data analysis is the process of systematically organizing the field notes, interview transcripts, and other accumulated materials until you understand them in such a way as to address the research questions and can present that understanding to others. Several techniques can be used to analyze qualitative data; the technique chosen depends on the goal of the study. For example, if you wish to generate new theories about devalued people living in group situa-

tions, the grounded theory approach and its attendant techniques would be suitable; if you wish to understand what participants perceive to be the curative factors in a helping group (Schultz, 1994), you could appropriately use a priori or a posteriori coding. Naturalistic researchers may even select specific techniques from different approaches for the same study, using their experience to judge what will best serve the goals of the project.

Report Writing

Naturalistic reports generally take the form of long narratives, sometimes interspersed with pictorial presentations. There are many formats to choose from. Again, what you plan to produce with the data will lead you to the appropriate choice. If you are writing a thesis or dissertation, certain format and style conventions will prevail. If you are producing an article or research report, there may be more flexibility. However, as Bogdan and Biklen (1982) point out, you will still need a beginning, a middle, and an end.

The beginning portion of the report should include a general background to help readers understand the focus of your paper. The introduction often concludes with a description of the design of the rest of the paper. The description should include a discussion of the research methods and techniques used, the time and length of the study, the number of settings and subjects, the nature of the data, where and how the documents were located, researcher-subject relations, checks on data, and other information that might help the reader evaluate the soundness of your study.

The middle of the paper makes up the bulk of the work. This is where you argue your thesis, present your theme, and illuminate your topic. Everything in the core of the paper should relate to the focus specified in the introduction. The material comes from the data analysis and can be organized around the patterns, themes, and relationships that arose from coding and categorizing the data. Use the most salient quotations you can find judiciously to illustrate the main points of the thesis.

The end section should be written as a conclusion. Often the focus is decisively restated, the arguments reviewed, and the implications elaborated. For more pointers, read Harry F. Wolcott's excellent booklet *Writing Up Qualitative Research* (1990).

Descriptions of Qualitative Designs

It is difficult to demarcate types of qualitative research designs in the same clear-cut manner in which quantitative designs can be specified and described. Qualitative designs do not have strict boundaries; the same researcher may use one set of procedures in one study and a different set in another, depending on the purpose of the study. However, some qualitative designs have distinguishing characteristics and can be discussed as discrete entities. For an ethnography or historical study, for example, researchers may begin with different mindsets but may use the same data collection and data analysis techniques.

The designs we will consider are:

1. The ethnographic research design, studying the culture within a program, institution, or other group setting

2. The case method research design, studying an individual person, program, or institution

3. The historical research design, studying a past event, a person or group of persons in the past, or the development of a phenomenon such as a profession or an organization

4. Unstructured interviewing as a research design in which open-ended interview questions are used to gain an in-depth individual perspective on an issue

The Ethnographic Research Design

Strict ethnography, as opposed to simply applying ethnographic techniques and approaches, is the art and science of describing a group and its culture. The description may be of the health care system in another country or of an inner-city clinic in urban America. Ethnography is characterized by the concept of culture as the organizational or conceptual principal for interpreting data.

The ethnographic research design originated in the field of anthropology and has occasionally been borrowed by health scientists to describe such settings as hospitals, special schools, sheltered workshops, and group homes. Schmid (1981) states that

> . . . among health professionals there has been a growing interest in a research paradigm that is responsive to questions of a holistic nature, questions that generate complex knowledge about how an individual, for example a client, perceives himself and the environment in which he selects his mode of life and adapts to it. (p. 105)

She goes on to say that the paradigm found in anthropology, sociology, and social psychology that emphasizes an understanding of the meaning of human behavior in social and cultural settings can satisfy such an interest.

Ethnographers, of course, have biases and preconceived ideas about the group under study, just as other researchers do. Controlled biases can focus and limit the study, whereas uncontrolled biases can undermine the quality of the research. The first task of ethnographers is to make specific biases explicit to themselves and, eventually, to the readers. Ethnographers try to achieve an open mind before going into the field because they are vitally interested in understanding and describing events and perspectives from the study participants' point of view, the emic perspective. This is crucial to ethnography.

Research Design

The research design for ethnography will list each step of the study in sequence, guiding the investigation toward an effective solution to the identified problem. Each step will build knowledge and understanding about the nature of the people or organization under study. Fieldwork is the main element of any ethnographic research design. The researcher will go out to the scene to meet the informants in their own setting, to observe events in context, and to view the environment itself. All fieldwork is exploratory, aimed at finding out as much as possible about the site and the participants and their lives.

Fieldwork

The early stages of fieldwork are concerned with learning the basics about the culture.

Let's say the culture under study is a particular rehabilitation department where an innovative, complex treatment regimen has been introduced. The ethnographer is trying to determine the long-term effect on the staff, the patients, and the overall functioning of the department, including its relationships with the rest of the facility and with other similar facilities. In the initial fieldwork, the researcher would focus on learning about the basic structure and function of the culture (the department, facility, and similar facilities), how many people are involved and something about their demographics, the relationships between all the people involved in the program, the language used by patients, staff, and administrators, and some historical data about the department and previous treatments.

The first few sessions at a fieldwork site can be awkward and painful for a researcher. Bogdan and Biklen (1982) have some suggestions to make this an easier time:

1. Do not take what happens in the field personally. What you are going through is a typical part of the fieldwork process.

2. Set up your first visit so someone is there to introduce you. One of the people who gave you permission [would be a good person to] do it. . . .

3. Don't try to accomplish too much the first few days. Ease yourself into the field. Have your first day be a short visit (an hour or less); use it as a time to get a general introduction and overview. . . .

4. Remain relatively passive. Show interest and enthusiasm for what you are learning, but do not ask a lot of specific questions, especially in areas that may be controversial. . . .

5. Be friendly. The first days in the field, subjects will ask about why you are here. Repeat what you told the people who gave you permission, . . . but try to use abbreviated explanations. Most suggestions on how to behave in the field parallel the norms governing nonoffensive behavior in general . . . (p. 127)

Once the ethnographer feels comfortable with baseline data on the culture, data collection and analysis begin in earnest. A distinct line is rarely drawn between baseline data gathering and "real" data collection; all of the information is usually used in the data analysis. How long baseline data collection takes varies enormously, depending on the investigator's previous knowledge of the culture, the complexity and size of the culture, and the complexity of the problem being studied.

Similarly, the amount of time spent in overall fieldwork varies significantly, depending on the same factors. The data for some very simple studies may be collected during 1 day per week for 6 weeks, for example, whereas a comprehensive study of a complex culture may take 2 or 3 years full-time in the field. The latter are typical anthropological studies of foreign cultures in distant lands, whereas the former are more typical of the recent ethnographic studies, sometimes called microethnographies, being undertaken by our colleagues in therapeutic environments. Most ethnographic studies probably fall on a timeline somewhere between the two.

Ethnographers in the field do their best to be unobtrusive. They try to blend in with the routines and appearance of the "natives," be they members of a foreign culture or therapists in a rehabilitation facility. Although ethnographers attempt to minimize their effect on the setting, a stranger who is asking questions and watching activities will always have some impact. Investigators need to keep a careful record of their own behavior to assess its possible influence on informants and the ensuing data collection.

The first problem in fieldwork is to gain access to the population under study. If it is impossible to get permission to enter the field, some researchers conduct covert or undercover research, collecting data without the subjects' knowledge. This approach was used very successfully in a classic study of a mental hospital in which the researchers had themselves admitted as patients. This approach is not recommended for new ethnographers, however; you will be more successful reaping the advantages of being free from the constraints of a regular participant, gaining access to a variety of informants, and perhaps most importantly, not having to deceive others and risk the embarrassment of being caught.

As to the degree to which you should participate in the activities of the setting, you may choose from a continuum ranging from one of a complete observer role to one of an active participant observer role. The complete observer does not participate in any activities and looks at the scene as though through a one-way mirror. At the other end of the continuum is the field-worker who is deeply involved in the site activities, with little discernible difference between the observer and the informants. Most field-workers settle on a role somewhere between these two extremes. If you are observing a classroom or a treatment setting, it is often inappropriate to take part in the teaching or treating. On the other hand, informants may ask you to act as an assistant; this may be perfectly suitable and not distract you from your task of observing. In the latter case, though, the students or patients will view you in a certain way—as other than solely an observer—and this must be accounted for in the data analysis.

Data-Gathering Techniques

There are several ways to gather information during ethnography fieldwork. The two most important techniques are observation, together with the resulting field notes, and interviews. Others include photography and examination of written documents and artifacts.

An important consideration is how to decide what and when to observe, whom to interview, how many and which documents and artifacts to examine, and what to photograph. In ethnography, this is the question of **participant selection** or **internal sampling.** If the focus of the study is narrow, you may be able to talk to all the subjects in the setting, review all the documents, or observe all the important events. If you are unable to do this, it is important to sample a range of people and materials, so that you have a diversity of perspectives on the setting.

Some informants are more willing to talk, have a greater experience in the setting, or are especially insightful about what goes on. These people become **key informants** and probably will be interviewed more frequently and for longer periods than other participants. Events and activities that are deemed important because they offer insight into the culture will be selected for observation; they are called **key events.** Some examples might be dinnertime in a group home for mentally retarded adults or the weekly staff meeting in a physical therapy department. Similarly, some documents, such as treatment plans or minutes of staff meetings, may be extremely fruitful and deserve more time

than other documents. Photographs can be used to take inventories of objects in a setting, and are also useful in reducing the need for descriptive field notes of those objects. They might include such things as a bulletin board, the writing on a blackboard, or the arrangement of furniture.

Often the timing of the ethnographer's visits affects the nature of the data collected. It is important during the initial field work period to find out as much as possible about routines, when certain events happen, and who attends. Selecting when to observe and interview, or **time sampling,** will depend on the purpose of the study. If the goal is to gain a perspective on the overall functioning of a rehabilitation department or of a group home, then the investigator should sample widely from different times of the day, week, and year. If, on the other hand, the goal is to gain insight into the morning meeting on a psychiatric ward, sampling should obviously occur during the morning meeting, perhaps 5 days per week over a several-week period.

Choices about sample selection are always made in the context of the study, with an eye toward achieving the goals for this particular study. The researcher often steps back during the study and asks, "If I go in now, if I talk to this person, what will I miss? What will I gain?" Ethnographers realize that choices are being made throughout the study that will affect the data collected and, therefore, the results of the analysis. They simply use their best judgment in making those choices.

Leaving the Field

During the first few days in the field, you will probably feel awkward. As time progresses, you will become more comfortable and can do your job more easily. Eventually you will have accomplished your goal and the time will come for you to leave the field. Leaving can be quite difficult. You will probably have become interested in the setting and fond of the participants. It is not uncommon to feel as if you are deserting people you have come to know well, especially if they are working under difficult conditions with a devalued population, or you may feel that you will miss something important to the study as soon as you stop visiting the site.

In any event, you must eventually tear yourself away. As therapists, we can use our knowledge of the termination process to leave gracefully, giving the informants due warning and easing out of the setting gradually. Frequently, ethnographers are asked to return to the setting at a later date to report on the findings, and occasionally it is necessary to return to collect some missing data. Otherwise, researchers need to recognize when they have reached the point of data saturation (when any new data collected simply repeats data they already have) and to say their good-byes.

The Case Method Research Design

In occupational and physical therapy, case studies are used when we want to learn from individual clients, understand certain issues and problems in our clinical practice, and form professional and managerial policy. A case is a unit of study. This unit is often an individual, but may also refer to a situation, a family, a hospital ward, a nursing home, or any group setting that can be considered a unit. Some recent case studies include:

"The experience of spinal cord injury: The individual's perspective—implications for rehabilitation practice" (Carpenter, 1994)

"A manual therapy approach to evaluation and treatment of a patient with a chronic lumbar nerve root irritation" (Koury & Scarpelli, 1994)

"Physical therapy management of peripheral vestibular dysfunction: Two clinical case reports" (Gill-Body, Krebs, Parker, & Riley, 1994)

"A task-oriented approach to the treatment of a client with hemiplegia" (Flinn, 1995)

"Approaches to improving student performance on fieldwork" (Kramer & Stern, 1995)

"Job site analysis facilitates work reintegration" (Canelon, 1995)

Novice researchers are often advised to choose a case study as their first research project because case studies tend to be more "doable" than some other types of qualitative research. Although case studies vary in complexity, it is possible to design one that is confined to one site or one person, that has a time limit, and that has a limit on the sources of data (such as the participant, records pertaining to the participant, and the participant's therapist). This keeps collected data to a manageable amount so that analysis can be accomplished in a relatively short

time. Also, the smaller volume of resulting material permits the study to be written up more easily than would a study generating a large volume of data.

Perhaps most commonly, the single-client case method design uses an ethnographic approach. The goal is to gain an understanding of that particular client's issues and circumstances, frequently concerning his or her disability and how it was overcome, so that our colleagues can better treat other clients in similar circumstances. **Data-gathering techniques** for a case method study are the ones that have been previously described, such as observation, interviewing, videotaping treatment sessions or the client's achievements, and reviewing related artifacts such as assistive technology. Documentary evidence is likely to play an important part in a case study; it may consist of patients' charts, minutes of meetings, reports of case presentations, patients' assessments and progress reports, or even institution newsletters and administrative memoranda.

Bogdan and Biklen (1982) describe the design of a case study as best represented by a funnel, the beginning of the study being the wide end, represented by researchers scouting around for possible sites or people they might wish to study and finding a few possibilities. They make a wide search to increase their chances of finding just the right case. Once they have found several possible sites, they collect some initial data, perhaps documents or an initial interview and observation. They then study the data, focusing in on the more promising aspects of the site. They make decisions about the direction of the study, whom they might eventually interview, which documents to access, and which events to observe. They may discard some initial ideas and formulate new ones as they go along, modifying the design and choosing procedures that will enable them to learn more about the topic. Eventually, they decide which individual or event will be studied; now they have developed a focus. The data collection narrows at this point to the particular topic under study—putting the researcher at the narrow end of the funnel.

When conducting an ethnographic case study, the investigator must follow the same overall strategies described in the section on qualitative research designs in Chapter 4. These include studying the case in its naturalistic setting; being concerned with meaning from the participants' point of view; viewing the case from a longitudinal perspective; using multi–data-gathering techniques; reviewing the data, both alone and with the participant(s) to explicate the ways by which these particular people understand, account for, take action, and manage their day-to-day lives; decontextualizing the data according to the goals of the study; and finally, analyzing and recontextualizing the data ready for presentation to colleagues.

Data are analyzed using the usual qualitative research analysis techniques. However, in a strictly ethnographic approach, analysis is more than an intensive, holistic description of a person's circumstances. Rather, concern will be shown for the client's cultural context. Wolcott (1980) has made a distinction between simply using ethnographic techniques to study a case and performing an ethnography:

> Specific ethnographic techniques are freely available to any researcher who wants to approach the problem or setting descriptively. It is the essential anthropological concern for cultural context that . . . makes genuine ethnography distinct from other "on-site-observer" approaches. (p. 59)

See Box 9–C for an example of an ethnographic case study.

Sometimes the major data-gathering technique in case studies is participant observation. If the focus of the study is an organization, the researcher must decide which aspect of the organization to study. For ex-

ample, if the organization under study is a rehabilitation hospital, the researcher may decide on a particular place within the hospital (such as the ward for people with quadriplegia); a specific group of people within the organization (such as the people with quadriplegia on that ward); or a specific activity or event within the organization (such as the daily routine of the people with quadriplegia on that ward).

The Historical Research Design

The goal of the historical research design, or historiography, is the same as those for many other qualitative research designs (i.e., to present a holistic description and analysis of a specific phenomenon whether it be event, person, or organization). Current behaviors or attitudes can often be better understood if the past is reviewed and examined in the light of current events. Thus, historical research is undertaken to test hypotheses or to answer questions about past events that may shed light on present behaviors or practices (Box 9–D).

Schwartz and Colman (1988) presented the debate about whether individuals other than historians can perform historical research in their own professions. They held that therapists can learn historiography and are thus in a good position to examine the development of their own professions. A number of excellent historical studies have been recorded in occupational and physical therapy literature. Loomis (1983) and Litterst (1988) have described the historical development of two schools of occupational

---

Box 9–C

In *Socialization to the culture of a rehabilitation hospital: An ethnographic study,* a group of occupational therapists examined the rehabilitation process from the insider's perspective, that of an individual patient with spinal cord injury. Daily interviews with Russell revealed that, in addition to learning how to function in the local world of the rehabilitation hospital, he also learned a new identity as a person with a long-term disability. "A central theme was the patient's ongoing attempt to figure out how his future was related to his life before the injury and how he could use previous competencies in adapting to disability."

(Spencer, Young, Rintala, & Bates, 1995, p. 53)

Box 9–D

In her APTA Presidential Address in Cincinnati in 1994, Moffat asked, *"Will the legacy of our past provide us with a legacy for the future?"* She presented a short history of the evolution of physical therapy, then used that information to determine if learning from that history would "eventually thwart our dreams and aspirations of professionalization" or if physical therapists could "chart a course to . . . soar to the heights that [their] profession should attain."

(Moffat, 1994, p. 1063)

therapy. Oral histories exploring the occupational and leisure history of women leaders have been used to identify the qualities that contribute to women's emergence as leaders (AOTA, 1977–1980). Colman (1986) has written a history of the formation of educational values in occupational therapy, and Gutman (1995) has described the influence of the U.S. military and occupational therapy reconstruction aides in World War I on the development of occupational therapy. One therapist has proposed that the origins of graded activity in occupational therapy lay in tuberculosis sanatoria of the late 1800s (Creighton, 1993). Another researcher posited that 19th-century practices of moral treatment and phrenology contributed to a loss of caring attitudes and actions in the treatment of mental illness (Peloquin, 1993). In physical therapy, Moffat (1994) has proposed the idea that therapists look to the evolution of their profession to decide whether they can move on to achieve their professional dreams or whether their past will thwart those dreams.

Historical research uses prescribed techniques for the collection, organization, and analysis of historical data. These include critical investigation of past events, careful weighing of evidence regarding the validity of sources, and interpretation and documentation of the investigation (Kerlinger, 1979). The historical researcher asks open-ended questions of individuals (or examines documents or artifacts) about a past event; uses thorough prior knowledge of the event to interpret the answers; and recontextualizes and documents the event in an interwoven narrative, thus providing the reader with a new explanation from which current events can be understood.

Thus, a historical study involves much more than making a chronology of an event. To understand an event and apply one's knowledge to present practice means knowing the context of the event, the assumptions behind it, and perhaps the event's impact on an institution or participants, both then and now (Box 9–E). A good historiography, like any good research design, relies on asking well-formulated questions, identifying reliable sources of information, verifying evidence, and accurately interpreting data.

At the basis of the historical study lies a clearly formulated, precisely worded **research question** clarifying what informa-

---

Box 9–E

Levine makes a graphic case for the importance of viewing the early development of occupational therapy within its social context. Both the Arts-and-Crafts Movement and the medical profession had a huge impact on the treatment modalities used in the profession:

> Thus occupational therapy survived the 1930s but was moored to the values of a forgotten social movement. Meanwhile, the medical profession had shifted from a holistic to a reductionistic focus. During World War II, the occupational therapy profession struggled with the same unresolved tension between craft proponents and therapists, but the context had changed. Younger physicians no longer understood or valued the arts-and-crafts philosophy. Since occupational therapy did not seem scientific or theory based, they tended not to take it seriously. . . . Few acknowledged that the context for health services had changed.

(Levine, 1987, p. 252)

---

tion the researcher is seeking. Historical research questions tend to have several components, dividing the topic under study into its various parts. As with other research designs, care should be taken not to have more questions than can comfortably be answered in one study and not to ask questions outside the scope of the particular study (Box 9–F).

Box 9–F

Levine's paper, *The Influence of the Arts-and-Crafts Movement on the Professional Status of Occupational Therapy,* asked the research question: "Why do occupational therapists use arts and crafts as therapeutic modalities?" Levine answers this question at various chronological checkpoints during the first 50 years of the 20th century. In order to arrive at the answer to the original question, she poses related questions: From where did arts and crafts arise? What is the Arts-and-Crafts Movement? What ideas in the movement were parallel to ideas expressed by occupational therapists?

(Levine, 1987)

The data for a historiography come from primary sources and secondary sources. A **primary source** is an original account of an event, such as an eyewitness account, minutes of a meeting, a photograph, or a treatment plan and progress notes written by a client's therapist (Box 9–G). A **secondary source** is a source of information at least one step removed from the original source, for instance, a newspaper account (if the reporter did not actually observe the event), a book by another historian, a clinical consult by a consultant who has not seen the client (see Box 9–G). A basic rule of historiography is that data sources should be predominantly primary sources, though an occasional secondary source may be used for back-up. Facts get biased and altered in the telling from one person to the next; the greater the distance from the original source, the more distorted the story. The historian lacks the accuracy and perspective of the eyewitness; even the veracity of the primary source should be checked, as far as that is possible.

At the core of historical research is **hermeneutics,** the study of historical texts, from the Greek *hermeneutikos,* meaning the clarification of what is unclear. Often, written documents are the only source of data available for historical research. If this is the case, it is particularly important that the investigator conduct an initial search to be sure there are sufficient primary sources to support a worthwhile study.

There are various ways of obtaining historical documents. Reviewing a town's newspapers or an institution's newsletters are easy ways to get started. However, you will probably get access to even more material by letting it be known, perhaps in your association newsletter, that you are interested in old letters, scrapbooks, minutes of meetings, and so on. Once you have found the first source, that person will lead you to others and you will soon find yourself with a network of informants. Libraries, archival collections, museums, government offices, and private papers are all good sources of primary data (Schwartz & Colman, 1988). Those interested in the history of occupational therapy would do well to consult the archives of the American Occupational Therapy Association, housed in the Moody Library of the University of Texas Medical Branch in Galveston (Truman G. Blocker, Jr., History of Medicine Collection).

One of the first tasks of the historian is to determine which data in the primary sources are actually facts and which are opinion or distortion. Facts are seldom stated in their pure form; they are usually mingled with the opinions of the source. The historical researcher must also assess the veracity of the data, while selecting only data that are relevant to the research question.

Interpreting data is an exceedingly difficult process, but doing it well is critical to the success of the study. The researcher needs a sound understanding of the data, based on well-formulated inferences and logic, in order to formulate a good analysis. Because historical researchers cannot go to first-hand informants for verification of their analyses, as other qualitative researchers can, the burden is on them to check their work for integrity and logic.

When documents are the only source of data, the researcher cannot confirm that one event in the past caused another to occur. In this case, the investigator must make assumptions or draw inferences that assign **causality.** The more information uncovered about an event, the more likely the possible cause of the event will become known. Investigators must be careful to restrict interpretations about causes to the evidence gathered. Of course, if the investigator is fortunate enough to have access to persons who

---

Box 9–G

In a paper on the historical basis for the use of graded activity by occupational therapists, Creighton (1993) proposed that graded activity originated in German tuberculosis sanatoria in the late 1800s. As a source of information, the author used a book written in 1887 by the physician who established the first such sanatorium. In this *primary source,* Brehmer gives a first-hand account of the reasons why he felt the hospital should be situated where it was, and describes the actual treatment used to strengthen the cardio-respiratory system (walking on hilly land with varying grades or degrees of slope). In the same study, Creighton also used an article written in 1985 by a nurse, another historian, who describes the history of tuberculosis. This would be described as a *secondary source.*

were involved in the event being studied, then triangulation can be used—checking one source of data against another for accuracy. Causality is a controversial subject among historians; studies obviously cannot be conducted under the controlled conditions of experimental research, and all variables are *ex post facto*. Most historical researchers confine themselves to describing conditions surrounding events and exploring associations that suggest emerging patterns and themes (Schwartz & Colman, 1988) (Box 9–H).

Two further tasks of historians are generalization and argumentation. What distinguishes a historian from a collector of historical facts is **generalization**—the ability to discern commonalities or patterns in the data and to infer a general principle from them. This is achieved through a similar process to that used by Glaser and Strauss (1967) in their description of formulating grounded theory. Like the grounded theoretician's approach, the historian must make logical generalizations that are based on sufficient data and do not go beyond the scope and nature of the data.

Historical researchers will make inferences from the data that will form the basis of an argument. **Argumentation** is their way of proceeding from an initial premise to an end argument (using inferences along the way) in an orderly and rational manner. The argument represents the researcher's understanding of the data. It is expected that the historian will approach the data with an open mind and let the facts shape the argument. The argumentation forms the major portion of the written report resulting from a historiography. Schwartz and Colman (1988) feel that a final report should include an introduction, a statement of the problem,

an identification of the assumptions and limitations of the research, a literature review, and a discussion of the findings (the argumentation). The report should take the form of a narrative and should describe and analyze the answers to the research question.

Recently, the volume of historical research in health care professions, particularly in physical and occupational therapy, has increased. These professions' rich heritage offer many opportunities for historical explorations. The more we probe our background, our roots, the more we will understand and be able to put into context our present practice.

Unstructured Interviewing as a Research Design

Although some may not regard unstructured interviewing alone as a full qualitative research design, it is presented here because it can be much more "doable" than longitudinal field studies. Unstructured, open-ended interviewing is often chosen as a sole data collection technique by students or therapists who have limited time and resources. These investigators can obtain a great deal of useful information, perform an in-depth data analysis, and produce a most useful account of an individual's or a group of people's perspective on an important issue in their lives (Box 9–I).

The design used in this method is a free-flowing, unstructured (or sometimes semi-structured) interview. Interviewers have a clearly defined set of topics in mind (and perhaps even some questions that are always

---

Box 9–H

In her article describing the visions that educational progressives and founders of occupational therapy expressed for their respective professions, Schwartz states that "a possible influence of the progressive education movement on the development of occupational therapy is suggested."

(Schwartz, 1992, p. 12)

Box 9–I

For her master's degree thesis, Courtney (1993) interviewed therapists concerning their personal feelings and ideas from recent "endings" (or terminations) they had experienced with clients, both those they considered successful and those that were unsuccessful. Courtney's goal was to analyze the data from several therapists and to recontextualize it in a way that would be useful for other therapists. She hoped that therapists could gain a perspective on termination from a therapeutic relationship, which might help them during their own "endings" with clients.

asked in the same words) that will allow them to achieve the overall goals of the study. The interviewee is told the topic and the goal of the interview and is then allowed to direct the flow of the conversation. Questions need not be asked in the same order from interview to interview, as in a structured interview, but may be interjected as they best fit that interviewee's line of thought. The interviewee is encouraged to engage in a far-ranging discussion of the topic at hand, to give copious examples, and to offer personal feelings and opinions about the topic. This type of interviewing takes a great deal of skill and practice; it is easy to get sidetracked and miss addressing the goals of the interview. The interview should be tape-recorded and transcribed before data analysis begins.

Once the material is in written form, it can be coded and analyzed, using one of the usual qualitative data analysis techniques. The outcome can be very useful in giving therapists the phenomenological perspective of their patients or colleagues. This design is particularly effective for probing sensitive issues that are difficult to talk about and that are usually written about only in an objective, impersonal manner (Box 9–J).

Some people try to use this type of qualitative research design by asking open-ended questions on a written survey. The written method tends not to be as successful as the face-to-face interview, because the personal rapport is lost that allows the interviewer to individualize the pace and style of the interview and because most respondents are unwilling to write several pages of narrative describing personal events and feelings. They have to be extremely invested in the topic to be persuaded to respond in a useful manner.

Box 9–J

Heeremans (1993) interviewed therapists who had recently experienced the death of one of their patients. She wished to understand this experience from a phenomenological viewpoint. Her findings are reported in her thesis entitled *Confronting Death and Dying: An Analysis of the Therapeutic Relationship between Occupational Therapists and Dying Patients.*

Validity and Reliability of Qualitative Research

Some critics feel that qualitative research, by its very nature, cannot be reliable, that is, replicated to produce similar findings from study to study. Others find that validity, determining the extent to which conclusions effectively represent subjects' reality, is difficult to assess in a qualitative study. Some ethnographers ignore such criticisms while others recognize that the credibility of their findings may be called into question and develop ways to address the criticism.

Validity

Many ethnographers feel that, contrary to the criticisms raised, validity is the strength of an ethnographic study. This is especially true when one compares ethnography with experimental studies, surveys, and other quantitative designs. Typically, the quantitative researcher gathers data in an "unreal" setting, asking subjects to perform in a contrived manner for a relatively short period of time. The ethnographer, on the other hand, goes to the subjects, observes them in their natural environment over a long period of time, and asks for their thoughts and opinions. Frequently, questions and observations are guided by what the informants feel is important and relevant, and data analysis is shared with informants to see if it "feels right." Thus, the qualitative study is more likely to achieve validity than the quantitative study.

Steps can be taken to further the likelihood of a valid study. Qualitative researchers must decide, first, how much confidence to place in their own analysis, and second, how to present their analysis so that readers can validate and verify the findings for themselves. It is important to remember that, through a data analysis, one presents only a perspective on the data, and not the "Truth." There are several ways to go about the task of validating and verifying that perspective. The seven ideas presented here are based on the work of Patton (1990) and Guba (1978).

Rival Explanations. Once the analyst has identified and described patterns, themes, and linkages from the data, it is important to look for rival or competing themes and linkages. This can occur inductively, by looking for other ways to organize the data that might lead to different findings; or it might be done logically, by thinking of other logical possibilities and seeing if these possibilities can be supported by the data. Failure to find strong supporting evidence for alternative themes or linkages helps increase the analyst's confidence in the original findings. There is unlikely to be clear-cut support for the alternative themes; but rather, one must consider the weight of the evidence and look for the best fit between the data and analysis. Alternative themes that were considered should be noted in the write-up, as this will lend credibility to the final findings.

Negative Cases. Once patterns have been described, our understanding of those patterns can be increased by studying the instances and cases that do not fit within the patterns—the negative cases. For example, in a large rehabilitation program in which the majority of the participants complete the program and return to work, the most important analysis may be an examination of the program dropouts. Readers may then decide for themselves the plausibility of the reasons why dropouts do not fit the usual patterns.

Triangulation. Triangulation is the process of using different data-collection techniques to study the same program. Two kinds of triangulation contribute to validating and verifying qualitative data analysis: (a) checking for consistency of findings generated by different data collection methods, such as a survey and an interview; and (b) checking for consistency of different data sources using the same data collection method (e.g., obtaining verbal accounts of the same event from two people). Triangulation tests the quality of information gained and may be useful in putting findings in perspective. Box 9–K gives an example of a study using triangulation, field notes, and peer debriefing to enhance credibility.

Design Checks. The validity of findings in qualitative research may be compromised if there were flaws in the data-collection techniques. Nontypical events or occasions may have been observed when the intent was to observe typical activities; problems may have been caused by the people who were selected for observations or interviews; and problems may have been caused by the time

---

Box 9–K

Quigley conducted a qualitative study "to explore and describe the role experience of five women whose lives were disrupted by a traumatic spinal cord injury and who later returned to their communities after completing intensive rehabilitation programs" (p. 780). In a section labeled "Credibility," she said, "Three methods, triangulation of data, field notes, and peer debriefing, were used to enhance the trustworthiness of the data collection and analysis" (p. 782).

(Quigley, 1994, pp. 780 and 782)

---

periods used for observations. It is important to acknowledge any such flaws in the write-up and to limit conclusions to those situations, people, and time periods sampled in the study.

Researcher Effects. The researcher can affect the findings of a qualitative research study in four ways:

1. **Program participants behaving differently because of the presence of the researcher.** There may be a "halo effect," so that staff perform in an exemplary manner, or there may be so much tension and anxiety that staff perform below par.

2. **Investigators becoming personally involved with participants during the study.** Should this happen, researchers may lose their sensitivity to the full range of events occurring in the setting.

3. **Researcher predispositions or biases.** Researcher biases definitely influence data analysis and interpretations, particularly because the outcome of a qualitative study is the presentation of a perspective. Qualitative research *is* subjective by definition; subjectivity, however, is not negative, as many critics would have us believe. It contributes to the quality of the observations made by the investigator and allows the investigator to employ the phenomenological approach desirable in most qualitative research. Guba (1978) suggests that the problem is one of vocabulary, and that using the word

"neutral" eliminates the biases instilled by using the words "subjective" and "objective." The answer is for investigators to be aware of their predispositions and biases, to note them in their field notes, and to inform readers about them.

4. **Researcher competence.** Competence can be demonstrated by using the verification and validation methods listed earlier to establish the quality of the data analysis; by showing fairness and responsibility in the write-up; and by not going overboard in the interpretations of the findings.

Participant Reactions to the Analysis. Investigators can learn a great deal about the accuracy, fairness, and validity of their data analysis by having the people in the study react to what has been described. The analysis is credible only if it "feels right" to the participants. The participants' reactions can be included in the final write-up as an indication of the validity of the study findings.

Intellectual Rigor. The thread that runs through the previous suggestions for verifying and validating qualitative data analysis is the investigator's intellectual rigor. The effective investigator returns to the data over and over again to confirm categories, patterns, themes, and linkages, and to re-examine any interpretations to see if they really reflect the nature of the program or activity being studied. To quote Patton (1990)

> Creativity, intellectual rigor, perseverance, insight—these are the intangibles that go beyond the routine application of scientific procedures. (p. 339)

Reliability

Study reliability is more difficult to achieve than is validity. Generally speaking, reliability is concerned with replicability; it requires that a researcher using the same data collection and analysis techniques can obtain the same results as those of a previous study. External reliability addresses the issue of whether two different researchers would arrive at the same final themes and theories in the same study setting; internal reliability refers to the extent to which other researchers, given a set of previously generated codes

and constructs, would match them with interview data and field notes in the same way the original researcher did.

Because ethnographic research is concerned with naturalistic behavior (which is seldom repeated in the same way) in a unique setting and occasion (which will never be repeated because it *is* unique), replication for the purpose of establishing reliability is a tall order. Problems with uniqueness and idiosyncrasy could lead to the claim that ethnographic studies can never be replicated; however, there are ways in which researchers can acknowledge and address issues of reliability. The following suggestions are based on the work of LeCompte and Goetz (1982).

External Reliability

Qualitative researchers can enhance external reliability by addressing five major problems: researcher status position, informant choices, social situations and conditions, analytic constructs and premises, and data collection and analysis techniques.

RESEARCHER STATUS POSITION

No ethnographer can completely replicate the findings of another because different ethnographers hold different social roles within the studied group and begin with different knowledge bases about the studied group. This problem can be eased by clearly identifying in the study report the researcher's role and status within the group investigated and the degree to which the researcher becomes involved with informants (i.e., where they fall on the spectrum between nonparticipant observers, with no personal relationships with informants, and participant observers who develop friendships that provide access to special knowledge).

INFORMANT CHOICES

This concerns the problem of identifying the informants who provide the data. Different informants represent different interest groups within the study group. When researchers associate with one particular group, they may forfeit information from people in other groups, who may not be comfortable associating with the first group. Additionally, people who gravitate toward researchers or are sought out by researchers to be informants may be atypical of the rest of the group. For instance, they may be chosen because they are introspective and insightful about their own lives, a characteristic that might not be found in other members of the group. Threats to reliability posed by informant bias can be handled by careful description in the research report of those who provided the data. Such descriptions should include personal characteristics relevant to the research, as well as those that make the informants similar to or different from the rest of the group.

SOCIAL SITUATIONS AND CONDITIONS

The social context in which data are gathered may influence external reliability. Informants may not feel free to reveal certain information in some social environments. For instance, a patient interviewed may give one set of information while receiving treatment in the hospital but other information when interviewed at home after discharge. The informants may also be influenced by whether they are interviewed alone or in a group. Thus, it is important to state the social setting in which the data are gathered.

ANALYTIC CONSTRUCTS AND PREMISES

Even if a subsequent researcher were to reconstruct the relationships and duplicate the informants and social contexts of a previous study, replication would be impossible if the constructs, definitions, or units of analysis of the former study were unclear. Analysts writing up their research must make clear the underlying assumptions, theoretical base, choice of terminology, and data collection and analysis techniques if a later researcher is to be able to replicate the study successfully.

TECHNIQUES FOR DATA COLLECTION
AND ANALYSIS

Replicability is impossible without precise identification and thorough description of the strategies and techniques used to collect data. It is tempting to use shorthand descriptors because of the brevity that journals often require in manuscripts. Unfortunately, shorthand descriptors are not yet universally accepted by qualitative researchers; consequently, their use can lead to serious misunderstandings. More importantly, the strategies used for analyzing data are often poorly defined or not described at all. This is probably because the analytic process used

with ethnographic data is often vague, personal, intuitive, and idiosyncratic to the analyst. There have been some efforts to codify techniques for data analysis (Glaser & Strauss, 1967; Goetz & LeCompte, 1984; Lofland, 1971), but these are not yet universally accepted or used. Unless researchers specify their data collection techniques and their analytic strategies, reliability will be impossible to achieve.

Internal Reliability

Internal reliability in an ethnographic study concerns whether, within a single study, multiple observers agree. The issue is particularly important when several researchers plan to investigate the same problem at different sites. The important issue within internal reliability is that of interrater or interobserver reliability—the extent to which meanings held by multiple observers are sufficiently congruent that they describe phenomena in the same way and arrive at the same conclusions about them. Agreement is sought on the description or composition of events rather than on the frequency of events. The following five strategies are commonly used to reduce threats to internal reliability: low-inference descriptors, multiple researchers, participant researchers, peer examination, and mechanically recorded data.

LOW-INFERENCE DESCRIPTIONS

Most guides to the construction of ethnographic field notes distinguish between two types of field notes. Low-inference descriptions, phrased in terms as concrete and precise as possible, are mandated for all ethnographic research. These include verbatim accounts of what people say as well as narratives of behavior and activity. The second category of notes may be any combination of high-inference interpretive comments and varies according to the analytic scheme chosen for the study.

Low-inference notes provide researchers with their basic observational data. Interpretive comments are then added, deleted, or modified, but the basic record of who did what under which circumstances remains unchanged. This basic material is analyzed and presented in excerpts to substantiate inferred categories of analysis. Studies rich in primary data, which provide the reader with multiple examples from the field notes, are generally considered most credible.

MULTIPLE RESEARCHERS

The most effective guard against threats to internal reliability in qualitative research is the presence of multiple researchers. Ideally, investigations are conducted by a team whose members discuss the meaning of what has been observed until agreement is reached. The discussion period is regarded as training in interobserver agreement. However, most ethnographic studies are conducted by pairs of researchers rather than larger teams or single researchers, because of funding constraints and because ethnographic research is often considered too time-consuming and labor-intensive for lone researchers. Two researchers who achieve interobserver reliability are considered preferable to a sole researcher for achieving internal reliability.

PARTICIPANT RESEARCHERS

Some researchers enlist the help of informants to confirm that what the observer has seen and recorded is being viewed identically and consistently by both subjects and researcher. Sometimes participants serve as arbiters, reviewing the field notes to correct researcher misperceptions and misinterpretations. Other researchers work in partnership with participants, keeping two sets of accounts of observations and comments. Quite commonly, ethnographers ask for re-actions and feedback to their ongoing analyses from informants.

PEER EXAMINATION

Researchers may corroborate their findings with other researchers in three ways. First, they may integrate descriptions and conclusions from other researchers in their final report. Second, findings from studies conducted concurrently at multiple sites may be analyzed separately, then compared. Similar findings across sites would support the reliability of observations. Last, the publication of study findings indicates that the material is offered for peer review and a debate of the findings is encouraged.

MECHANICALLY RECORDED DATA

Qualitative researchers use a variety of mechanical devices to record data, such as audiotape and videotape recorders and cameras. The idea is to record and preserve as much of the data as possible, so that the veracity of the conclusions can be checked by other researchers.

In this chapter, the main principles in qualitative research have been discussed and some of the qualitative designs have been described. If you are planning to engage in qualitative research, now is the time to decide which design and data collection and analysis techniques will best serve your purpose. Completing the following worksheets will help you make this decision.

WORKSHEETS

Think about your project.

Do you wish to find out about your informants' viewpoint on an issue meaningful to them? In other words, are you interested in a phenomenological approach to a topic?

If the answer to these questions is yes, a qualitative design based on ethnographic principles is probably appropriate for your study.

You will need to have formulated:

A problem statement

A theoretical base for your study

A research question

Review these portions of your study now. If necessary, rewrite them so they are clearly stated.

Choose one of the following qualitative designs:

1. **Ethnography**—you wish to study a group and its culture; you are able to go into the field; you will gather data via observation, interviews, and examination of documents; you will be able to select key informants and key events.

2. **The Case Method Research Design**—you wish to study one unit (person, situation, group setting); you have access to that unit; you will gather data via observation, interviews, videotaping, and examining documents; you will analyze the unit in its environmental context.

3. **The Historical Research Design**—you wish to study a past event or person in order to better understand the present; you have access to adequate primary sources; you are able to adhere to the principles of causality, generalization, and argumentation.

4. **Unstructured Interviews**—you have limited experience with qualitative research and limited time to conduct your study; you wish to address sensitive issues; you have access to key informants.

After you have selected the design for your study, answer the following questions:

1. Do you have access to an appropriate site for the study?

   Name the site:

   How will you gain permission to enter the site?

2. Are there appropriate participants for your study?

   List the criteria for participants who would be appropriate for your study:

   How many people will you be able to choose from?

   How will you gain their permission to be participants?

3. Data collection:

Can you enter the field often enough to gather data?

How often do you calculate that will be?

What data collection techniques will you use?

a. Observation: Which people, interactions, or behaviors do you wish to observe?

b. Interviews: Which participants do you wish to interview?

Outline the topics you wish to gain information or opinions about:

c. Audiotape recording (do you have equipment?)

Videotape recording (do you have equipment?)

Do you need separate permission for this activity?

If yes, how will you get that permission?

Which events, interactions, or behaviors do you wish to record?

d. Artifact review: what kinds of documents or objects will you need to examine?

Where will you locate such artifacts?

e. Client record review: Do you need separate permission for this activity?

If yes, how will you get that permission?

Which client records will you need to review? What are the selection criteria?
How many records will you need?

References

AOTA, (1977–1980). *The visual history series.* Bethesda, MD: Archives of the American Occupational Therapy Association.

Bogdan, R.C. & Biklen, S.K. (1982). *Qualitative research for education: An introduction to theory and methods.* Boston: Allyn and Bacon.

Canelon, M.F. (1995). Job site analysis facilitates work reintegration. *American Journal of Occupational Therapy, 49*(5), 461–467.

Carpenter, C. (1994). The experience of spinal cord injury: The individual's perspective—implications for rehabilitation practice. *Physical Therapy, 74*(7), 614–629.

Colman, W. (1986). History of the formation of educational values in occupational therapy. In *Occupational therapy education: Target 2000 Proceedings* (pp. 12–18). Rockville, MD: American Occupational Therapy Association.

Courtney, E. (1993). *Termination of the therapeutic relationship: Themes and techniques in occupational therapy.* Unpublished master's thesis, Tufts University, Medford, MA.

Creighton, C. (1993). Looking back. Graded activity: Legacy of the sanatorium. *American Journal of Occupational Therapy, 47*(8), 745–748.

Fetterman, D.M. (1989). *Ethnography step by step.* Newbury Park, CA: Sage Publications.

Flinn, N. (1995). A task-oriented approach to the treatment of a client with hemiplegia. *American Journal of Occupational Therapy, 49*(6), 560–569.

Gill-Body, K., Krebs, D., Parker, S., & Riley, P. (1994). Physical therapy management of peripheral vestibular dysfunction: Two clinical case reports. *Physical Therapy, 74*(2), 129–142.

Glaser, B.G. & Strauss, A.L. (1967). *The discovery of grounded theory: Strategies for qualitative research.* New York: Aldine De Gruyter.

Goetz, J.P. & LeCompte, M.D. (1984). *Ethnography and qualitative design in educational research.* San Diego, CA: Academic Press.

Guba, E.G. (1978). *Toward a methodology of naturalistic enquiry in educational evaluation.* CSE Monograph Series in Evaluation No. 8. Los Angeles: Center for the Study of Evaluation, University of California, Los Angeles.

Gutman, S.A. (1995). Looking back. Influence of the U.S. military and occupational therapy reconstruction aides in World War I on the development of occupational therapy. *American Journal of Occupational Therapy, 49*(3), 256–262.

Heeremans, S. (1993). *Confronting death and dying: An analysis of the therapeutic relationship between occupational therapists and dying patients.* Unpublished master's thesis, Tufts University, Medford, MA.

Kerlinger, F.N. (1979). *Behavioral research.* New York: Holt, Rinehart & Winston.

Koury, M. & Scarpelli, E. (1994). A manual therapy approach to evaluation and treatment of a patient with a chronic lumbar nerve root irritation. *Physical Therapy. 74*(6), 548–560.

Kramer, P. & Stern, K. (1995). Approaches to improving student performance on fieldwork. *American Journal of Occupational Therapy, 49*(2), 156–159.

LeCompte, M.D. & Goetz, J.P. (1982). Problems of reliability and validity in ethnographic research. *Review of Educational Research, 52*(1), 31–60.

Levine, R.E. (1987). The influence of the Arts-and-Crafts Movement on the professional status of occupational therapy. *American Journal of Occupational Therapy, 41*(4), 248–254.

Litterst, T.A. (1988). *Boston School of Occupational Therapy.* Unpublished paper.

Lofland, J. (1971). *Analyzing social settings: A guide to qualitative objectivity and analysis.* Belmont, CA: Wadsworth.

Loomis, B. (1983, April). *Professional occupational therapy education in Chicago, 1908–1920.* Paper presented at the Written History Committee Symposium, American Occupational Therapy Association Annual Conference, Portland, OR.

Moffat, M. (1994). Will the legacy of our past provide us with a legacy for the future? *Physical Therapy, 74*(11), 1063–1066.

Patton, M.Q. (1990). *Qualitative evaluation and research methods.* (2nd ed.). Newbury Park, CA: Sage.

Peloquin, S.M. (1993). Looking Back. Moral treatment: How a caring practice lost its rationale. *American Journal of Occupational Therapy, 48*(2), 167–173.

Quigley, M.C. (1994). Impact of spinal cord injury on the life roles of women. *American Journal of Occupational Therapy, 49*(8), 780–786.

Schmid, H. (1981). The foundation. Qualitative research and occupational therapy. *American Journal of Occupational Therapy, 35*(2), 105–106.

Schultz, C. (1994). Helping factors in a peer-developed support group for persons with head injury. Part II: Survivor interview perspective. *American Journal of Occupational Therapy, 48*(4), 305–309.

Schwartz, K.B. (1992). Occupational therapy and education: A shared vision. *American Journal of Occupational Therapy, 46*(1), 12–18.

Schwartz, K.B., & Colman, W. (1988). Looking Back. Historical research methods in occupational therapy. *American Journal of Occupational Therapy, 42*(4), 239–244.

Spencer, J., Young, M., Rintala, D., & Bates, S. (1995). Socialization to the culture of rehabilitation hospital: An ethnographic study. *American Journal of Occupational Therapy, 49*(1), 53–62.

Taylor, S.J. & Bogdan, R. (1984). *Introduction to qualitative research methods: The search for meanings.* New York: John Wiley & Sons.

Wolcott, H. (1980). How to look like an anthropologist without really being one. *Practicing Anthropology, 3*(2), 6–7, 56–59.

Wolcott, H. (1990). *Writing up qualitative research.* Qualitative Research Methods Series, Vol. 20. Newbury Park, CA: Sage Publications.

Additional Reading

Block, J. (1971). *Understanding historical research: A search for truth.* Glen Rock, NJ: Research Publications.

Coffey, A. & Atkinson, P. (1996). *Making sense of qualitative data: Complementary research strategies.* Thousand Oaks, CA: Sage Publications.

Depoy, E. & Gitlin, L.N. (1994). *Introduction to research: Multiple strategies for health and human services.* St. Louis: CV Mosby.

Fetterman, D. (1989). *Ethnography: Step by step.* No. 17 in Applied Social Research Methods Series. Newbury Park, CA: Sage Publications.

Hammersley, M. & Atkinson, P. (1990). *Ethnography: Principles in practice.* New York: Routledge.

Kielhofner, G., & Burke, J.P. (1977). Occupational therapy after 60 years: An account of changing identity and knowledge. *American Journal of Occupational Therapy, 31*(10), 675–689.

Merriam, S.B. (1988). *Case study research in education: A qualitative approach.* San Francisco: Jossey-Bass.

Silverman, D. (1993). *Interpreting qualitative data: Methods for analyzing talk, text, and interactions.* Thousand Oaks, CA: Sage Publications.

Spradley, J.P. (1979). *The ethnographic interview.* New York: Holt, Rinehart and Winston.

West, W. (1979). Historical perspectives. In *Occupational Therapy: 2001 AD.* Rockville, MD: American Occupational Therapy Association, (pp. 9–17).

Yin, R.K. (1989). *Case study research: Design and methods.* No. 5 in Applied Social Science Research Methods Series. Newbury Park, CA: Sage Publications.

10

Analyzing Qualitative Data

Although there are diverse approaches to qualitative data analysis, Miles and Huberman (1994) have proposed a fairly typical sequence of analytic procedures. With some modification, they are as follows:

- [Assigning] codes to a set of field notes drawn from observations, interviews, [study of documents and artifacts]
- Noting reflections or other remarks in the margins
- Sorting and sifting through these data to identify similar phrases, relationships between variables, patterns, themes, distinct differences between subgroups, and sequences
- Isolating these patterns, . . . commonalities and differences, and taking them [back into] the field [for] the next wave of data collection
- Gradually elaborating a small set of generalizations that cover consistencies identified in the database
- [Comparing] those generalizations with [existing theoretical constructs and properties] (p. 9)

It may be misleading to have a separate section on data analysis, because in qualitative research, data collection and data analysis go hand in hand. Throughout observation, interviewing, and other data collection methods, researchers continually read through their notes and transcripts, noting any themes, patterns, or questions that occur to them. They return to the field to get answers to emerging questions and hunches, and develop tentative concepts and propositions as they go. Early formulation of ideas may alter the proposed course of the data collection; thus there is no definite moment when data collection stops and data analysis begins. It is only for convenience that data collection techniques and data analysis are discussed separately here.

Qualitative data are generated from descriptive research such as the types described in Chapter 9: the case method, ethnographies, and historical research. These types of studies often generate large amounts of descriptive, nonquantifiable data that need to be organized and synthesized in a useful manner. The data collection method employed, such as observation or interviewing, will determine the type of data generated. For example, data from interviews and questionnaires may be straightforward and simple to tabulate and analyze if they are generated from closed-ended questions, but if generated from open-ended questions, they may yield a mass of data in no particular format that will be difficult to reduce in a meaningful way for analysis and interpretation.

By its very nature, qualitative data analysis is inductive analysis, meaning that the patterns, themes, and categories of analysis come from the data; they emerge out of the data rather than being imposed on them before data collection (Patton, 1980). There are two ways of representing patterns: First, the analyst can use the categories developed and articulated by the people in the program being studied, *in vivo* codes. Second, the analyst may become aware of categories or patterns for which the people in the program do not have labels or terms, and the analyst must develop terms to describe these categories, **analyst-constructed typologies.** The recommended way to find out if analyst-constructed typologies are accurate is to ask the participants to check them to see if they make sense.

There are several ways to derive meaning from data. One is to look for patterns, categories, and descriptive units as ways to describe data and to deduce causes, consequences, and relationships (Lincoln & Guba, 1985; Patton, 1980). A second way is to use a variety of coding and linking mechanisms, with the goal of generating theory grounded in that particular data, rather than verifying existing theory (Glaser & Strauss, 1967). A third way is to represent the data with coding and display methods such as charts and drawings, in an attempt to order and explain the data, to generate meaning from the data, and to verify resulting conclusions (Miles & Huberman, 1994). A fourth method is to describe and interpret the data to test a hypothesis provisionally, using a priori and a posteriori coding (Bogdan & Biklen, 1982; Herzberg, Mausner, & Snyderman, 1959). Some qualitative researchers use combinations of these methods, and others use entirely different ways to analyze their data.

The style of qualitative research and data analysis method you choose will depend on whether your ultimate goal is to inform policy, describe situations in a novel manner, or generate theory. The following is an outline of each of the four methods just mentioned, but you will want to supplement your knowledge with more in-depth sources (see the references at the end of this chapter) to carry out a successful qualitative research project.

Patterns, Categories, and Descriptive Units

This is a summary of Patton's (1980) and Lincoln and Guba's (1985) methods for qualitative data analysis. Although Patton was writing about evaluation research, his data analysis methods can be applied to most types of qualitative research studies.

As stated previously, there is no clear point at which data gathering ends and data analyzing begins. While you are still collecting data, you will have some ideas about how to analyze it, and you must be sure to make those ideas part of the field notes and refer to them during the continuing analysis. Patton believes that the investigator should look for both evidence to confirm the initial hypotheses and alternative explanations that would refute them, strengthening the validity of the study. Thus, there will be two sources of information for you to consider during the final data analysis: the research questions you formulated during the conceptualization of the study, and the analytic insights and interpretations you made as you collected the data.

Patton describes data analysis as a "painstaking process requiring long hours of careful work, going over notes, organizing the data, looking for patterns, checking emergent patterns against the data, cross-validating data sources and findings, and making linkages among the various parts of the data and the emergent dimensions of the analysis" (p. 297). This process will be described next.

Organizing and Describing Data

First, organize the data by reading through and making sure that they are all present, filling in any gaps by returning to the field, if necessary. Get a feel for how much data there are, including transcriptions of interviews, field notes from observations, memos to yourself, formal documents, descriptions of artifacts, and so on. Then make four copies of everything: one to be put away in a safe place, one for writing on, and two for cutting and pasting.

Read through all the field notes and transcripts, and make comments in the margins, attaching notes if needed, with initial ideas on how the data will be categorized into topics. Patton likens coming up with topics to constructing an index for a book or labels for a file system. One looks at what is there and gives it a name or a label. Many passages can serve several different topics, which is why multiple copies of the data are needed for cutting and pasting. You will need to read the materials several times before they are completely indexed. In this initial step, the data are being "classified" or "coded." The copy on which the topics and labels, or codes, are written becomes the indexed copy of the field notes or interviews.

The primary purpose of writing in the margins and developing typologies (codes, categories, themes, patterns) is to *describe* the data. (See Box 10–A for examples of margin-writing.) Later you will use typologies to make interpretations about the nature of the program under study, but for now it is important to have an accurate description of the program. Simplifying the complex data into some manageable classification scheme is the first step of content analysis—getting the data under control.

Rather than margin-writing, Lincoln and Guba (1985) suggest writing on index cards as an alternative method for the first step of content analysis. They summarize their method as unitizing, categorizing, and filling in patterns. By **unitizing,** Lincoln and Guba are referring to units of information that will serve as the basis for the categories. These are phrases, sentences, or paragraphs that have some meaning to the analyst, and must "be the smallest piece of information about something that can stand by itself" (p. 345). Units are found in the transcripts and field notes. Initially, it is better to err on the side of overinclusion; it is easier to reject irrelevant information later than to recapture discarded information.

Having located a unit, the analyst enters it onto an index card, or directly into a computer using one of the many qualitative research database management programs now available. Each computer program has its own method for allowing units of data to be identified and coded (see Appendix F). Here we will assume that index cards are being used, although the principles may easily be applied to computer analysis methods.

The back of each index card should be coded in multiple ways: the source of the information (e.g., interview transcription, treatment plan, observation notes) by page and paragraph number; the particular episode during which the information was collected (e.g., interview with rehabilitation director, team meeting); the type of respondent (e.g., staff person, administrator); the site where the information was gathered (e.g., school classroom, rehabilitation clinic, supervisor's office).

You will probably produce a large number of index cards at this initial stage. Later stages of analysis will require fewer and fewer cards, as the study becomes more focused. The quality of the rest of the analysis and the final product of the study depends on careful initial unitizing.

The next step is **categorizing.** Here you will group cards that relate to the same provisional category, devise rules that describe those categories, and finalize a set of categories that are internally consistent (that do not overlap each other and include all relevant data). The following steps are outlined by Lincoln and Guba (1985, pp. 347–349):

1. From the more-or-less haphazardly arranged pile of cards that has resulted from the unitizing process, select the first card from the pile, read it, and note

---

Box 10–A

The following are examples of initial margin-writing from an unpublished study (Bailey, 1996) of occupational therapy managers and their decision-making strategies in the face of ethical dilemmas. Codes have not yet been refined or ordered.

Establishes trust	Allies with staff
Orderly thinking	Conscientious
Looks for those having interests in the outcome	Feels a responsibility
Creative response	Looks for power source
Takes actions on himself or herself	Honest
Advocacy role with staff	Emphasizes the positive
Has faith in staff	Educates staff
Frustrated at lack of power	Puzzled about what to do
Feels defeated by "system"	Reassured by facility support

its contents. This first card represents the first entry in the first yet-to-be-named category. Place it to one side.

2. Read the second card and note its contents. Determine on tacit or intuitive grounds whether this second card is a "look-alike" or "feel-alike" with card 1; that is, whether its contents are essentially similar. If so, place the second card with the first and proceed to the third card; if not, the second card represents the first entry in the second yet-to-be-named category.

3. Continue with successive cards. Decide whether each card is a "look/feel-alike" of cards that have already been placed in some provisional category or represents a new category. Proceed accordingly.

4. After some cards have been processed, you may feel that a new card neither fits any of the provisional categories nor seems to form a new category. You may also recognize other cards as irrelevant to the developing set. Place these cards into a miscellaneous pile. Instead of being discarded at this point, they should be retained for later review.

As the process continues, new categories will emerge rapidly at first, but the rate of emergence will diminish sharply after 50 to 60 cards have been processed. At this point, some of the "look/feel-alike" categories will have accumulated a substantial number of cards, about six to eight, and you may begin to feel pressed to start on the memo-writing task leading to the delineation of category properties and devising of a covering rule. To proceed:

5. Take up cards that have accumulated in such critical-size categories. Attempt to make a propositional statement about the properties that seem to characterize the cards. Combine these properties into a rule for inclusion. Write the provisional rule on another index card and place it beside the category. Give the category a name or title that catches as well as possible the "essence" of the rule, to make later sorting easier.

6. Continue with steps 3 and 4, and with step 5 as other categories approach critical size, until all the cards have been

sorted. Whenever a card is now assigned to a category for which a provisional rule has been devised, the card should be included or excluded *not* on the basis of its "look/feel-alike" quality but on the basis of whether it fits the rule.

7. When all the cards have been sorted, review all the categories. First, look again at the cards assigned to the "miscellaneous" pile. Now that the full category set is apparent, you may find that some of these cards fit in somewhere after all. Some cards may be judged to be clearly irrelevant and may be discarded. Others may still not fit into any of your categories. As a rule of thumb, these unassignable (but not discardable) cards ought not to exceed 5 to 7 percent of the total; a higher percentage probably signals a serious deficiency in the category set.

Second, review the categories for overlap. The set is inadequate if there are ambiguities about how any particular card might have been categorized. You may find that some unit cards were prepared inappropriately, with dual content.

Third, examine the set of categories for possible relationships among categories. Certain categories may be subsumable under others; some categories may be unwieldy and should be further divided; and some categories may be missing, a fact made evident by the logic of the category system as a whole. Further, other categories may be incomplete, showing sufficient presence to have been included but not sufficient to be definitively established. Missing, incomplete, or otherwise unsatisfactory categories should be earmarked for follow-up as part of the continuous data collection and processing sequence.

Finally, Lincoln and Guba address **filling in patterns.** Categories that require fleshing out may be pursued in subsequent data collection efforts through the use of extension (building on items of information already known), bridging (making connections among different items), and surfacing (proposing new information that ought to fit and then verifying its existence).

The descriptive phase of the analysis has

ended when you feel that sources of data have been exhausted, categories have been saturated (any new categories seem redundant), clear patterns have emerged, and analysis "overextends" the original boundaries of the study.

Writers who advocate this approach to data analysis tend to acknowledge that the process described thus far is difficult. Patton feels that it is "arty" and "intuitive." Formulating codes, patterns, and themes into an eventual category system requires careful decisions about what is truly significant and meaningful in the data. Even with great experience, judgment, and intelligence, the analyst can decide something is significant when it is not, or miss identifying a really significant event in the data.

Once the data have been unitized and categorized, Patton suggests two more ways to organize data, a cross-classifying matrix and a process/outcomes matrix.

Cross-Classifying Matrix

Some categories lend themselves to being described as dimensions; they can represent a continuum of events from one extreme to another (Box 10–B). The content of each continuum is taken directly from the data and will become evident to you during the coding process. Once the two continua are placed on the matrix, however, new categories will become apparent in the resulting cells (Box 10–C). The purpose of the cross-classifying matrix is to generate new categories as a way to explain the data. All parts of the resulting typology may or may not be represented in the data. The content of some cells may result from logical construction on the part of the

---

Box 10–B

Cross-classifying matrix

Patients' behaviors might range from one extreme of taking great initiative in their treatment to the other extreme of shifting initiative to the therapist. This dimension of initiative could be placed on one axis of a matrix, while the other axis might contain the continuum of a dimension concerning patients' desire to attain independence.

Desire for independence		Initiative-taking		
Great desire	(Fill cells with quotes)		"I know the OT could have come to my house, but I wanted to practice using the bus"
Average desire			
Some desire			
No desire	"I expected the OT to come to my house to see me"		
	None	A little	A great deal

Box 10–C

Categories generated from cells of a matrix

Here is an example of a map of categories at one end of a continuum (Fred is an "egghead" who always studies in the library, works too hard, and doesn't fit in with his classmates). Other components of the map indicate the opposite end of the continuum with categories generated from the cells of a cross-classifying matrix (Fred goofs off, is friendly, and fits in). These will be looked for in the data to see if there is a construct to be made regarding Fred's accessibility.

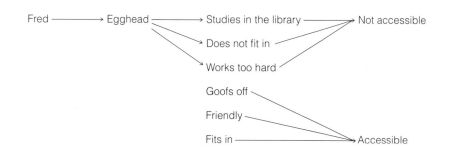

The typology constructed in the cells of a cross-classifying matrix often is represented by metaphors. Patton feels that metaphors are powerful and clever ways of communicating findings because a great deal can be conveyed by a single phrase. However, he cautions that the investigator must be sure that the major connotation of the metaphor is appropriate to the particular data, and that an investigator should not try to force data to fit an extra-clever metaphor just because he or she wants to use it. (See Box 10–D for an example of a study metaphor.)

Process/Outcome Matrix

Uncovering links between process and outcome is often invaluable in understanding

Box 10–D

In a study of occupational therapists' clinical reasoning, Mattingly and Fleming coined the term "underground practice." The term referred to therapists' actions in treatment that were not reflected in their record keeping because they thought those actions might not be considered proper therapy by supervisors or insurers.

the program under study and can be effectively achieved by using process/outcome matrices. In this type of matrix, a process continuum (such as encouraging patients to formulate their own treatment goals) is placed along one axis, and an outcome (such as degrees of success at returning to independent living) along the other axis. The categories for the process and outcome continua are generated from the data. The information in the resulting cells describes linkages, patterns, themes, or program content that lead to an understanding of the relationships between processes and outcomes. These relationships may be generated directly from the data or may be logically derived by the analyst.

Using the example just given, the blank cell created by crossing the process (encouraging patients to form their own treatment goals) with the outcome (patient success at returning to independent living), creates a data analysis question: What types of treatment goals do patients come up with that lead to their return to independent living? The analyst then carefully reviews the transcripts, looking for data that will answer that question. By describing actual treatment goals patients make in that particular program, we can make judgments about the strength or weakness of the link between this process and the desired outcome. The eventual purpose is for the analyst to offer interpretations and judgments about the nature and quality of this apparent process/outcome connection.

Causes, Consequences, and Relationships

Once the data have been organized and described, the next step in data analysis is to consider causes, consequences, and relationships in the data. However, Patton cautions that any causal theorizing in qualitative research is tentative.

> Statements about which things appear to lead to other things, which parts of the program produce certain effects, and how processes lead to outcomes are areas of speculation, conjecture, and hypothesizing (p. 324).

He notes that investigators must not make the mistake of picking out of context isolated variables that are mechanically linked together, thus falling into a quantitative mindset.

Patton does not give further directions for seeking out causal relationships, so the analyst must turn to other theorists for assistance in this task. The goal of the **Patterns, Categories, and Descriptive Units** method of data analysis is to provide useful, meaningful, and credible answers about a program. To see if this goal has been reached, the data analysis findings must be validated and verified using some of the techniques presented in Chapter 9.

Grounded Theory

The qualitative research method of grounded theory developed by Glaser and Strauss (1967) is one of the most commonly described and referred-to methods, yet it may be the most difficult to carry out. You should follow Glaser and Strauss's (1967) book *The Discovery of Grounded Theory: Strategies for Qualitative Research* if you plan to undertake this type of research.

The following description of the grounded theory approach is based on Glaser and Strauss's original work and Turner's (1981) interpretation of their method. Because Glaser and Strauss have not given detailed guidelines for the handling of data, Turner has set out a series of nine stages for analyzing qualitative data in order to arrive at grounded theory. His nine stages are used here to describe the process.

As in other qualitative approaches, the data for grounded theory can come from various sources: interviews, observations, government documents, videotapes, newspapers, letters, and books. Each of the latter sources can be coded and analyzed in the same way as interviews or observations. One copy of the transcripts and field notes should be kept intact, and you should have several other copies for writing on and for cutting and pasting.

1. **Develop categories.** The first stage is to use the field notes and transcribed interviews to label tentatively the phenomena that are felt to be relevant to the study. First, number each paragraph sequentially for reference purposes throughout the analysis. Turner (1981) asks himself, "What categories, concepts or labels do we need in order to describe or to account for the phenomena discussed in this paragraph?" (p. 232). Write each label on an index card together with the number of the paragraph, and file the card. Several cards are usually needed for each paragraph. Continue this procedure until you are satisfied that all features of significance are labeled before moving on to the next paragraph. (Glaser and Strauss suggest writing the labels directly on the transcripts, in the margin, so that the transcripts can be cut up and paragraphs with like labels grouped together.)

   At this point, the labels may be long and ungainly phrases, not necessarily in their final form. The most important point to remember is that the label should fit the phenomenon described exactly. If you are not satisfied with the fit, change the words until the fit is exact.

   As the cards mount up, you can begin a system of cross-referencing. Each card can be numbered and titled with a category that encompasses relevant labels. The paragraph numbers together with a brief reminder of the content generating that label are listed on that card. At the bottom of the card is the cross-reference note; for example, that this particular card can be linked with card 9 and card 11. The note will indicate that the labels listed on this card have some sort of connection with labels in another category.

This first stage is perhaps the most difficult and may be quite time consuming. It may be done alone or by pairs of analysts, or in groups. It is worth taking time over, however, because the meaningfulness of the theory eventually developed depends on the accuracy of initial labeling.

2. **Saturate categories.** This term refers to the process of adding examples to each category until you feel confident that you really know what that category means. At this point, you should feel comfortable each time a new piece of data is classified into a particular category. The point of saturation may be reached at different times for different categories.

During this stage, the **constant comparative method** is used. It is the defining activity of the grounded theory approach to data analysis. While labeling an incident or piece of data for a category, compare it with the previous incidents that have been put in that category to be sure it is similar. The constant comparison of incidents and labels will soon start to generate ideas about the theoretical properties of the category. You begin thinking in terms of a range of continua for the category, "its dimensions, the conditions under which it is pronounced or minimized, its major consequences, its relation to other categories, and its other properties" (Glaser & Strauss, 1967, p. 106) (Box 10–E). This leads to the next stage, defining the categories.

3. **Abstract definitions.** Write a definition for each category that explicates the qualities being recognized when a new case is being added to a category. The definition will be abstract and several sentences long (Box 10–F).

While producing category definitions, the analyst often develops a deeper and more precise understanding of the exact nature of each category. As a result, it is possible to find that more than one category is being subsumed under one

---

Box 10–E

In *An Explorative Study of How Occupational Therapists Develop Therapeutic Relationships with Family Caregivers,* Clark, Corcoran, and Gitlin used thematic analysis on their audiotapes and field notes. They used open coding and axial coding to conceptualize and compare related phenomena within the data.

The transcriptions from the treatment sessions were first reviewed with the use of open coding in which the first author searched the data for emerging themes. This review required labeling the phenomena, discovering categories, and naming the categories. . . . Once the initial categories emerged, axial coding was used for further analysis and creation of subcategories. This analysis involved examining the various categories for specific properties and dimensions such as *who* was involved, *when* did it happen, *what* was the meaning, and *why* did it occur.

(Clark, Corcoran, & Gitlin, 1995, p. 588)

---

title, or that two categories embrace the same theme.

4. **Use the definitions.** Once the definitions have been produced, they can be used to help the researcher recognize other areas of the study that could be pursued. Stimulating further ideas for investigation is the point of this close

---

Box 10–F

One of Turner's cards produced the title: "Battle for control over marginal territory."

The definition produced for this category read:

Many forms of authority relate to territorial areas: this leads to particular attention centering upon the boundary areas between two authorities' territories. This category refers to a situation in which a marginal territory, not clearly under the control of either of the two parties adjacent to it, forms the basis of a power struggle between the two parties.

(Turner, 1981, p. 236)

scrutiny of the data. Glaser (1978) refers to the "drugless trip," the productive intellectual journey that occurs when the writing of definitions spills over into interesting ideas about the data—the nature of patterns, links between data, and insights into data. Glaser suggests strongly that the researcher write these ideas down rather than "dissipating" them by talking about them. Once they are in writing, *then* talk to your colleagues about them.

5. **Exploit categories fully.** At this stage, the categories can be developed further by generalizing from the specific people in your category to others who might experience something similar. Glaser and Strauss (1967) were studying nurses working with dying patients. At this point in their analysis, they discovered that their theoretical categories could be generalized to the care of all patients (not just dying ones) by all staff (not just nurses).

Also, properties of categories other than people might be investigated to see if the definition still applies when they are changed. For instance, "territory" used in the example in Box 10–F, might not have to refer to physical territory, but could refer to such features as "personal autonomy" or to "time." The investigator could examine situations using personal autonomy or time as marginal territories to see if the category definition holds true.

What we are doing here is building speculatively upon a single category, producing a number of related possible categories, exploring some directions of thought, and producing a number of provisional hypotheses. Although this is a somewhat arbitrary exercise, it does free analysts from the concrete instance in the data and allows them to look for similar clusters of properties at a higher conceptual level. The exercise will suggest a number of logically related categories, but of course there will be no actual data in them. The investigator can now keep an eye out for relevant data that does occur, or may choose to return to the field to investigate the potential categories.

This stage may seem quite a leap for some beginning qualitative researchers, but the aim in using this method of data analysis is to create theory. As Turner (1981) says, ". . . grasping the possibility of constructing a series of abstract elaborations" while learning to see "similarities between phenomena which were initially regarded as different and non-comparable is the step which helps [new researchers] to begin to think theoretically. It might be suggested that the ability to construct a range of abstract variations upon a given concrete piece of evidence is one of the skills that the theorist must learn to develop" (p. 238).

6. **Note, develop, and follow up on links between categories.** When you have worked through stages 1 to 5 for several categories, various links will become apparent. Causal connections may be confidently assigned to some of these links, whereas others will be more tentative and need further investigation.

7. **Consider the conditions under which the links hold.** This line of thought raises the question of the conditions under which one outcome occurs rather than another. In this way, the analyst has "spilled over" into postulating hypothetical links between categories. If any of these links seems useful to the purpose of the study, you can look for data to confirm the link. For example, in a study of occupational therapy managers (Bailey, 1996), it quickly became apparent that demands for increased productivity from their bosses led the managers to meet with their staff to "brainstorm" ways to see more clients, an apparent causal link. At a slightly higher level of abstraction, this link could be expressed as one in which "administrative pressure" led to "planning meetings." This conceptualization, in turn, leads to the possibility of other links such as, are there other outcomes arising from administrative pressures, are group planning strategies the only way to deal with administrative pressures or might there be alternatives such as individual mandates from the manager, or setting up a competitive

atmosphere to encourage individual therapists to increase their productivity?

The analyst could set up typologies based on the data, about the varieties of administrative pressure and the varieties of resulting group or individual strategies. In this way, each new condition would strengthen the hypothesis that certain administrative pressure will lead to certain planning strategies.

8. **Make connections to existing theory and build grounded theory.** You now have sufficient information to decide whether existing theory has anything useful to contribute to the problem. Assess the suitability of existing theory, based on the various conditions elicited from the analysis. Many qualitative researchers wait until this stage in their analysis to read relevant literature, so as not to bias their thinking thus far.

When the approach outlined here is applied to an area that is new to the researcher, a large number of categories is likely to be developed in the early stages. But after intense interaction with the data, the researcher forms a vocabulary describing the basic categories and concepts to express what is important and relevant about the research question. As the analysis proceeds, the need to add new vocabulary diminishes. At this stage, links that are seen or suspected between sets of categories begin to clarify and can be readily sorted into clusters. Various physical activities, such as sketching diagrams of the links, writing memos about them, or sorting file cards into groups, may be helpful in this stage of crystallization. When the relationships become clear, they form the basis for the emerging theory that is now grounded in the study data, grounded theory.

You will find two important characteristics of your newly formed theory. There should be a closeness of fit between the theoretical constructs and the area being studied that makes the analysis understandable to the study participants. Participants should be consulted to be sure there is a closeness of fit. You will also find a degree of complexity, so that theoretical constructs are unlikely to fall readily into a set of simple logical propositions. Most participants recognize that their "slice of life" is complicated. Again, their responses to the theory should be sought and modifications made, if necessary.

9. **Determine the strength of the emerging theory.** This is the second level of what Glaser and Strauss refer to as the constant comparative method. In order to test the limits of the propositions developed in the emerging theory, an active search should be made for confirming and disproving instances. This can be done by identifying the central propositions of the theory, specifying the variables and dimensions that are likely to affect those propositions, and seeking out situations in which the variables are pushed to their limits, to see if the original effects still hold.

There are several other ways researchers can test the strength of their propositions. They can look for large numbers of similar cases to confirm propositions that were developed on a small number of cases. Alternatively, researchers who have developed a complex theory that is comprehensible to the participants in the study may want to solicit feedback from those participants, from investigators working in similar areas, and from lay people familiar with the area under study. Another method is for researchers to conduct several small-scale investigations to check out propositions of which they are unsure.

Properties of Theories Developed Using the Grounded Theory Approach

A theory that has been generated using the constant comparative approach to data analysis, grounded theory, will probably have several properties. It will be a **complex theory** that corresponds closely to the data. The analyst will have compared each incident in the data with other incidents for similarities and differences, considering the diversity of the data. This is in contrast to simple coding, which establishes only whether an incident indicates a property in the category.

The constant comparative method tends to result in the creation of **developmental theory,** theories that show process, sequence, and change and that are relevant to social organizations, people's positions, and social interaction. This is an inductive method of theory development in which the analyst is forced to develop ideas on a higher level of conceptual abstraction than the actual data being analyzed. The underlying similarities and differences in the data are brought to light and presented at the abstract level. This process will result in either substantive theory or formal theory.

If analysts start with their own raw data, they will end up with **substantive theory;** for example, the nature of patient care provided by nurses, or decision making by therapy managers. If analysts start with findings drawn from several existing studies, they will end up with **formal theory;** for example, how professional people give service to clients, or decision making by people in power. Substantive theory can be raised to formal theory, but this move requires additional analysis of the substantive theory and the inclusion of other relevant studies.

Coding and Displays as Methods for Qualitative Data Analysis

The type of data analysis advocated by Miles and Huberman (1994) is typified by specific methods for coding and by the use of displays to show the results of the data analysis. Their method has been referred to as a quasi-experimental approach to qualitative data analysis. Much of Miles and Huberman's work has been informed by the methods of social anthropology. By their own admission, however, they "have gravitated to more fully codified research questions, more standardized data collection procedures, and more systematic devices for analysis" (p. 8). It is these systematic devices for analysis that concern us here.

Miles and Huberman view data analysis as consisting of three concurrent activities: data reduction, data display, and conclusion drawing and verification.

Data Reduction

Data reduction refers to the process of selecting, focusing, simplifying, abstracting, and transforming the data contained in field notes or transcriptions. Its activities may include writing summaries, coding, teasing out themes, making clusters, making partitions, or writing memos. Data reduction occurs throughout the life of the study and continues until the final report is complete. Most importantly, data reduction is not separate from data analysis; it is part of analysis.

Data Display

Data display

is an organized, compressed assembly of information that permits conclusion drawing and action. . . . Looking at displays helps us to understand what is happening and to do something—either analyze further or take action—based on that understanding (Miles & Huberman, 1994, p. 11).

The most common form of display in qualitative research is text. Miles and Huberman feel strongly that text is extremely cumbersome; it is dispersed, sequential, poorly structured, and bulky, and may lead investigators to hasty, poorly formed conclusions. They advocate other forms of displays, such as matrices, graphs, charts, and networks, feeling that these assemble information into an immediately accessible, compact format so that the analyst can see what is happening. As with data reduction, data displays are not separate from analysis but rather part of it.

Conclusion Drawing and Verification

The third concurrent stream of data analysis is conclusion drawing and verification. From the start of data collection, the analyst is making decisions about what the data mean, noting patterns, explanations, possible causal flows, and propositions. At first, these conclusions are held lightly, but as the evidence grows, they become increasingly explicit and grounded. Although "final" conclusions may not appear until the end of the study, they have often been in the researcher's mind from the beginning. Verification is the other half of this stream of data analysis;

conclusions need to be verified as the analysis proceeds. Verification may be as brief as a quick recheck of the data to confirm a current idea, or as lengthy as a thorough review of data among colleagues or an attempt to replicate a finding in another data set.

Early Data Analysis

The following methods, typically used in the early stages of data analysis, help the researcher think about existing data and generate strategies for collecting new, often better, data. Field notes and interviews should already have been transcribed.

Contact Summary Sheet

A contact summary sheet is a one-sheet series of questions and answers about a particular field contact. Your questions are formulated ahead of time, and might include such ideas as:

What people, events, or situations were involved?

What were the main themes or issues in the contact?

Which research questions and which variables in the initial framework did the contact bear on most centrally?

What new hypotheses, speculations, or hunches about the field situations were suggested by the contact?

Where should the field worker place most energy during the next contact, and what kinds of information should be sought? (Miles & Huberman, 1994, pp. 51–52).

Contact summary sheets should be completed as soon after the field contact as possible, while events are fresh in your mind. Contact sheets may be used: to guide planning for the next contact; to suggest new or revised codes; to reorient you when returning to the write-up; and to help with further data analysis, because the contact sheets themselves can be coded and analyzed.

Start Codes and Definitions

Codes are labels that assign meaning to the descriptive data. They are usually attached to "chunks" of data of varying size (words, phrases, sentences, or paragraphs) and may take the form of a straightforward assigning label or a more complex metaphor. Codes are used to organize and retrieve chunks of data and to categorize, cluster, and display the data. Codes may be descriptive, in which you simply assign a label that describes a segment of text; or interpretive, in which you assign a more complex, underlying meaning to the text when you have learned more about the dynamics behind the data.

Miles and Huberman prefer the a priori method of creating codes. They recommend that the researcher create a provisional "start list" of codes before beginning the data collection. The list is generated from the preparatory work for the study, when the researcher goes through the written materials and pulls out codes from issues identified in the conceptual framework of the study, from research questions or hypotheses, and from problem areas and key variables. A start list can have from a dozen or so up to 50 to 60 codes.

The list should be kept on a single sheet of paper so that it is readily at hand during coding. The suggested format is a list of code words placed in categories, a corresponding list of the actual code letters that will be used on the transcripts, and a notation as to which research question or hypothesis (if any) the code was drawn from (Box 10–G).

The next step is to write "start-definitions" for the codes and categories, knowing that these definitions will be revised as the study proceeds. Now you are ready to start coding the transcripts, writing the codes in the left margin next to chunks of data.

The codes will need to be changed as the coding progresses, because you cannot possibly predict, during the compilation of the start list of codes, all the issues that will come up during data collection. Codes will need revising for several reasons: some codes do not fit, or they merely decay (these should be discarded); some flourish and grow out of bounds, and will need to be broken into subcodes; some new codes emerge in later data collection and need to be added to the code list within the appropriate category. All of this activity leads to the relabeling of the codes written on the transcripts and a reexamination and possible revision of the categorical structure for the codes.

It is most important that the codes have a categorical structure in order to bring order to the mass of data. Codes should relate to

---

Box 10–G

A priori list of code words and code letters linked to research questions

Categories of Code Words	Code	Research Question
Manager's Behavior	MB	2.1
MB:controlling	MB-cont	2.1.1
MB:facilitating	MB-fac	2.1.2
MB:encouraging	MB-enc	2.1.3
Manager's Attitudes	MA	3.1
MA:optimistic	MA-opt	3.1.1
MA:pessimistic	MA-pess	3.1.2
MA:encouraging	MA-enc	3.1.3
MA:superior	MA-sup	3.1.4
MA:sup:other managers within facility	MA-sup-omwf	3.1.4.1
MA:sup:other managers outside facility	MA-sup-omof	3.1.4.2
MA:sup:own staff	MA-sup-os	3.1.4.3
MA:inferior	MA-inf	3.1.5
MA:inf:other managers within facility	MA-inf-omwf	3.1.5.1
MA:inf:other managers outside facility	MA-inf-omof	3.1.5.2
Manager's Relationships	MR	4.1
MR:with own staff	MR-os	4.1.1
MR:with staff in rehab dept	MR-wsrd	4.1.2
MR:with staff outside rehab dept	MR-sord	4.1.3
MR:os:boss	MR-os-bos	4.1.1.1
MR:os:peer	MR-os-pr	4.1.1.2

---

one another in a coherent manner that is relevant to the study. Miles and Huberman refer to the structure as a "conceptual web, including larger meanings and their constitutive characteristics" (p. 63). Coding with a poorly designed structure makes the codes difficult to remember and makes retrieval and organization of the data burdensome. Sometimes, partway through the coding, a researcher will realize that the start-code structure doesn't work for this set of data. It is better to start another structure from scratch than to try to force the data into the existing structure. It may seem time-consuming, but it will improve the eventual quality of the study immeasurably.

Clear, operational definitions of the codes are absolutely necessary, and redefinition should occur whenever a code or category is changed. The definitions are crucial to making it possible to apply the codes to the data consistently over time, and to enable more than one coder to apply consistent codes to the same data. Definitions will be improved and become more focused as the coding proceeds, and the meanings of the data will become more apparent in the context of the study.

Reflective Remarks

Reflective remarks are notes made of reflections and commentary that occur to you while you are writing up the field notes from the day's activities. As you write, reflect on the items already mentioned in the discussion about processing field notes in Chapter 7.

- What your relationship with the informant feels like, now that you are off the site
- Thoughts on the meaning of what a key informant was "really" saying during an exchange that seemed somehow important

- Doubts about the quality of some of the data; second thoughts about some of the interview questions and observation protocols
- A new hypothesis that might explain some puzzling observations
- A mental note to pursue an issue further in the next contact
- Apparent connections to material in another part of the data
- Reactions to some informants' remarks or actions
- Elaboration or clarification of a previous incident or event that now seems of possible significance (Miles & Huberman, 1994, p. 66)

When a thought like one of these occurs to you, it is useful to enter it directly into the write-up, identifying it as a reflective comment by using double parentheses.

Marginal Remarks

Marginal remarks made during the coding process should be made in the right margin of the transcripts (the actual codes are in the left margin). They are ideas and reactions that frequently occur in response to the data. These ideas are important for suggesting new interpretations and connections with other parts of the data, and often point toward questions and issues to look into during the next phase of data collection.

Pattern Coding

Pattern coding is a secondary level of coding that identifies emergent themes or patterns in the data, grouping the earlier codes into a smaller number of constructs. This activity gets the researcher into analysis during data collection, so that later fieldwork can be more focused. It also helps the researcher construct a cognitive map for understanding incidents and interactions. To move the analysis along, you may want to produce some "maps" at this stage to assist in the formation of the constructs.

Memoing

Coding is so engrossing that a coder is likely to become overwhelmed with the flood of de-

tails and ideas that arise: the poignant remark, the particular personality of an informant, the gossip after a key meeting, certain telling body language of an informant. Writing memos to yourself and theorizing connections and relationships is one way to keep track of these ideas.

Memos are conceptual in content; they do not merely report data but tie together different pieces of data into a cluster, which is often the beginning of a later study construct. They are your way of making sense of the data in the first flush of formulating ideas. Memo writing should be fun and "often provides sharp, sunlit moments of clarity or insight—little conceptual epiphanies" (Miles & Huberman, 1994, p. 74; see Box 10–C).

Memos should always be dated, titled with key concepts being discussed, and linked to particular data in the transcripts and to relevant codes. Always give priority to memoing; stop whatever else you are doing when an idea strikes, and get it down. Memoing can occur throughout the data analysis process. Usually the ideas raised in memos start to stabilize and repeat themselves about two thirds of the way through the data collection. Memoing contributes strongly to the development and revision of the coding system.

Interim Case Summary

During the data collection phase of the study, data analysis is typically done on the run, in spare moments, and is carried out only on some of the material collected. It is easy to lose sight of the big picture, to wonder what is really going on with the study, and to be unsure of the patterns and themes that are emerging. For all of these reasons, it is useful to write an interim case summary, which provides a synthesis of what the researcher knows about the study so far and what remains to be found out. The summary is a review of findings, a careful look at the quality of data supporting them, and the agenda for the next phase of data collection. In summary, it is a first attempt to pull together what you know about the case—to write a coherent, overall account of the study.

Typically, an interim case summary will include such items as information about the site (geography, demographics of community, organizational chart); a brief chronology of events being studied (what has occurred so far and what events are anticipated); the current status of the research questions (which ones have been addressed, have changed, or are yet to be investigated); a list of uncertainties or puzzles; any causal networks that have come to light; and notes about the methodology used to date (how the analysis was done, problems encountered, suggested changes for next analysis).

Later, Deeper Analysis: Systematic Displays

In the deeper descriptive analysis of qualitative data, Miles and Huberman (1994) advocate the use of data displays for drawing and verifying conclusions. These methods can be used either during or after data collection. By *display,* Miles and Huberman mean "a visual format that presents information systematically, so the user can draw valid conclusions and take needed action" (p. 91). Displays fall into two major categories: matrices, with defined rows and columns, and networks, which are a series of "nodes" with links between them. Data entries on the displays can take many forms; they can be short blocks of text, quotes, phrases, ratings, abbreviations, symbolic figures, labeled lines and arrows, and so on.

A matrix is the crossing of two lists, set up as rows and columns. Matrices can be time-ordered but need not be. Networks take various free-flowing forms. They are useful for focusing on more than a few variables at a time, are easily set up, can hold a great deal of readily analyzable information, and can be time-ordered or not.

Creating and revising formats for matrices and networks is quick work. What takes time is the data entry itself. Appropriate, coded data must be located in the transcripts and extracted, condensed, and summarized. Further data transformation may also be necessary, such as selecting ratings, making judgments, or picking representative quotes. The time taken depends on the method of data storage used, the number of variables in the display, and the kind and number of transformations made to the data.

You will need to write an analytic text to explain the displays. The text draws attention to features in the display, makes sense

of display data, knits display data together, and permits the analyst to draw conclusions and to add interpretations.

> The act of writing text as you ruminate over the meaning of a display is itself a focusing and forcing device that propels further analysis. . . . Writing, in short, does not come after analysis; it *is* analysis, happening as the writer thinks through the meaning of data in the display. Writing is thinking, not the report of thought (Miles & Huberman, 1994, p. 101).

Display Methods

Miles and Huberman's display methods will be briefly mentioned here; you will want to refer to their book for more specifics on the methods.

1. **Partially ordered displays:** These are useful in the exploratory, opening-up stage of a study, when variables are not yet clearly specified.
   a. **Context chart:** This is a network, mapping in graphic form the interrelationships of people's roles and behavior, in a context (Box 10–H).
   b. **Checklist matrix:** This is a matrix for analyzing data about a major do-

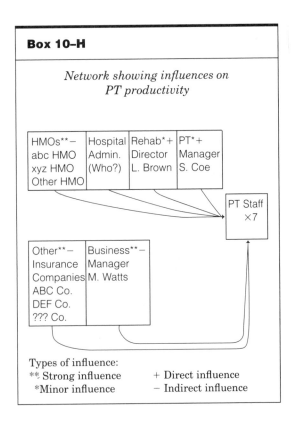

Box 10–H

Network showing influences on PT productivity

Box 10–I

Matrix showing presence of supporting conditions for new Rx technique

Condition	For Clinician	For Dept. Managers
Commitment	Strong—"wanted to make it work"	Weak—"no one cared if we did it"
Understanding	Basic—"felt I could do it but wasn't sure"	Absent—"admin didn't know we were doing it"
Materials	Inadequate—"it was ordered too late to use"	N/A
Training	Spotty—some had courses, some not	None

---

main of interest in the study that includes several components about the single variable (Box 10–I).

2. **A time-oriented display:** This is used when time is a crucial aspect of a study, and you need to describe the flow of events and processes carefully.

   a. **Event listing:** This is a matrix that arranges a series of concrete events chronologically, sorting them into several categories. Figure 2 in the Introduction is an example of a very simple event listing with a time axis. It could be made more complex by making categories for more than one study on the vertical axis and noting blocks of time when the whole group had completed the task on the horizontal axis.

   b. **Critical incident chart:** This is a matrix limited to events that are viewed as critical, influential, or decisive in the course of the case being studied (Box 10–J).

   c. **Event-state network:** This is a matrix or network using phrases to describe the "state" or "condition" that links events together. Events can be enclosed in squares or rectangles and states in circles for a more quickly grasped presentation (Box 10–K).

   d. **Activity record:** This describes a specific recurring activity, limited in time and space (e.g., an activity of daily living such as putting on a shirt). Nodes in the network are linked with arrows indicating direction (Box 10–L).

3. **Role-ordered matrices:** These describe the interaction of people in their roles (Box 10–M).

4. **Conceptually oriented displays:** These are used when studies are less exploratory, are nearing their end stages, and have clearly defined sets of key variables; displays rely on concepts.

   a. **Conceptually clustered matrix:** This matrix is useful for a study with many research questions or variables or concepts, and can clus-

---

Box 10–J

Matrix showing critical events for introduction of new hospital record-keeping system

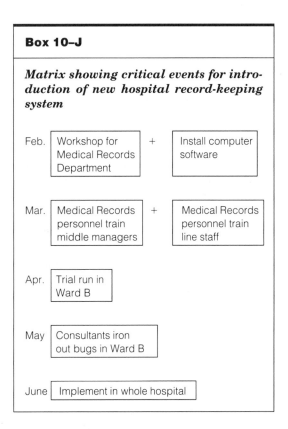

Box 10–K

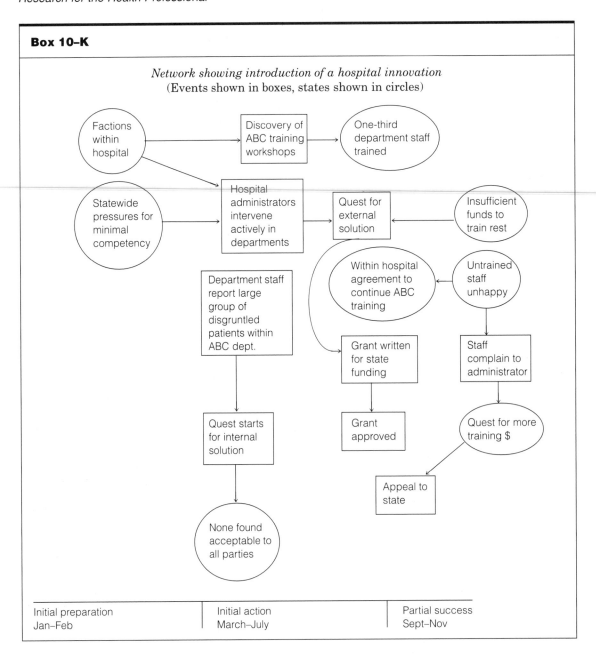

Network showing introduction of a hospital innovation
(Events shown in boxes, states shown in circles)

| Initial preparation Jan–Feb | Initial action March–July | Partial success Sept–Nov |

Box 10–L

Network showing steps in putting on a shirt

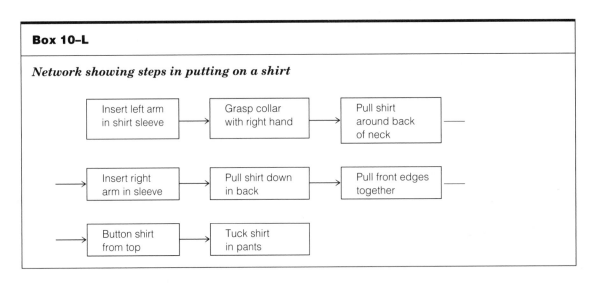

Box 10–M

Matrix showing first reactions to innovation

Role		*Personal*	*Past Experience*	*Anticipated Changes*
Line staff	Smith PT	Flexible Pt.-oriented	"Never tried it"	"Shouldn't make much difference to my job"
Line staff	Brown OT	Creative Pt.-oriented	"Tried it once in another setting—it was OK"	"Not sure it will improve things here"
Dept. Manager	Murphy Med. Records	(Etc.)		
Administrator	(Etc.)			

ter several research questions so that meaning can be generated more easily. The questions or concepts may be decided upon before the study starts, or may be generated from the data after a period of data collection (Box 10–N).

b. **Cognitive map:** This displays an individual participant's ideas about a particular issue, showing the relationships among the ideas (Box 10–O).

c. **Effects matrix:** This matrix displays the outcome or effect of some intervention. It focuses on the dependent variable(s) of the study (Box 10–P).

Qualitative Causal Analysis

Some researchers may choose to end their analysis at this point, presenting a useful representation of the study data to readers, while others will choose to go further and

Box 10–N

Matrix showing innovation of new record-keeping system

PARTICIPANTS	*Greatest impact on whom?*	*Tenure: Leave or stay?*	*Attitude: Pos. or neg?*	*Pt. care: affected or not?*
		RESEARCH QUESTIONS		
Line staff	(fill cells with quotes)			
Dept. managers				
Medical Records staff				
Administrators				

Box 10–O

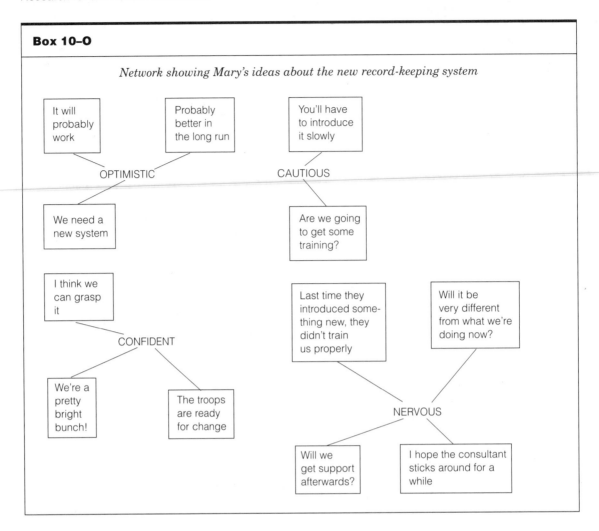

Network showing Mary's ideas about the new record-keeping system

Box 10–P

Matrix showing changes after implementation of record-keeping system

Effect on	Early Changes*		Later Changes†	
	Primary	Secondary	Primary	Secondary
Personnel				
Patients				
Patient records				
Other paperwork				
Communication with other facilities				

*Jan–July, 1996
†Aug–Dec, 1996

conduct a causal analysis. Miles and Huberman (1994) consider qualitative analysis a powerful method for getting at causality. Once a hypothesis is supported by one case, they recommend that the analytic procedure be repeated through a series of cases, lending greater confidence to the evolving hypothesis.

They describe displays, matrices, and networks that can support explanation-building and assist the researcher in making causal links within the data. Some of these displays include the following.

Explanatory Effects Matrix

This matrix asks, "Why were these outcomes achieved? What caused them, either generally or specifically?" (Miles & Huberman, 1994, p. 148). The matrix helps clarify an issue in conceptual terms, understanding things temporally. However, because each row is looked at one at a time as a causal sequence, it is difficult to grasp complexity and interactions between rows. More thorough causal analysis requires other display methods.

Case Dynamics Matrix

This matrix displays a set of forces for change and traces the resulting processes and outcomes. It addresses the problem of trying to understand why specific things happen as they do, and how the people in the study explain why things happen as they do.

Causal Network

This is a display of the most important independent and dependent variables in the study and of the relationships among them, showing directionality of the relationships. A causal network needs an associated analytic text describing the meaning of the relationships among variables.

Making and Testing Predictions

Predicting what will happen in your case after 6 months or a year has elapsed is a useful way to test the validity of your analysis. The anticipated implications or consequences should be spelled out and operationalized, then checked out with a new field contact. The result is the qualitative researcher's equivalent of the predictive validity coefficient that a quantitative researcher might use.

In summary, "Displays such as the *explanatory effects* matrix and *case dynamics* matrix are helpful in beginning to sort out what leads to what over time, but *causal networks* are better at dealing with the complexity of causal processes. They can be verified via informant feedback, but the strongest test of their accuracy is whether *predictions* based on them are confirmed or not" (Miles & Huberman, 1994, p. 171).

A Priori Coding

In a relatively simple study, such as describing the results of a survey of less than 50 respondents, first-step coding may be the only type of data processing necessary. If your survey contains several open-ended questions and you wish to portray an overall picture of respondents' views, you may choose to use the a priori coding method. In this method, named categories are decided upon before coding begins, and data obtained are then sorted by these categories. Loosely speaking, then, **a priori** refers to having named categories before data collection, whereas **a posteriori** coding refers to generating named categories from the data after it has been collected.

The categories selected during the design phase of the research project usually take the form of research questions. You perform a thorough review of the literature on the topic under study (just as occurs in quantitative research), and formulate questions that address your specific areas of interest. The list of research questions is often extensive, perhaps 10 or 15 questions, and addresses detailed specifics about the overarching study hypothesis (Box 10–Q).

Word Coding

When using the a priori method, one must have a way to look for equivalency or representation of the material in the transcripts to the content of the research questions. Some people choose to break down their research questions into component words or short phrases, which are then considered to represent the variables of interest in the study. These investigators then engage in

---

Box 10–Q

Schwartzberg interviewed patients with psychiatric problems to elicit their own perspectives on their treatment. Her overarching hypothesis was that they would have views on what blocked or facilitated their performance in work, leisure, and self-care activities. She also wished to shed light on what constituted their particular performance deficits and assets. She analyzed the patients' responses to identify patterns that responded to the following preformulated questions:

(a) what motivates a patient's involvement in occupational behaviors (the human activities of work, play, education, leisure, and self and environment care)?, (b) what contributes to the patient's lack of involvement in occupational behaviors?, (c) what is the relationship between a sense of well being and occupational behavior, for the patient?, (d) what is the potential relationship between values and type of involvement in daily life activities, for the patient?, (e) is there a perceived relationship between values and how the patient spends time? What is the nature of this relationship?, (f) do patients inherently value activities of daily living? If so, why and which activities? If not, why and which activities?, and (g) what configuration of daily life activities does the patient value and why?

(Schwartzberg, 1982, p. 12)

---

word coding, in which the analysis consists of going through the transcripts looking for the occurrence and frequency of the identified words and phrases. However, if the analyst simply uses the frequency of occurrence of words or phrases to suggest the degree of importance of that issue to informants, the study has been reduced to a quasi-quantitative study and will generally not be highly regarded. This technique is rarely used in recent times. Rather, the analyst must use judgment and experience with the group under study, to decide the relevance and import of the informant's responses in relation to the variables. The analyst should use such items as the tone of voice, body language, and emotional responses of informants to supplement their actual words during interviews.

Concept Coding

Another way of analyzing data when using the a priori approach is by concept coding. Here the researcher has a concept or idea in mind, as represented by each of the research questions, and notes when that concept is mentioned by respondents. This process is more difficult than word coding because the concept can be elusive, and it takes great concentration to decide if specific groups of words in the data comprise the concept. A priori concept coding requires training, expertise, patience, and perseverance.

Managing Data

Once the transcripts have been word-coded or concept-coded, it is left to the analyst to decide if there was sufficient occurrence of each research question theme, either in weight or frequency, to consider the topic important or relevant to the informant and to provide an answer to that research question. A priori coding uses mechanical techniques for managing data similar to those described earlier in this chapter. For instance, the a priori research questions may be assigned numbers, and those numbers may be inserted in the margin of the transcripts as they occur. The labeled transcripts may be cut and pasted or sections with like numbers may be inserted in separate folders for closer inspection.

Further analysis of the material represented by a single number or theme might yield other themes or patterns which can, in turn, be resorted and coded according to the new system. If you choose to proceed in this manner, you are now engaging in a posteriori coding methods, even though you began the project using the a priori approach.

Feasibility

Many researchers new to qualitative methods find the a priori method "doable" and less formidable than some of the previously described methods. They feel secure in having their research variables present and clearly articulated from the start. The coding techniques are manageable, and it is relatively easy to decide on an end point to the analysis. This is most important for students who need to keep graduation dates in mind or for clinicians who do not have the time to engage in long-term studies. Probably for these reasons, there seem to be many studies that loosely follow the a priori approaches described here, even though there is very little written about this method in research texts. Bogdan and Biklen (1982) described something roughly akin to the a priori approach in a section of their book entitled "Modified Analytic Induction," although they point out that analytic induction "has had a long and controversial history" (p. 65).

Summary

This chapter has presented several important strategies for analyzing qualitative data. Some potential analytic difficulties can be reduced if you have a general strategy for the analysis. With this strategy in mind, you are encouraged to "play with the data" in order to define the specific strategy that is most appropriate (e.g., pattern matching or coding). Skill and patience are required to execute most of these methods well. Qualitative data analysis is definitely a skill that improves with practice.

References

Bailey, D.M. (1996). *Occupational therapy managers' responses to ethical dilemmas.* Unpublished paper.

Bogdan, R.C. & Biklen, S.K. (1982). *Qualitative research for education: An introduction to theory and methods.* Boston: Allyn and Bacon.

Clark, C., Corcoran, M., & Gitlin, L. (1995). An exploratory study of how occupational therapists develop therapeutic relationships with family caregivers. *American Journal of Occupational Therapy, 49*(7), 587–594.

Glaser, B.G. (1978). *Theoretical sensitivity: Advances in the methodology of grounded theory.* Mill Valley, CA: Sociology Press.

Glaser, B.G. & Strauss, A.L. (1967). *The discovery of grounded theory: Strategies for qualitative research.* New York: Aldine De Gruyter.

Herzberg, F., Mausner, B., & Snyderman, B. (1959). *The motivation to work.* New York: John Wiley & Sons.

Lincoln, Y.S. & Guba, E.G. (1985). *Naturalistic enquiry.* Beverly Hills, CA: Sage Publications.

Miles, M.B., & Huberman, A.M. (1994). *Qualitative data analysis: An expanded sourcebook* (2d ed.). Thousand Oaks, CA: Sage.

Patton, M.Q. (1980). *Qualitative evaluation and research methods.* Newbury Park, CA: Sage.

Schwartzberg, S. (1982). Motivation for activities of daily living: A study of selected psychiatric patients' self-reports. *Occupational Therapy in Mental Health, 2*(3), 1–26.

Turner, B.A. (1981). Some practical aspects of qualitative data analysis: One way of organising the cognitive processes associated with the generation of grounded theory. *Quality and Quantity, 15,* 225–247.

Additional Reading

Gladwin, C.H. (1989). *Ethnographic decision tree modeling.* No. 19 in Qualitative Research Methods Series. Newbury Park, CA: Sage Publications.

11

Final Preparation Before Implementing the Research Plan

Now you are almost ready to conduct your project. Just two more items need to be dealt with before you begin. First, you must gain permission from the relevant human subjects committee(s) to put your study into practice. Second, you should consider running a pilot study.

Human Subjects Committee Procedures

Before you carry out your research intervention, you must submit a proposal describing your study to the human subjects committee that is responsible for safeguarding the rights of the subjects you will be studying. (These committees may be known by other names, such as institutional review board or research protocol review committee.) If you are a student, you will address the committee within your university; if you are a therapist, you will approach the committee within or connected to your facility. Students planning to study patients frequently need consent from the human subjects committees of both the university and the treating facility.

The purpose of human subjects committees is to ensure that individuals participat-

ing as subjects in research studies are protected and that ethical research standards are employed. This concern for the welfare of human subjects in medical research studies was organized into a worldwide system in 1964, at the 18th World Medical Assembly in Helsinki, Finland. At that meeting, what has come to be known as the Declaration of Helsinki was adopted by the assembly and has since provided the guiding principles for human subject research. The Declaration of Helsinki is reprinted in Appendix G.

Before embarking on your study, you must present a proposal to the appropriate human subjects committee(s) outlining the purpose, hypotheses, background, definitions of terms, and methodology of the study, as well as describing procedures you will use to ensure the safety of the subjects. When committee members are satisfied that their requirements have been met, they will give you permission to go ahead with the research study. The committee will review the proposal to see if it meets the following criteria:

1. The scientific logic on which the study is constructed is sound.
2. The study is worthwhile.
3. The proposed methodology is sound.
4. Procedures are safe.

5. The investigator has the skills to perform the study.

6. There is provision for informed consent by subjects.

7. The benefits of participating in the study outweigh the risks.

8. Subjects may withdraw their consent to participate at any time.

9. Subjects' confidentiality will be protected.

10. Necessary treatment will not be withheld.

Let's review these items in more detail:

1. **Sound scientific logic:** This issue will be addressed by the material you present to the committee on the background, literature review, and scope of the study. These sections of the proposal have already been prepared from the work you did in Chapters 2, 3, and 6, and a summary of these sections will explain the scientific logic of the study to the committee.

2. **Study is worthwhile:** This issue can be addressed by a summary of the sections you prepared on the purpose and significance of the study, following Chapter 3.

3. and 4. **Sound methodology, safe procedures:** These items are addressed by the material in Chapters 5 to 10 containing the research design and the techniques for collecting and analyzing data. The committee will decide whether the method is appropriate to the study and whether it will achieve the purpose of the study.

5. **Your skill:** Your qualifications for conducting the research may be substantiated by submission of a resume or by your presence before the committee to present your credentials.

6. **Informed consent:** Subjects and participants must understand the nature of the project, what procedures will be used, and to what use the results will be put (Box 11–A). Any explanation of the study must be made in lay terms. In survey research, subjects have given their tacit consent to participate if they return the survey. In experimental, quasi-experimental, and qualitative studies, subjects or participants give their consent in writing and must be offered a copy of the form they have signed. Samples of informed consent forms are given in Appendices H and I. If you feel that a subject is unable to give informed consent by virtue of cognitive or physical incapacity or age, the consent of the legal guardian must be obtained. If the subjects are children, the consent of the parents or guardians must be obtained (see Appendix K). If the nature of the research dictates that you cannot tell subjects the purpose of the study (because the knowledge

---

Box 11–A

The following excerpt from the 1994 Occupational Therapy Code of Ethics pertains to research behavior.

Principle 2. Occupational therapy personnel shall respect the rights of the recipients of their services. . . .

B. Occupational therapy personnel shall fully inform the service recipients of the nature, risks, and potential outcomes of any interventions.

C. Occupational therapy personnel shall obtain informed consent from subjects involved in research activities indicating they have been fully advised of the potential risks and outcomes.

D. Occupational therapy personnel shall respect the individual's right to refuse professional services or involvement in research or educational activities.

E. Occupational therapy personnel shall protect the confidential nature of information gained from educational, practice, research, and investigational activities.

(Commission on Standards and Ethics, 1994, p. 1037)

might bias results or responses), that must be explained honestly.

7. **Benefits outweigh risks:** In the consent form, any risks or benefits that may result from participating in the study must be explained to subjects (see Appendices H, I, and K; and Box 11–A). The committee will expect that the benefits will outweigh the risks. Possible side effects of the study should be pointed out, and precautions that will be taken by the researcher to prevent harm to subjects should be discussed. The place and length of time for the study sessions should be explained.

8. **Withdrawal of consent:** Included in the informed consent form should be a statement that there will be no reprisal, regardless of the subject's willingness to participate (see Box 11–A). Occasionally, clients may fear that their treatment may be compromised in some way if they refuse to participate in a study; perhaps they feel they will not receive the same quality of care as the study participants. This is a problem especially if the therapist carrying out the study is also the clients' treating therapist. It must also be made clear in the written consent form that subjects can terminate participation in the study at any point without fear of reprisal (see Appendix H).

9. **Confidentiality:** If there has been any audiotape or videotape recording of subjects' behavior or output, such as samples of subjects' writing or art work, the document must state how these materials will be used and what will happen to them at the conclusion of the study (see Box 11–A). It is usual to offer participants, subjects, or their guardians an opportunity to view the materials if they wish. Subjects must be assured that materials will be kept in a secure place during the study and told who will have access to them (see Appendices H and J).

If the results of the study are to be published, subjects need to know that their anonymity is guaranteed. Separate written permission must be gained if photographs are to be used in the published material (see Appendix J).

Survey respondents also need to be assured that their anonymity will be guarded. This is usually accomplished by having them return the surveys anonymously. Survey respondents are not asked to sign a consent form, because responding to the survey is considered as consent to participate.

If subjects are to be paid for their participation in the study, payment should be based on work and time considerations rather than as compensation for any risk involved or as inducement to poor subjects to participate.

10. **Treatment will not be withheld:** If there are to be experimental and control groups in the study, subjects might not be told to which group they are assigned. If the study is conducted to test a new procedure with the experimental group, the control groups may receive either the standard treatment or no treatment. Some facilities don't allow subjects to be in control groups that do not receive treatment, which is understandable, as these individuals are usually in the facility for the express purpose of being treated. This expectation will dictate the activity of the control group, and investigators must abide by the facility's regulations.

Ethics

Researchers are expected to behave ethically in all areas of their practice. It is the responsibility of the investigators themselves to know the rules of conduct. Professional associations each have a code of ethics: a public statement of the values and principles expected of practitioners in that profession. Some of these ethical principles pertain to therapists' research behavior (see Box 11–A). Researchers must show integrity and be guided by ethical principles that include respecting the rights of subjects, abiding by the research design, and reporting results as they are found.

It is particularly important to guard zealously the rights of subjects who are in institutional environments such as facilities for the mentally retarded, mental hospitals, and prisons. People in these settings are particularly vulnerable and are not usually in a position to serve as their own advocates; researchers must be especially careful not to take advantage of them. There is often an ombudsman or client advocate in these types of facilities, and researchers would do well to include such persons in the consent process.

Another ethical consideration is that investigators must abide by the research design as it was presented to and approved by the human subjects committee. Unexpected issues may arise that cause researchers to redesign their study. If this is the case, the revised design must be submitted to the committee to ensure that it still meets requirements. If any of the changes affects the agreement signed by the subjects, they too must be informed and a new agreement signed.

Finally, there are definite ethical standards involving the reporting of research results. Sometimes, some findings support the hypotheses while others do not. All findings must be reported. If findings are not at the identified level for statistical significance, they must be presented as found. The highest integrity must be maintained in reporting on all phases of the study, exactly as they occurred (see Box 11–A).

The above codes of behavior tend to fit issues raised in experimental research better than those raised during naturalistic inquiries. Ethical issues in qualitative research take a slightly different twist. In qualitative research, investigators must consider ethical issues raised when they become closely involved in the events or situations under study; confidentiality of data that may be extremely personal; anonymity of participants who may provide idiosyncratic and identifiable data; readers' ability to distinguish between data and the researchers' interpretations; possible long-term effects of in-depth interviewing about personal issues; and knowledge gained from participants' unselfconscious acts during participant observation. Some sources to help you think about these issues are suggested in the Additional Reading section at the end of this chapter.

Pilot Studies

Several times throughout this book, the pilot study has been suggested as a way to check on the feasibility of various components of the project. We now examine what a pilot study should include, how it is done, and what can be learned from it.

The pilot study is a preliminary trial of the study, or a ministudy, and should be performed before the final study. Most of the steps in the final study should be included in the pilot study, but on a smaller scale. The number of subjects used will be considerably smaller than the final sample size, but they should be selected from the target population, so that results are likely to be representative of those of the final study. The process will be that proposed for the major study, even including analysis of the data generated from the pilot group. As a result, the pilot study provides an evaluation of the proposed process and may be used to remove flaws.

A pilot study may reveal fundamental problems in the logic that leads to the hypotheses, in which case a major revision of the research questions may be in order. Lesser flaws may require only simple changes in the measuring instrument or subject selection criteria to make the project satisfactory. Some modifications of the original proposal are almost always necessary, so pilot studies invariably improve the design and data of the final project. It is always worthwhile to take the time and effort to perform a pilot study.

The items that may be tested in a pilot study concern methods and scientific logic. Those concerning scientific logic might include:

- Has the problem under study been too broadly or too narrowly defined?

- Are the variables suitable?
- Will the resulting data address the purpose of the study?

Methodological issues might include:

- Are the survey questions clearly stated and unambiguous?
- Will the investigative methods generate information suitable for answering the research question?
- Are appropriate subjects available?
- Are the variables discrete and can they be measured meaningfully?
- Is the measuring instrument accurate and practical?

Typically, certain items in each type of research design can be best evaluated by a pilot study. For example, in survey research, the way in which questions are composed is all-important. A pilot study will tell the investigator if respondents understand the questions, if the questions elicit the information desired, and whether the survey is too long or too short. Respondents should know that they are answering a pilot study instrument and that they will be asked if they have any suggestions for improvements in the questions and the cover letter and how long it took them to complete the survey.

Performing a pilot study can be difficult in experimental research because the investigator may have access to only a few subjects who meet the selection criteria. If subjects are used for a pilot study, there may not be sufficient subjects for the final study. In behavioral research, subjects often cannot be used twice (once in the pilot study and again in the final study) because the effects of the pilot treatment could influence the results of the final study treatment. Sometimes one can deal with this problem by using a pilot sample of suitable individuals from another facility or by using a slightly different population. This solution is often preferable to eliminating the pilot study altogether.

Sometimes experimental and quasi-experimental research studies are performed on very small samples with no pilot studies. Lacking a pilot study, the researchers undertake these studies with uncertain methodology and unclear justification for the study. The results of such projects are inevitably published with a list of limitations and disclaimers. These investigators would have

done better to regard the project as a pilot study, then pursue a second study, amending philosophy and procedures to escape the limitations of the first. The results of the second study would then be more valid, meaningful, and publishable (Boxes 11–B and 11–C).

Case study research is often conducted as a pilot study, in the sense that the individual case is used to generate hypotheses that will later be tested experimentally on a large sample of similar subjects. However, if the investigator does not intend the case study to be a pilot for a larger study, portions of the study may be piloted ahead of time. Portions

---

Box 11–B

"In a dental study conducted several years ago, the first batches of data collected were incomplete and ratings were remarkably similar across patients. The problem was that dental hygienists who were collecting the data had not been included in the decision-making process and did not appreciate data collection requirements. Piloting in that case should have included not only a sample of patients similar to the proposed subjects, but a sample of dental hygienists similar to those who would be collecting data. In the end, the inadequate data had to be treated as a pilot and discarded [from the final study]."

(Grady & Strudler Wallston, 1988, p. 148)

Box 11–C

In discussing the design of qualitative research, Marshall and Rossman state that:

. . . use of a pilot can lend credence to the researcher's claim that he can conduct such a study. He can illustrate his ability to manage qualitative research by describing initial observations or interviews. . . . A description of initial observations demonstrates not only the ability to manage this research, but also the strength of the approach for revealing enticing research questions. Inclusion of a description of a pilot study or initial observations can strengthen the proposal.

(Marshall & Rossman, 1989, p. 51)

that may be pretested include the use of equipment, the validity of a measuring instrument, or the usefulness of a data-gathering technique.

Historical research does not lend itself to the use of a pilot study because it involves only one event or chain of events being studied. If the method of data collection proves unsatisfactory, no harm has been done to the historical event and other methods may be explored. Generally, it is considered part of the study method to try different forms of data collection and data analysis until satisfactory methods are found.

Ethnographic research is similar to historical research in this respect. One culture or program is under study, and data can be collected and analyzed in many ways until the process is considered satisfactory. Sometimes an event within the culture or treatment program will occur only once (such as an unusual ceremony or a patient trying a rare treatment); in that case the investigator must be ready with the best method to capture that event exactly when it occurs. This may require preparation by testing certain techniques ahead of time; in other words, running a pilot study, perhaps in a simulated situation. It is almost always methodology, rather than scientific logic or philosophical issues, that needs testing in this type of once-only research. In fact, in ethnographic research, proposing and rejecting philosophical issues in the data analysis is one of the main ways of interpreting data, as was described in Chapter 10.

In methodological research, the pilot study is built into the research process at the stage when the newly developed measure is tested on a sample, changes are made, and the revised measure is tested again. The process may occur several times before the researcher feels satisfied with the results. This test/retest procedure serves the same purpose as a pilot study and may be considered as such.

In the summative component of evaluation research, the survey instruments used to garner data about the program under study may appropriately be subjected to a pilot study. This ensures that the questions will elicit needed data and be understood by respondents.

Finally, another important purpose of performing a pilot study is that it gives you a chance to practice conducting research. Like most things, research becomes easier and improves in quality with practice. A pilot study gives the novice researcher a good opportunity to gain skill while achieving the all-important goal of improving the research design.

Implementing the Project

You are finally ready to carry out your research project. As you can see, it takes an enormous amount of work to prepare for the treatment or action component of a research study. Yet often this is the only component that people equate with the term "research."

Practical issues must now be arranged. Depending on the type of research, these may be as varied as setting up times and places to meet with participants or subjects, arranging access to rooms and equipment, training raters or data gatherers, copying and mailing surveys, locating suitable client records for review, or arranging to videotape a group procedure.

Stumbling Blocks

Investigators often underestimate the length of time needed to gain permission from a human subjects committee. This process can take anywhere from 1 to 4 months, depending on the frequency of committee meetings and whether all materials have been submitted correctly and completely. If the protocol needs to be revised, it may take even longer. You should probably submit the proposal to the committee just about when the research protocol is being written. This will allow sufficient time for notification by the committee before the start of data collection.

Much time and aggravation can be saved by finding out ahead of time the exact requirements of the committee to which you are applying. Some committees have detailed written instructions, whereas others merely give a verbal outline. The packet of instructions for the Harvard Committee on Human Studies (1995), for instance, is about 30 pages long, whereas the submission requirements for a day activity program with which I am familiar are not defined in writing at all. A sample of guidelines for informed consent for a children's hospital is given in Appendix K.

I strongly recommend that you take the time to get to know the administrator of the human subjects committee. If you do, you are likely to be informed of exact requirements or of any changes in plans (such as meeting dates) and that your material will be processed quickly.

When describing a study to potential subjects in order to obtain their consent to participate, it is sometimes difficult to know if the explanation has been fully understood. This may be especially true when talking to clients who are mentally retarded or mentally ill. If there is any doubt about the client's comprehension, it is a good idea for the person who knows the client best to be present to assess how much is understood and perhaps to reword the explanation so that it is meaningful to the client. Some human subjects committees require that a member of the committee be present on such an occasion, whereas others have a human rights officer, an ombudsman, or an advocate who will serve this purpose.

WORKSHEETS

PROPOSAL FOR HUMAN SUBJECTS COMMITTEE

Find out which human subjects committee is responsible for the subjects or participants you intend to study. Request a copy of that committee's requirements. Following the guidelines, prepare a proposal for the committee. The committee may want the following information:

1. A general description of your study, including its background. Detail the problem you will be addressing and your purpose (what you hope to achieve). Define the terms you will be using and spell out the research questions or hypotheses. You should state the importance or significance of the project. Describe the method you will use, including subjects, research design, and data collection techniques. All of this material is available from the worksheets in previous chapters.

2. An informed consent statement for subjects.

Prepare an informed consent statement (see samples in Appendices H and I). Remember to:

- Include the purpose of the study
- Include the place and the amount of time the study will require of subjects
- Include a description of the procedure to be used
- State that participation is voluntary
- State that participation can be withdrawn at any time without fear or reprisal
- List the risks and benefits of the study
- Cite any costs that may be involved
- Describe how confidentiality will be protected
- Give the name of someone who will be available to answer questions about the research
- State that a copy of this statement will be offered to subjects
- Provide a space for the subject's signature, a witness's signature, and, if needed, a parent/guardian signature
- Provide a space for the date of the signatures

3. The names of all the investigators involved in the study. List your qualifications as head of the research team, and state why you are qualified to carry out the proposed research project.

Find out if you may be present at the meeting to answer questions about your proposal.

Find out when and in what manner you will be advised if your proposal is accepted.

PILOT STUDY

Decide whether your study lends itself to a pilot study. Will methodological issues, scientific logic issues, or both need to be piloted? List the parts you think could be improved by a pilot study and say why.

Methodological issues:

Scientific logic issues:

Can you afford to use some of the target population for the pilot study sample?

If so, how will you select them?

If not, where can you find pilot study subjects?

Write a protocol for a pilot study. It will resemble the protocol you wrote earlier and should contain the following:

- Subject criteria
- Subject selection method
- Research questions or hypotheses
- Variables
- Procedures for treatment (if quantitative research)
- Data collection techniques (if quantitative research)
- Data analysis methods (if quantitative research)
- Procedures for data collection and analysis (if qualitative research)

References

Commission on Standards and Ethics, AOTA. (1994). Occupational Therapy Code of Ethics. *American Journal of Occupational Therapy, 48*(11), 1037–1038.

Grady, K.E., & Strudler Wallston, B. (1988). *Research in health care settings.* No. 14 in Applied Social Research Methods Series. Newbury Park, CA: Sage Publications.

The Harvard Committee on Human Studies. (1995). *Policies and Procedures of the Harvard Committee on Human Studies:* Policies and procedures governing the conduct of research, development, or related activities involving human subjects carried out at the Harvard Medical School or Harvard School of Dental Medicine or under their aegis in the facilities of an affiliated institution. Cambridge, MA: Harvard Medical School and Harvard School of Dental Medicine.

Marshall, C., & Rossman, G.B. (1989). *Designing qualitative research.* Newbury Park, CA: Sage Publications.

Additional Reading

American Occupational Therapy Foundation: Research Advisory Council. (1986). *Ethical considerations for research in occupational therapy.* Rockville, MD: Author.

Berger, R.M., & Patchner, M.A. (1988). Chapter 7: Research ethics. In *Implementing the research plan: A guide for the helping professions* (pp. 143–154). No. 51 in Human Services Guides Series. Newbury Park, CA: Sage Publications.

Bogdan, R.C., & Biklen, S.K. (1982). *Qualitative research for education: An introduction to theory and methods.* Boston, MA: Allyn and Bacon.

Currier, D.P. (1984). Chapter 4: The proposal and ethics. In *Elements of research in physical therapy* (pp. 51–73). Baltimore: Williams & Wilkins.

Glesne, C. & Peshkin, A. (1992). Chapter 6: But is it ethical? Learning to do it right. In *Becoming qualitative researchers: An introduction* (pp. 109–125). White Plains, NY: Longman.

Merriam, S.B. (1988). Chapter 10: Dealing with validity, reliability, and ethics in case study research. In *Case study research in education: A qualitative approach* (pp. 163–184). San Francisco: Jossey-Bass.

Noonan, M.J., & Bickel, W.K. (1981). The ethics of experimental designs. *Mental Retardation, 19*(6), 271–274.

Schwartzberg, S.L. (1980). The Foundation: Issues in human subject occupational therapy research. *American Journal of Occupational Therapy, 34*(8), 537–538.

12

Reporting Results and Drawing Conclusions

Now that you have conducted your experimental study or been in the field gathering and interpreting qualitative data about your informants, you are ready to write the final report. This chapter discusses various formats for presenting your findings, depending on whether you have conducted quantitative or qualitative research.

Quantitative Research

In quantitative research, the results of the study and the discussion and conclusions about the study are presented in separate sections. In a thesis they are in two separate chapters. First, the results are presented in numerical form. They may also be displayed pictorially. Then interpretations are made and conclusions drawn.

Reporting the Data

In the results section of a paper, only the facts of the study are presented, with no interpretation. Authors must be careful not to include their own biases or conclusions in the results section. Rather, they must keep to a factual recording of what actually happened and what was actually found.

All the results must be mentioned in the results section of a report, not only the ones that substantiate the hypotheses or suit the investigator's needs. Even though you will later present your own interpretations and conclusions from the results, readers must be able to decide for themselves the efficacy of these conclusions by having all the data at hand. At the end of the results section, it should be clearly stated which of the hypotheses were or were not supported. In the case of inferential statistical results, the reader should be told if the significance level established at the start of the project was reached.

First, you need to describe the subjects numerically (Box 12–A). From this information, it will be possible for readers to gain a clear picture of the study sample, so that later they may superimpose the findings of the study on that picture. No matter what type of research design you have used, you will want to describe the sample. It is usual to present frequencies, percentages, a range, and some sort of central tendency (such as the mean) for the data. This information will give readers solid information about what your subjects looked like and how they performed in the study (Box 12–B).

If you have conducted experimental, quasi-experimental, or correlational research, your study will have yielded quantitative data, and you may have used inferential statistics to determine if there are meaningful differences or similarities between groups. The probability ratios will provide that information and will indicate if the

---

Box 12–A

"A convenience sample of 20 consumers at a community support services program participated in the study. . . . The sample consisted of 11 men and 9 women, with 9 being Caucasian and 11 African-American. The mean age was 37 years. Six of the participants lived alone in their own apartment, 5 lived with a roommate, 8 lived with family, and 1 lived in a group home."

(Brown, Moore, Hemman, & Yunek, 1996, p. 203)

---

hypotheses have been substantiated. At this point, go back to each of the hypotheses and check them against the statistical results (Box 12–C). For each hypothesis, inform readers if the hypothesis was substantiated, give the probability level, then report the details of the findings. It is customary for results to be reported from the general to the specific.

If you have conducted a survey, case study, or evaluation research, you will probably have garnered descriptive quantitative data. The data will continue to be reported in a manner similar to that used to describe the sample; that is, using frequencies, percentages, ranges, and central tendencies.

Box 12–B

"Twenty-one subjects were selected (12 men and 9 women). Their ages ranged from 51 to 78 years, with a mean age of 64.5 years ($SD = 8.9$). Fourteen subjects had experienced a first onset of CVA and 7 a second onset. The duration from the most recent onset until data collection ranged from 23 days to 176 days, with a mean duration of 81.6 days ($SD = 46.5$). The sample consisted of 7 subjects with left hemiplegia and 14 with right hemiplegia. The period of data collection was 69 days.

". . . . Brunnstrom's upper extremity stage for the 21 subjects ranged from 2 to 6, with a mean stage of 3.9 ($SD = 1.0$); the lower extremity stage was from 3 to 6, with a mean stage of 4.4 ($SD = .8$)."

(Hsieh, Nelson, Smith, & Peterson, 1996, p. 12)

Box 12–C

A study was conducted comparing younger subjects (aged 20 to 60 years) with older subjects (aged 61 to 80 years) on body image, as measured by a semantic differential scale of attitudes toward various body parts. Therapists subjected data from the two groups to the Mann-Whitney U test to test the hypotheses that elderly and younger adults would have significantly different perceptions of their trunk, arms, hands, and legs. The level of significance was set at $p < .05$. The study showed that elderly subjects perceive only their hands as substantially different from those of younger adults.

To determine in which direction the difference lay, the investigators turned to the means of scores on the semantic differential. They found that the mean for the older group was smaller (less positive) for hands than the mean for the younger group; thus they had a finding: that community-based elders had a less positive body image regarding their hands than did younger adults.

(Van Deusen, Harlowe, & Baker, 1989)

In a descriptive study reporting on the incidence of upper extremity discomfort among piano students, Revak (1989) used a survey to generate data. Revak describes the results concerning the respondents' discomfort as shown in Box 12–D. He continues to report the results in this fashion, listing frequencies and percentages for each finding in the study so that readers gain a graphic picture of the pianist respondents and their upper extremity discomforts. This is a typical and most effective method for reporting descriptive research findings. Having such a complete roster of data about respondents allows readers to form their own opinions and draw their own conclusions concerning the sample.

In a nonexperimental study, you may have subjected some data to one or more of the coding procedures. The results of the coding must be presented as clearly and simply as possible. In this type of presentation, it is the weight of the evidence that will determine if the hypotheses have been substantiated—a judgment the investigator must make because it is not possible to subject the evidence to statistical significance testing.

Box 12-D

"Eighty-three percent of the respondents with physical discomfort reported more than one symptom. Pain or aching of the upper extremities was the predominant discomfort experienced. . . .

"The respondents were divided into two groups, those who sought treatment and those who did not. The discomforts reported by each group differed. Pain/aching (82%) was the only physical discomfort reported by more than half of the students who sought medical treatment. Students in this group also frequently complained of tenderness (47%). Over half of the students not seeking medical treatment reported pain/aching (71%), fatigue (65%), weakness (59%), and muscle cramp (53%). . . .

"Fifteen (50%) of the students that experienced physical discomfort reported it in both hands and/or arms. Eight students reported discomfort only on the right side, and six students reported discomfort only on the left. As shown in Table 2, the most frequent regions of discomfort were the hand (49%), the forearm (19%), and the wrist (16%). Discomfort was reported nearly equally on the dorsal and volar surfaces of the wrist and forearm."

(Revak, 1989, pp. 150–151)

Pictorial Display of Data

Sometimes it is useful to display data pictorially. This allows readers to gain an immediate and overall concept of the results and lets them make sense of quantities of data at a glance; as the old saying goes, "A picture is worth a thousand words," or in this case, a thousand numbers. Tables, graphs, or charts can eliminate many complicated or boring sentences, but they should be used judiciously; too many become confusing.

Many pictorial means exist for presenting data. The following are some of the most commonly used. Simple lists of frequencies and percentages are probably best presented in tabular form. Use tables to consolidate and present data, such as numbers of pounds squeezed on a goniometer. If scores were arranged in order from highest to lowest (rank ordering), for example, readers could easily gain an overview of a group of responses. They could see the range of scores—the high-

est, lowest, and middle scores—and could compare one person's scores against the others. Table 12–1 shows the rank ordering of two types of values reported by 385 occupational therapy administrators and clinicians.

Tables are especially useful for condensing large quantities of data so that the reader can make sense of the information more readily. Suppose a study yielded 50 scores of degrees of elbow flexion for a group of patients. Even presenting the 50 scores in order of magnitude would be difficult for a reader to digest and think about usefully. In this case, grouping the scores, say into units of 20, would reduce the data and allow the reader to grasp its implications more efficiently (Table 12–2). From this table it is possible to understand quickly the spread of scores; that most patients had flexion in the midrange (60 degrees to 120 degrees), whereas few patients had flexion at the greater and smaller angles. Even though some detail is lost in this type of grouping, it is generally a useful and efficient representation of data.

Tables are commonly used to illustrate the findings from descriptive and inferential statistics. In this case, they can present detailed materials more easily and in less space than would be required by narration. It is not necessary to repeat all the table data in the text; the investigator should merely highlight important points. Tables 12–3 and 12–4 present data generated from descriptive statistics and inferential statistics.

Although tables are invaluable for communicating concisely a large set of numbers, many people find it difficult to get the "big picture" from a table. This is why we turn to graphs to convey a visual image of a distribution of items or events, or changes in numbers of items over time, or how several items compare.

There are many types of graphs, one of the most popular being the frequency polygon, illustrated in Figure 12–1, where a single line joins frequency points of occurrence. There is traditionally a y-axis noting the frequency of items or events and an x-axis charting the item under study. In Figure 12–1, the hours per week a student requires supervision are entered on the graph. All of the points are joined to form a continuous line on the graph. The bar graph or histogram is illustrated in Figure 12–2 and is

TABLE 12–1   **Rank Ordering of Terminal and Instrumental Values by Occupational Therapy Administrators and Clinicians (N = 385)**

	Administrators' Rank Ordering (n = 201)	Clinicians' Rank Ordering (n = 184)	Total Group Rank Ordering
Terminal values:			
Self-respect	1	2	2
Health	2	1	1
A sense of accomplishment	3	5	4
Inner harmony	4	3	3
Freedom	5	6	5
Wisdom	6	4	6
Mature love	7	7	7
An exciting life	8	8	8
A comfortable life	9	9	9
Equality	10	10	10
Social recognition	11	12	12
Pleasure	12	11	11
Instrumental values:			
Capable	1	3	3
Honest	2	1	1
Responsible	3	2	2
Independent	4	4	4
Loving	5	5	5
Helpful	6	6	6
Courageous	7	9	9
Broad-minded	8	7	7
Loyal	9	8	8
Imaginative	10	10	10
Ambitious	11	11	11
Obedient	12	12	12

similar to the frequency polygon, except that it is formed by drawing a vertical bar at each frequency gained, across the width of the score interval. The number of students achieving each test score forms a solid block on the graph; in this way, the histogram offers a strong visual impact.

When one group of scores is compared with another, such as scores from 1989 and scores from 1990, both types of graph may be used, but the histogram is particularly visually effective. Figures 12–3 and 12–4 illustrate this point. A pie chart is often used to depict a breakdown of some quantity; for example, expenditures for a program or types of employees in a facility, as shown in Figure 12–5.

These are just three of the many possibilities for displaying data pictorially. For further ideas, you may refer to the books mentioned in the Additional Reading list at the end of this chapter.

If you use pictorial methods for presenting data, be sure to refer to specific tables or figures in the text. Label them correctly—tables are called "tables;" whereas graphs, charts, drawings, photographs, and so forth, are called "figures." In the text, tell readers what to look for in the tables and figures, picking out salient features. You do not need to repeat all the material shown in the pictorial, but you should highlight the most important points.

TABLE 12–2   **Degrees of Elbow Flexion Following Treatment (N = 50)**

Degrees of Elbow Flexion	Frequency of Occurrence
20–40	2
40–60	4
60–80	9
80–100	10
100–120	12
120–140	9
140–160	3
160–180	1

TABLE 12–3   **Distribution of Demographic Characteristics for Occupational Therapy Administrators and Clinicians (N = 385)**

Demographic Characteristic	Administrators (n = 201)		Clinicians (n = 184)		Total Group	
	Frequency	Percent	Frequency	Percent	Frequency	Percent
Age:						
20–25 years	0	0	2	1	2	0.5
26–30 years	17	9	46	25	63	16
31–35 years	56	28	52	28	108	28
36–40 years	33	16	26	14	59	15
41–50 years	53	26	40	22	93	24
51 + years	42	21	18	10	60	16
College degrees:						
BA or BS in OT	95	47	113	61	208	57
Certification in OT	13	10	17	9	30	8
MOT	10	6	8	4	18	6
MA or MS in OT	21	11	4	2	25	7
Non-OT MA/MS	47	25	19	15	66	17
Doctorate	4	2	0	0	4	1
When subject decided to become an OT:						
Jr. high school	20	10	11	6	31	8
Sr. high school	60	30	61	33	121	31
First 2 years of college	80	40	71	39	151	39
Second 2 years of college	18	9	16	9	34	9
After college	12	6	14	8	26	7
Other	11	5	11	6	22	6
Age when took first job as an OT:						
20–25 years	178	89	156	85	334	87
26–30 years	14	7	14	8	28	7
31–35 years	4	2	5	3	9	2
36–40 years	2	1	5	3	7	2
41 + years	5	2	4	2	9	2
Specialty within OT:						
Psychiatry	60	30	49	27	109	29
Pediatrics	31	15	59	32	90	24
Physical disabilities	95	47	63	35	158	41
Geriatrics	15	8	11	6	26	7

TABLE 12–4   **Differences Between Administrators and Clinicians on Demographic Characteristics (N = 385)**

Role by Characteristic	Pearson Chi-square	Significance Level
Role by age	31.22	0.00*
Role by degree	31.22	0.00*
Role by age when decided to become an OT	2.68	0.75
Role by age at taking first job	2.24	0.69
Role by specialty in OT	18.20	0.00*
Role by mother's education	3.71	0.81
Role by father's education	7.73	0.36
Role by mentor	6.22	0.10

*$p < .001$

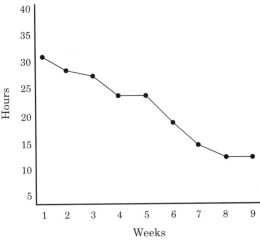

FIGURE 12–1   Hours per week during which a student requires supervision.

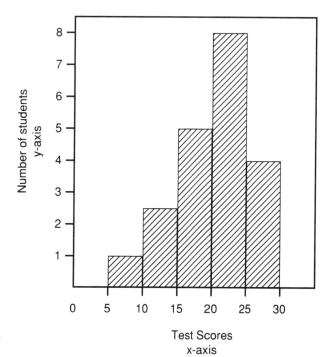

FIGURE 12–2 Histogram showing students' test scores.

With accurate and complete titles, column headings, axes labels, and footnotes, tables should be understandable on their own, without text. Titles should be concise and describe exactly the information included. If a table is to be studied without any text, the title should be complete enough for readers to know what to expect and to be able to read the contents.

Interpretations and Conclusions

Now go back to the literature review. It is time to compare your results with those of

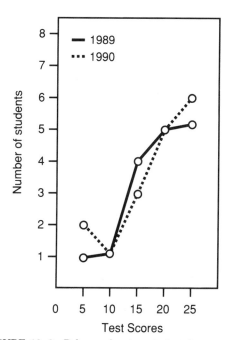

FIGURE 12–3 Polygon showing students' test scores for 1989 and 1990.

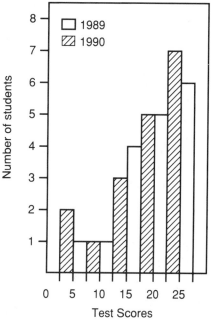

FIGURE 12–4 Histogram showing students' test scores for 1989 and 1990.

others who have studied the topic. Integrate your findings with those of previous studies, and note points of agreement and departure. You might have suggestions as to why you found different results, as pointed out by the authors in the study described in Box 12–E. The purpose of comparing your findings with those of similar studies is to put your study in a context with work that has already been done on the topic. Ideally, your study should be contributing to a larger body of work, adding one more brick to the wall of knowledge about that topic and perhaps adding evidence that will tip the scales in one direction or the other concerning theory about a particular issue.

At this point, you may speculate and draw your own conclusions about what the results mean. You are interpreting the results. Start by discussing the similarities and differences between the results of your study and those of other studies. Keep adding to the reader's understanding of the entire problem under investigation with each new statement you make, relating your findings to other people's theories about the problem. Any finding is fair game for comment, as long as it was reported in the results section. However, you should not discuss a finding that was not reported. This is also true of theorists. If an author was not mentioned in the literature review section, that person's name may not be introduced in the conclusion section.

Findings that do not support the hypotheses or do not conform with other findings from the study should be commented upon. It is customary to speculate as to why they occurred and what they might mean, as shown in Box 12–F. Notice that the author does not apologize for the fact that the finding does not conclusively support the hypothesis. She merely makes the statement, conjectures as to why this result may have been found, and suggests that a different approach should be taken with this type of subject in future studies on upper-extremity weight bearing.

This brings us to the topic of what to do about the study that generates few data in support of the proposed hypotheses. Should this study be reported and published? Sometimes it is important that health professionals be given access to the results of such studies because of one of the following:

- They may put to rest a popular myth that needs to be dispelled (Box 12–G).

- They may show that a particular methodology or research design is not a useful way to investigate a particular problem, thus saving others from making the same mistake.

- Others may learn from the flaws and problems in the studies, which may then be redesigned to achieve the original purpose.

In the final section of the paper, it is customary to remark on the shortcomings of the study, but it is not necessary to dwell on them. A simple acknowledgment is sufficient. Sometimes an instrument may have proved unreliable; subjects may have dropped out of the study; or there may have been some unforeseen interference with the study procedure. Whatever the problem, the reader will assume that you did what you could to correct it and that you ran the study to the best of your ability. Giving readers the information will allow them to decide for themselves if the integrity of the study has been compromised (Box 12–H).

Summary of the Quantitative Report

Once you have interpreted your findings and drawn conclusions, it is customary to summarize what has happened during the study. In the summary, you are answering the questions:

1. What have I contributed?

2. How has my study helped to solve the original problem?

3. What conclusions and theoretical implications can I draw from my study?

If the study is being written as an article for a professional journal, a paragraph is usually all that can be devoted to the summary, owing to space constraints. Trying to answer the three questions above in a paragraph is a challenge, but it can be done. It should be noted that many journals require an abstract, which is printed at the beginning of the article. Some editors feel that this summarizes the article sufficiently and discourage authors from adding a summary at the end.

It is appropriate to suggest briefly improvements that could be made in the study procedures and design and to propose new research that may be appropriate based on

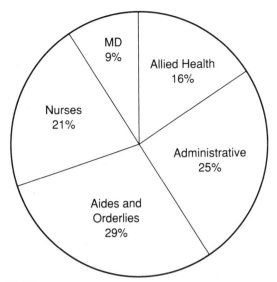

FIGURE 12–5   Pie chart depicting percentages of personnel employed in a hospital.

Qualitative Research

Writing up the findings from a qualitative study is quite a different proposition. Data collection and analysis tend to be cyclical, the researcher collecting and analyzing some data and then returning to the field to collect data with a more focused approach. This process may be repeated several times, as the analysis becomes more focused and the researcher has a clear image of the outcome of the study. Because of the integrated nature

---

Box 12–E

Van Deusen, Harlowe, and Baker (1989) report (a) similar findings to a study that used a wider age group than theirs and (b) inconsistent findings with a similar study in which the younger age group had been separated into two sections. The authors suggest that differences in findings in the latter case might have been due to the use of different measurement procedures. They also state that they cannot compare their project to a third study because the researchers had used different assessment tools.

Box 12–F

In Barnes's study on the relationship of upper-extremity weight bearing to hand skills of boys with cerebral palsy, the author states in the discussion:

> The data on the left arm of Subject 4 are inconclusive. Subject 4's performance may have differed from that of Subject 5 and 6 because of his bilateral elbow contractures. The weightbearing treatment technique may not be as effective with subjects with contractures as with those free of joint limitations; therefore, alternate strategies for such patients should be considered.

(Barnes, 1989, p. 241)

---

of data collection and data analysis, the results and discussion of a qualitative study are written as one. They make up the bulk of the qualitative research article.

Using Examples

Naturalistic research yields rich descriptions that are used throughout the discussion portion of the article, resulting in a lengthy nar-

---

Box 12–G

Some writers have suggested that splinting would be helpful in increasing function for patients with hand contractures due to progressive systemic sclerosis. Seeger and Furst's study showed that this was not the case with their sample. Their abstract reads:

> One of the major factors in the decreasing functional ability of patients with progressive systemic sclerosis is involvement of the patient's hands with secondary immobility and contractures. In a 2-month study of 19 patients, we assessed whether dynamic splinting could decrease proximal interphalangeal (PIP) flexion contractures. Of the eight patients who completed the study, one experienced a statistically significant improvement in PIP range of motion as a result of the splinting. There was no evidence that the use of splints served to maintain PIP extension when compared with the control hand.

(Seeger & Furst, 1987, p. 118)

Box 12–H

While investigating the relationship between oral sensation and drooling in persons with cerebral palsy, Weiss-Lambrou, Tetreault, and Dudley warn readers that their findings:

> ... should be interpreted with caution because of the following methodological limitations: (a) the small sample size; (b) the poor test-retest reliability of the tests of oral stereognosis and oral form discrimination; and (c) the lack of data on interrater reliability.
>
> The tests of oral sensation used in this study were not designed for persons with cerebral palsy; consequently, the major difficulty encountered in examining this parameter was the lack of oral sensation tests that are applicable with this population.

(Weiss-Lambrou, Tetreault, & Dudley, 1989, p. 160)

---

rative. Illustrative quotations are usually used to convey an understanding of what settings and people are like. Examples should each be short and to the point because most readers find it tedious to read through long quotes. Resist the temptation to overuse colorful data; no single quote should be used more than once. "Verbatim quotations are extremely useful in presenting a credible report of the research. Quotations allow the reader to judge the quality of the work—how close the ethnographer is to the thoughts of

---

Box 12–I

Davis and Bordieri not only suggest directions for further research based on their work, but also say why such research would be helpful to the profession:

> ... the next research step would be to identify strategies that foster perceived autonomy and that combat the disincentives reported by occupational therapists. This line of research would be invaluable to occupational therapy managers in today's competitive market who are seeking to attract, retain, and professionally motivate their staff members, and thus ensure the highest possible level of patient care.

(Davis & Bordieri, 1988, p. 595)

---

the [participants] ... and to assess whether the ethnographer used such data appropriately to support the conclusions. The ethnographer therefore must select quotations that are typical or characteristic of the situation or event described" (Fetterman, 1989, p. 22).

Using Pictorials

It is often appropriate to use charts, matrices, and graphs to display verbal data, particularly if the researcher is using Miles and Huberman's (1994) or Patton's (1990) data analysis techniques. These techniques have been described in some detail in Chapter 10. When used in a research article, they serve the same purpose as pictorial representations of numerical data from quantitative research: to help the reader understand large amounts of data by presenting it in an organized, accessible, and condensed format.

Writing Formats

The writing of the analysis, meanings, interpretations, and implications of a qualitative study may take different forms, depending on the naturalistic design that was used. For example, in an ethnography in which the prime purpose is to describe a culture, the report may be written chronologically in the order in which the information was gleaned and understood. Interpretations and supporting literature may be sprinkled throughout the write-up. In a phenomenological design, on the other hand, which focuses on the unique experience of a particular group of persons, the report may be written as a story, told from the perspective of the participants. Emphasis is placed on the participants' own words to depict their viewpoint and researcher interpretations are kept to a minimum.

Ringing True to the Participants

The success or failure of the analysis depends on the degree to which it rings true to participants and colleagues. Readers may disagree with the researcher's interpretations and conclusions, but they should recognize the details of the description as accurate. The researcher's task is not only to collect information from the emic or insider's perspective, but also to make sense of all the data from an etic or external social scientific perspective. A researcher's explanation of the group or event may differ from that of the participants or other professionals, but basic descriptions of events and places should sound familiar to both groups.

Reporting the results of your study, interpreting them, drawing conclusions or formulating new theories are the last components of the research process. All that remains is getting the written report into suitable shape for publication.

Stumbling Blocks

Some professional journals have a limit on the number of pictorial representations (tables and figures) that may be used, because of reproduction costs. The author's guide, which is provided by the publisher, will probably mention any such limitation.

When interpreting your findings from experimental studies, the temptation is to try to make too much of the results. Investigators sometimes fall into the trap of extrapolating information and drawing conclusions that are not really warranted from the available data. It is important to stand back and critically review the data, asking yourself, "Am I justified in drawing this conclusion?" and "Is this really what the data mean?" Sometimes a colleague can offer an objective view, should you become so embroiled in your own findings that you start drawing unwarranted conclusions.

Novice qualitative researchers, on the other hand, often end their data analyses too soon, losing the opportunity to develop their ideas about the topic fully. They often describe their findings in great detail but make only cursory mention of new thoughts about the group or event. Remember that most qualitative studies are made in an attempt to generate new theories or hypotheses, and extensive analysis of the data is needed to achieve this goal.

WORKSHEETS

REPORTING RESULTS

Describe the sample in numerical terms:

Total number:

If subjects are people, include:

Mean age:

Age range:

Number of male and female subjects:

Qualifications:

Other attributes relevant to your study:

or

If subjects are records or other items, describe relevant characteristics:

Tabulate the data from your data sheets (these may be measurements from tests or equipment, returned surveys, recordings from interviews, data from client records, notations on observation sheets, and so on).

If you are using descriptive quantitative data:

Code your results, using the method you proposed earlier:

If you are using quantitative data:

Perform the statistical analyses on your tabulated data using the methods you proposed earlier. If you are working with a statistician, this is the time to take your material to him or her.

List your research questions or hypotheses here:

A.

B.

C.

D.

Review the results of the data analyses.

If you are using inferential statistics:

Did the findings reach significance levels for:

Hypothesis			
	A.	____Yes	____ No
	B.	____Yes	____ No
	C.	____Yes	____ No
	D.	____Yes	____ No

For each hypothesis that achieved significance, go back to the tabulated raw data to see the direction of the result (e.g., positive or negative, more of or less of, greater than or smaller than).

Go back and note beside each hypothesis whether or not it was supported by the data.

If you are using descriptive data:

Following your coding, does the preponderance of evidence suggest support for the hypotheses?

Hypothesis			
	A.	____Yes	____ No
	B.	____Yes	____ No
	C.	____Yes	____ No
	D.	____Yes	____ No

INTERPRETATIONS AND CONCLUSIONS

Turn to the literature review section and state whether your findings agree with or differ from the findings of earlier studies you have mentioned.

Authors of study   Findings agree   Findings differ

For those findings that differ, speculate here as to what you think caused the difference.

Now, interpret your findings and draw conclusions for each hypothesis:

Hypothesis A

Hypothesis B

Hypothesis C

Hypothesis D

SUMMARY SECTION

Address the following questions:

What have I contributed here?

How has my study helped to solve the original problem?

What conclusions and theoretical implications can I draw from my study?

Mention any major shortcomings of the study:

Suggest improvements that could be made in the study design or procedures:

Propose new research that would build on your study:

References

Barnes, K. (1989). Direct replication: Relationship of upper extremity weight bearing to hand skills of boys with cerebral palsy. *Occupational Therapy Journal of Research, 9*(4), 235–242.

Brown, C., Moore, W.P., Hemman, D., & Yunek, A. (1996). Influence of instrumental activities of daily living assessment method on judgments of independence. *American Journal of Occupational Therapy, 50*(3), 202–206.

Davis, G., & Bordieri, J. (1988). Perceived autonomy and job satisfaction in occupational therapists. *American Journal of Occupational Therapy, 42*(9), 591–595.

Fetterman, D.M. (1989). *Ethnography step by step*. Newbury Park, CA: Sage Publications.

Hsieh, C., Nelson, D., Smith, D.A., & Peterson, C.Q. (1996). A comparison of performance in added-purpose occupations and rote excercise for dynamic standing balance in persons with hemiplegia. *American Journal of Occupational Therapy, 50*(1), 10–16.

Miles, M.B. & Huberman, A.M. (1994). *Qualitative data analysis: An expanded sourcebook* (2nd ed.). Thousand Oaks, CA: Sage Publications.

Patton, M.Q. (1990). *Qualitative evaluation and research methods* (2nd ed.). Newbury Park, CA: Sage Publications.

Revak, J. (1989). Incidence of upper extremity discomfort among piano students. *American Journal of Occupational Therapy, 43*(3), 149–154.

Seeger, M.W., & Furst, D.E. (1987). Effects of splinting in the treatment of hand contractures in progressive systemic sclerosis. *American Journal of Occupational Therapy, 41*(2), 118–121.

Van Deusen, J., Harlowe, D., & Baker, L. (1989). Body image perceptions of the community-based elderly. *Occupational Therapy Journal of Research, 9*(4), 243–248.

Weiss-Lambrou, R., Tetreault, S., & Dudley, J. (1989). The relationship between oral sensation and drooling in persons with cerebral palsy. *American Journal of Occupational Therapy, 43*(3), 155–161.

Additional Reading

Cox, R., & West, W. (1986). Chapter 7: Dealing with data. In *Fundamentals of research for health professionals* (pp. 67–87). Laurel, MD: RAMSCO Publishing Co.

Currier, D.P. (1990). Chapter 12: Revealing research. In *Elements of research in physical therapy* (3rd ed.). Baltimore: Williams & Wilkins.

Morris, B., Fitz-Gibbon, J., & Freeman C. (1987). *How to communicate research findings*. Newbury Park, CA: Sage Publications.

Oyster, C.K., Hanten, W.P., & Llorens, L.A. (1987). Chapter 15: Communicating research. In *Introduction to research: A guide for the health science professional* (pp. 190–207). Philadelphia: J.B. Lippincott.

Writing and Publishing

You have made it to the final stage, but don't sit back and think you have finished! No research project is complete until the results are shared. Unfortunately, this is often the point at which investigators run out of steam, and the material languishes in a drawer waiting to be written. Until colleagues are informed about the findings of the study, those findings are not useful. The only benefit up to this point is that you have had the opportunity to conduct a piece of research.

If you completed the worksheets in this book as you went along, you have done most of the work involved in writing the study. When carrying out future research projects, if you can bring yourself to do the writing as you conduct each phase of a project, producing the final report will be far less formidable. This does not mean that the material is written in its final form, but rather that the thinking and planning you went through are captured on paper. It is then a relatively simple matter to put those notes into a suitable form, either for publication in a journal or as a thesis. The format and amount of detail for journal publications and for theses are quite different, and the two will be addressed separately here.

Publishing in a Journal

If you wish to submit your work for publication in a professional journal, you will need to select an appropriate publication, find out about the required writing style, write up your work in that format, submit the article, wait for the review process, make requested revisions, and comply with copyright procedures.

Choosing a Journal

You may already have decided which professional journal you will submit your study to. Sometimes it is clear that one is more appropriate than another. For occupational therapists and physical therapists, the choices are usually the *American Journal of Occupational Therapy, Physical Therapy,* the *Occupational Therapy Journal of Research, Physical and Occupational Therapy Journal in Pediatrics, Physical and Occupational Therapy Journal in Geriatrics,* or *Occupational Therapy in Mental Health.* Other publications you might consider include *Physiotherapy Canada,* the *Canadian Journal of Occupational Therapy,* the *British Journal of Physiotherapy,* or the *British Journal of Occupational Therapy.* Other health- and sociology-related journals are included in Appendix L.

Look in back issues of the journals you are considering, for the aim and scope of the publication (often in the first or last issue of each year), so that you can see which organization is responsible for publishing the journal, its aim and purpose, which professional fields it addresses, what topics it covers, features of the journal (such as book and software reviews), and the type of review process to which articles are subjected. The circulation may be mentioned somewhere in the journal so that you can see how many of your colleagues the publication will reach.

Be sure to follow the guidelines in the journal's Author's Guide or Information for Authors. Author's guides are often printed at the end of a journal annually or more frequently. They will give information about the writing style used by the journal, how many manuscript pages are acceptable, and any specific requirements the publication may have regarding photographs, drawings, figures, and so forth. A sample of the Aim and Scope for the *Occupational Therapy Journal of Research* is given in Appendix M; the Instructions to Authors from *Physical Therapy* and the Author's Guide for the *American Journal of Occupational Therapy* are given in Appendix N.

Look through several copies of any journal you are considering to be sure it is the kind of publication in which you would like your article to appear. It may be helpful to browse in the journal room of a well-stocked library to get an idea of appropriate publications. Most libraries display the current month's journals in alphabetical order by title. The following publications also may be of assistance to prospective authors: *The Serials Directory: An International Reference Book* and *Ulrich's International Periodicals Directory*. These multivolume directories are available in the reference section of most libraries. They provide the name of the journal, the publishing organization, cost, frequency of publication, circulation, major topics covered, where the journal is indexed, and the document type (e.g., peer-reviewed, academic, or government document). *Magazines for Libraries* (Katz & Sternberg Katz, 1995) lists periodical titles alphabetically and by subject areas. The frequency of publication, price, circulation, suitable audience, publisher, and whether articles are peer-reviewed are listed for each periodical. The table of contents includes these topics: disabilities, rehabilitation, medicine and health, aging, psychology, sports medicine, sociology, and occupational health. A computer listing of periodicals can also be found on the EPIC/OCLC database through First Search in WorldCat.

Most editors request that you not submit your manuscript to any other journal while it is under their consideration. Once your article has been accepted for publication, you may be required to sign a copyright form.

Writing Styles

After you have selected a journal, you should find out which writing style is in use. Many journals of interest to therapists subscribe to the style described in the *Publication Manual of the American Psychological Association (APA)*. These journals include the *American Journal of Occupational Therapy,* the *Occupational Therapy Journal of Research, Occupational Therapy in Mental Health,* and *Physical Therapy and Occupational Therapy in Geriatrics.* However, *Physical Therapy* and *Physical Therapy and Occupational Therapy in Pediatrics* use the *American Medical Association (AMA) Manual of Style* (1995). Most journals accept an article for review only if it is written in the required style.

The format for writing a research article is detailed in the APA and AMA publication manuals; you should use these manuals during the writing process. Most libraries have the manuals, but I highly recommend that you obtain your own copies, because you will refer to them often as you write. The manuals give useful information about such general topics as quality of content; types of articles; parts of a manuscript; and length, headings, and tone. They also give guidelines for specific items such as nonsexist language, punctuation, abbreviations, quotations, tables and figures, references and reference lists, footnotes, and typing.

Format for an Article Describing Quantitative Research

The general format of scientific articles tends to be similar in most journals. Articles are usually divided into the following sections: problem, background, purpose, hypotheses, method, results, and discussion. Each section is described here. All of the material to be included in your paper can be obtained from the worksheets you have completed.

Problem

Present the problem that you described in the problem statement worksheet following Chapter 3. This is the major issue you wish to address by conducting your study. Tell readers why this is an important problem and why it needs a solution. Are there clients who will benefit or programs that will be improved? Using the material you wrote in the background section following Chapter 3, answer for readers the question, "What is wrong in society or a patient's life that this study will help?"

Next, summarize in a sentence or two how the hypotheses and experimental design relate to the problem; that is, how your particular study will address the larger problem. Finally, mention the theoretical implications of the study—what is likely to be improved as a result of your study. This whole section should not be more than a paragraph or two and should give the reader a firm sense of what was done and why.

Background

Most of the background section of an article will come from the literature review you conducted. Discuss the literature, but do not include an exhaustive historical review. This is the section that will be most condensed, given the amount of material you have amassed. Because of space constraints, most journals will not accept more than one or two paragraphs concerning the background literature. However, a publication that specializes in research papers, such as the *Occupational Therapy Journal of Research,* may allow more background material because the

journal allows considerable space for each article. The APA manual provides useful guidelines for writing the background section (Box 13–A). Point out the logical continuity between previous work and your work on the topic. Controversial issues should be treated fairly, and studies supporting both sides of the argument should be presented.

Purpose

Tell your readers your purpose in carrying out the study: what you hoped to accomplish and why your study, above all others, was worth doing. You have already written these statements in the purpose and significance sections of the worksheets following Chapter 3.

Hypotheses

In this section, you simply state the hypotheses or null hypotheses or research questions. A formal statement will lend clarity to the paper.

Method

This section describes in detail how the study was conducted. It should contain sufficient detail to allow other researchers to replicate the study and readers to assess both the appropriateness of your methods to the purpose of the study and the reliability and validity of the study. The method section of the article should contain the material you described following Chapters 4, 5, and 6 and may be divided into subsections covering subjects, materials and instruments, and procedures. You have already written information on these three items in the protocol at the end of Chapter 5.

Subjects

Subjects are data sources for research studies—the people or items from which you have gathered data. In writing the subject section, describe the criteria used to determine the population for the study, stating the literature that indicates that these criteria are necessary or desirable. Then, describe the method of sample selection (i.e., random or nonrandom). If nonrandom selection was used, was a convenience sample or some other technique used? The method of

---

Box 13–A

"A scholarly review of earlier work provides an appropriate history and recognizes the priority of the work of others. Citation of and specific credit to relevant earlier works is part of the author's scientific and scholarly responsibility. It is essential for the growth of a cumulative science. At the same time, cite and reference only works pertinent to the specific issue and not works of only tangential or general significance. If you summarize earlier works, avoid nonessential details; instead, emphasize pertinent findings, relevant methodological issues, and major conclusions. Refer the reader to general surveys or reviews of the topic if they are available."

(American Psychological Association, 1994, p. 11)

assigning subjects to groups should be addressed, if relevant. State the number of subjects in the study and how many were included in each group. If there was any subject attrition during the study, this also should be mentioned.

Instruments

All the data collection methods used should be listed in this section. The information can be obtained from the worksheets following Chapter 7. Include any information you found on reliability and validity. If you devised the measure specifically for the study, this should be mentioned, and it may be useful to include a copy of the instrument in the article. There should be a complete description of how the data collection methods were administered, including whether a pre-test and post-test were used, who administered the test, whether the test was administered in a group or individually, the environmental conditions, and how long the data collection took.

Procedures

This section should spell out each step undertaken during the study. The information can be found in the research protocol you wrote and in the method section of the Proposal for the Human Subjects Committee. Ideally, this section should be written in sufficient detail that the study could be replicated; however, journal space constraints often make this impossible. In most professional journals, the author's name and address are printed with the article so that interested readers can write and request further information.

Results

In the results section, briefly summarize the main findings, then report the data in detail so that you may justify the conclusions that will be drawn later. Discussing implications is not appropriate in the results section; just stick to the facts. For large sets of data, remember to use pictorial representations such as tables, graphs, and charts.

When reporting the findings from inferential statistics such as t tests, chi-squares, or f tests, include information about the significance level and the degrees of freedom. The style manuals give information on how to type statistical results (e.g., when to use upper and lower case letters, such as "N" for population and "n" for sample).

Discussion

Here is your chance to enjoy yourself and speculate on what the results mean. First, jot down all the ideas that come to mind about your findings; in later drafts you can expand on meaningful theories and discard those that are not useful or valid. Don't be afraid to interpret your findings, but remember that you can discuss an issue only if you mentioned its findings in the results section. Material for this final section will come from the worksheets following Chapter 12.

The opening statement of the discussion should inform the reader whether the hypothesis was supported or the research question was answered. Then you are free to draw on the literature, discussing similarities and differences in the findings of your study and the studies mentioned in the literature review. You must state findings that do not support your hypotheses and briefly speculate on why they might have come about and what they might mean.

At one time, it was customary to end with a paragraph reviewing the study and its main findings, but this is less necessary now because most journals print an abstract at the beginning of the article.

References

The reference list and referencing in the text are the most common places to make typographical errors and errors in style. In APA format (which has been used throughout this book), references are cited both in the text and in the reference lists.

In the text, cite the authors' last names and year of publication (or just the year if the names already appear in the text). In the reference list, give the author's last name, initials, year in parentheses, title of article or book (underline the title of the book), publisher of book or name of journal (underline the name of the journal), volume number (underlined), issue number, and page numbers of the article.

Box 13–B

Sample citation and reference from *Physical Therapy:*

Auricular TENS significantly decreased pain in fifteen patients suffering with various distal extremity disorders.[11]

[11]Longobardi AG, Clelland JA, Knowles CJ, et al: Effects of auricular transcutaneous electrical nerve stimulation on distal extremity pain: A pain study. Phys Ther 69:10–17, 1989.

Sample citation and reference from the *American Journal of Occupational Therapy:*

A major goal of occupational therapy is to enhance a person's ability to interact in the environment in a competent manner (Rogers, 1982).

Rogers, J.C. (1982). Guest Editorial—Educating the inquisitive practitioner. *Occupational Therapy Journal of Research, 2,* 3–11.

In AMA style, references in the text are indicated by superscript numerals which run consecutively throughout the text. The numbered references are listed at the end of the text. In the reference list, give the author's last name, initials, title of article or book, name of journal or publisher of book, page numbers, and year of publication. Samples are given in Box 13–B.

It is a good idea to have a colleague go through the entire manuscript with you, one of you reading the references in the text and the other checking the reference list, to ensure that names and dates or reference numbers match. Journal editors hold authors responsible for the accuracy of references.

Abstract

Most journals require an abstract of the article and specify a number of words the abstract may not exceed; for example, the *American Journal of Occupational Therapy* and *Physical Therapy* both have a maximum abstract length of 150 words. In summarizing your article, the content should be factual; that is, state only events that occurred, items that were used, or data that were found, rather than opinions or suppositions. Even if it is succinct by necessity and definition, an abstract also should be "sufficiently complete to enable the reader to grasp the essence of the paper quickly" (*American Journal of Occupational Therapy,* 1996, p. 73). Typically, an abstract will contain a statement of the problem, method of study, results, and conclusions. Boxes 13–C and 13–D give abstracts from the *American*

Journal of Occupational Therapy and *Physical Therapy.*

Format for an Article Describing Qualitative Research

The written format for qualitative studies is quite different from that for quantitative studies. Qualitative studies can be written in many styles and formats. A typical ethnography written by an anthropologist, for instance, is a lengthy document describing the history of the group under study, the geography of the location, kinship patterns, symbols, politics, economic systems, and educational or socialization systems. Specialized ethnographies, more often written by health professionals, may focus on specific elements of such events as absorbing disabled children into a school classroom or the role of a caregiver for a person with severe, permanent disability. In this book, however, we will concentrate on the therapist or student writing a qualitative study for a thesis or journal article.

Typically, these are ethnographically informed reports; in other words, they are specialized commentaries about a narrowly defined topic that have been conducted using naturalistic methods. They will be briefer than, though just as useful as, a full-blown ethnography; yet will be less credible because many of the built-in quality controls of ethnography will not have been included.

Qualitative articles are typically long, narrative reports. Journal editors who are unused to publishing naturalistic studies often object to the length of these reports; however,

---

Box 13–C

"*Objective:* Five styles of commercial static wrist extension orthoses were compared to determine whether any style, or styles, afforded better power grip strength or finger dexterity. Because wrist extensor orthoses are intended for use during functional tasks, their influence on hand function is of great importance.

"*Method.* Twenty-three right-hand dominant women without upper extremity dysfunction participated in this crossover study. Dominant-hand finger dexterity and power grip were evaluated while wearing each of five commercial orthoses—Kendall-Futuro #33 [Registered] (Futuro), AliMed Freedom Long [Registered] (AliMed Long), AliMed Freedom Short [Registered] (AliMed Short), Smith & Nephew Rolyan D-Ring [Registered] (Rolyan), and LMB Wrist Rest [Registered] (LMB)—and while using the dominant hand without an orthosis (free hand). Finger dexterity was assessed with the unimanual subtest of the Purdue Pegboard. Grip strength was assessed with a Jamar [Registered] hydraulic dynamometer.

"*Results.* Four of the study orthoses (Futuro, AliMed Short, Rolyan, and LMB) afforded finger dexterity that did not differ significantly from that of the free hand. The AliMed Long orthosis slowed finger speed when compared with the speeds afforded by both the LMB orthosis and the free hand.

"*Conclusion.* The five styles of commercial orthoses affect power grip and finger dexterity differently. When power grip or finger dexterity are priorities, differences among the orthoses furnish grounds for initial suggestions, although medical needs and patient preference should be the overriding factors in the final selection of an orthosis."

(Stern, 1996, p. 32)

Box 13–D

"The study was designed to provide a quantitative analysis of toe-walking in children with cerebral palsy (CP). The total internal moment developed about the ankle joint during locomotion and the passive component of this internal moment were measured. The contributions of the active and passive components were expressed as the ratio (R) between the passive moment and the total internal moment. Measurements were compared for 13 children with CP and 5 healthy children. For the data analysis, the children with CP exhibiting apparently similar toe-walking, were divided into 2 groups: 1) Group CPI and 2) Group CPII. Group CPI was characterized by a small ratio R value, which indicated the presence of excessive contractions of the triceps surae muscle during locomotion. In Group CPII, the ratio R value was abnormally high, which indicated that a contracture (ie, structural change of the muscle or the tendon) was entirely or at least partly responsible for toe-walking. Each group requires a different therapeutic strategy."

(Tardieu, Lespargot, Tabary, & Bret, 1989, p. 656)

---

qualitative researchers tend to agree that lengthy commentaries of thick description are necessary if the essence of the participants or event is to be presented adequately. The study will probably be received more positively if it is kept to a reasonable length and if a clear, easy-to-read writing style is used. Readers unfamiliar with the culture or topic of the study should find the report understandable and interesting.

Fetterman (1989) feels that ethnographic writing is difficult, yet satisfying.

From simple notes about small events . . . to efforts to describe an experience or explain a sudden insight, ethnographic writing requires an eye for detail, an ability to express that detail in its proper context, and the language skills to weave small details and bits of meaning into a textured social fabric. The ethnographic writer must recreate the varied forms of social organization and interaction that months of observation and study have revealed. The manifold symbolism every culture displays and the adaptiveness of people to their environment must somehow come to life on the page (p. 104).

The following basic elements should be included in the article.

Purpose

What was your original purpose in developing the study? How did this change over time?

Research Questions

State the research questions you asked as you went into the study, and relate how they changed as you gathered and analyzed the data.

Background

Tell the reader how you identified and selected settings, participants, and documents. Did theoretical sampling or analytical induction guide your selection? Did you know the settings or participants beforehand? (Box 13–E).

Procedures

Readers should know how much time was spent with participants, at the scene in general, and over what time frame. Mention the types of settings studied and how many there were. Who were the participants and how many of them were there? (Box 13–E). Discuss how and to what extent you established rapport with the participants. How did participants come to see you? How did your relationship with them change over time?

Data Collection and Analysis

It is important to tell readers how you collected and interpreted the data. They must know enough to decide for themselves

---

Box 13–E

The following excerpt is from the method section of an article by Taylor and McGruder entitled *The meaning of sea kayaking for persons with spinal cord injuries.*

Subjects were persons with SCI [spinal cord injury] who had participated in sea kayaking expeditions. . . . One woman and two men volunteered. . . . The three subjects were nonambulatory, and each had incomplete spinal cord lesions with some upper extremity function preserved. . . .

The subjects were self-selected by their apparent interest in the topic and willingness to participate in interviews. These subjects are not taken, therefore, to represent all persons with SCI or even all persons with SCI who have engaged in a new outdoor activity after injury.

There follows a detailed description of the three subjects.

(Taylor & McGruder, 1996, pp. 40–41)

Box 13–F

Pasek and Schkade describe their data collection and analysis methods in the abstract of their article, *Effects of a skiing experience on adolescents with limb deficiencies: An occupational adaptation perspective.*

Participant observation data collection methods included videotape, interviews, daily progress notes by ski instructors, and a 1-month posttrip questionnaire. Data were analyzed for evidence of efficiency, effectiveness, and satisfaction to self and others (properties of relative mastery described in occupational adaptation). Skier reports of positive effects were analyzed for implications of an impact on self-esteem. Three occupational therapists who have extensive experience working with adolescents also reviewed videotapes and written information.

(Pasek & Schkade, 1996, p. 24)

---

whether your research is credible, and to be able to understand your research in context. If information about the data collection methods is omitted, for example, the reader cannot know if your findings come from your own knowledge of the culture and direct personal experience of the activities studied, from other people's theoretical frameworks, or from actual fieldwork and interviewing.

Readers need to be informed about specific data collection techniques such as participant observation, in-depth interviewing, and document review, as well as any mechanical recording devices or covert recording used (Box 13–F).

How did you analyze the data? If a particular method was followed, such as Glaser and Strauss's grounded theory, this should be stated and explained. What checks did you impose on participants' statements? Did participants review your findings? What did they say about the findings? Did you use any triangulation methods? (Box 13–G).

Making It Interesting

Scientific writing is different from literary writing, but that does not mean it has to be boring. Although reporting on research in an interesting manner is a challenge, it can be done. The writing should not lack style or be

---

Box 13–G

In the study mentioned in Box 13–E, Taylor and McGruder used Guba's model of rigor in qualitative research to address the trustworthiness of their data. Several methods of triangulation were used. First, "a kayaking guide and a recreational therapist who accompanied the kayakers with SCI also were interviewed. A second triangulation compared interview data, the first author's field notes, and a published account of kayaking with a disability (Webre & Zeller, 1990). Neutrality was ensured at the level of data analysis through code-recording and member checking procedures. . . ." The authors also asked the participants to review and evaluate their analysis of the interview data, and the second author analyzed the middle half of the transcripts and recoded themes independently.

(Taylor & McGruder, 1996, p. 41)

---

dull. Present your research and your findings directly, but aim for an interesting and compelling style that shows readers how you are involved with the project. Your involvement should be infectious and make readers want to read on to see what happens. The *APA Manual* offers useful advice on the expression of ideas (Box 13–H).

The manual provides excellent suggestions for orderly presentation of ideas, smoothness of expression, economy of expression, precision and clarity in word choice, strategies to improve writing style, and grammar (*APA Manual,* 1994, pp. 23–26). Reading this section may prove inspir-

---

Box 13–H

"You can achieve clear communication, which is the prime objective of scientific reporting, by presenting ideas in an orderly manner and by expressing yourself smoothly and precisely. By developing ideas clearly and logically and leading readers smoothly from thought to thought, you make the task of reading an agreeable one."

(American Psychological Association, 1994, p. 23)

---

ing to the would-be author of an article. New guidelines on reducing bias in language and sections on gender, sexual orientation, racial and ethnic identity, disabilities, and age are particularly useful.

Procedures for Publication

Once you have selected the journal and prepared your article according to the appropriate format, you are ready to mail your work. Be sure to follow the directions for number of copies, typing style, page numbering, spacing, and so on. Include a cover letter stating the name of the article, together with any covering statements requested in the author's guide. These often include a statement to the effect that your paper is not under consideration by any other publication and that you are willing to sign a copyright form.

If your article is accepted for review, you will receive a card from the editor saying that the article has been received and the review process has begun. Be prepared for a long wait, probably several months. At this point, the editor will send copies of your article to three or four reviewers, usually experts in your field and in the area of specialization of the study. Often reviewers are asked a series of questions that will help the editor decide whether the topic is relevant to the readership, if it has been appropriately covered and is timely, and if the study was reasonable and of good quality. Once all the reviews are returned, the editor will make a decision as to whether to accept the article as it is, accept it with revisions, or reject it. As you can imagine, it takes several months for you to receive the letter containing this decision.

If your article is rejected for publication, you will usually be told the reason for this rejection. Perhaps the topic is unsuitable for the readership or is considered untimely, or reviewers do not consider the project of a standard worthy of publication. Do not be discouraged. Submit your work to another journal, perhaps one whose aim and scope are more compatible with your work.

Often editors accept an article but require the author to make some changes. It may be discouraging to see one's work covered with red pencil markings, but the requested changes are often not as major as they may first appear. If you believe that a requested revision would not improve the article or that it would alter your meaning or intent, merely note why the changes would not be beneficial, and perhaps suggest a rewrite that would better clarify your meaning. Make reasonable alterations quickly and send back the revised copy within a couple of weeks.

Do not be surprised if your article goes back and forth between you and the editor a few more times before it is acceptable. Above all, do not become so discouraged that you stop revising and resubmitting. If the editor considers the material suitable for publication, it is merely a question of time before you have it in publishable form.

When your article is finally ready, the editor may ask you to sign a copyright form stating that you are handing over the publishing rights of your article to that publication. You will also be informed that your article is being sent to the printer to be prepared for publication and that you will shortly receive proofs. When the proofs arrive, check them immediately for errors and mail them back. The time allowed for checking proofs may be so short that you may be asked to phone in your corrections. Only minor changes, such as spelling or punctuation corrections, should be made in proofs. It is too late to rewrite sentences or make any major changes in content.

Finally, nothing remains to be done except to sit back and wait to see your name in print. Some publications will send you a complimentary copy of the issue in which your article appears, whereas others will send you several copies of the article itself. Now you really have finished. You have something to show for all your effort, and you can be proud of your contribution to your profession.

Thesis Preparation

Preparing a thesis requires a somewhat different procedure and considerations. The steps involved usually consist of:

1. Preparing a thesis proposal and presenting it to your chosen thesis committee at a thesis proposal hearing; making required changes

2. Preparing materials for a human subjects committee review; presenting or submitting materials to the human subjects committee responsible for your facility; making required changes; presenting or submitting materials to the human subjects committee of the facility in which the research will be performed (if relevant); making required changes

3. Implementing the research project

4. Preparing the written thesis and defending it before your thesis committee at a thesis defense meeting; making required changes; preparing the thesis document for binding and presentation to the required sites, such as your department or college library

Although these are customary procedures involved in the preparation of a thesis, they may be different at your institution. You should follow the procedures used there.

Writing Style

As with journal articles, required writing styles vary from college to college. In occupational therapy and physical therapy programs, the style used is often that of the American Psychological Association or the American Medical Association, but you should check with your department to be sure. Again, I advise that you obtain your own copy of the relevant style manual, because you will probably need to refer to it frequently during the writing process.

Thesis Proposal Format

There may be a required format for a thesis proposal at your college. If so, it will probably be similar to the following format.

Front Page

Show the title of the study, the name of the researcher, the date of the proposal, and the names of the thesis readers.

Description and Rationale for the Study

INTRODUCTION

You may choose to have an introduction or you may move right into the Problem Statement. If you have an introduction, it should be brief and set the stage for the problem to be investigated.

PROBLEM STATEMENT

State clearly the problem your study will address. This material can be found on the problem statement worksheets following Chapter 3. A group of people, an issue, or an event will be substituted for a "problem" in qualitative research.

BACKGROUND

State the need for the study or why the problem is of pressing concern. The material comes from the literature review and generally will not exceed two or three pages. Include several people's opinions regarding the problem's importance and the need to study it, together with some general facts about the nature, extent, and seriousness of the problem.

PURPOSE

State how you wish to address the problem by carrying out your study. Gather the material from the purpose section of the worksheets following Chapter 3. For qualitative research, state what type of information you wish to find out about the participants and events under study and whether you plan to generate hypotheses.

SIGNIFICANCE

The "so what?" of your study. What will be changed as a result of your study? Use the material on the worksheets following Chapter 3.

LITERATURE REVIEW

At this stage of thesis preparation, you will probably have conducted only a preliminary literature review, so this section will contain a list of the topics your in-depth review will cover. However, try to include one or two studies that support your view that the problem is important as well as some studies using similar and dissimilar research methods to the method you propose to use.

Design of the Study

RESEARCH QUESTION OR HYPOTHESES

Simply state the research question(s) or hypotheses. A formal statement will clarify the proposal. Although research questions may change during a naturalistic study, it is important to have some starting questions to guide the design of the study.

ASSUMPTIONS

These are the assumptions you made while designing the study. Use the material on the assumptions worksheet following Chapter 6.

SCOPE AND LIMITATIONS

Describe the scope of your study and outline the limitations that are apparent so far. This material can be found on the worksheets after Chapter 6.

RESEARCH DESIGN

A simple statement of your decision about the research design you will use. For a quantitative study, this is the decision you made after reading Chapter 5. For a qualitative study, you will have made the decision after reading Chapter 9.

RESEARCH METHOD FOR
QUANTITATIVE RESEARCH

Subjects. Include the criteria you will use to define the population, the method you will use to select the sample, how many will be in the sample, and the method you will use to assign the subjects to experimental and control groups. All of this material will be found in the subject worksheet following Chapter 6.

Variables. Identify the dependent and independent variables if you are doing experimental or quasi-experimental research; identify the variables being correlated if you are doing correlational research.

Definition of Terms. Define the terms that will have a simple definition; then operationalize those terms that will play an important role in your study, usually those mentioned in the hypotheses. You did this task when you completed the worksheets following Chapter 6.

Procedures. This is the step-by-step account of your research project as you listed it in the protocol at the end of Chapter 5. Included here are the procedures to ensure subject confidentiality, to obtain subjects' informed consent, and to ensure that necessary treatment will not be withheld. Also, mention statements concerning the risk/benefit ratio to subjects and the safety of the study. You prepared this material for inclusion in the material for the human subjects committee on worksheets following Chapter 11.

Data Collection Instruments. These are the methods you will be using to collect data from the subjects. Describe the methods, tests, or measures, and give reliability and validity (if relevant). State when in the research process the tests will be administered. This material is found on the worksheets following Chapter 7.

Data Analysis. This is the method you propose to use for data analysis. Your methods may change once you have actually gone through the experience of collecting the data, but thesis committee members will want to see that you have thought about the analyses and that you have an idea of the procedures you will use. You have thought this process through on the worksheets following Chapter 8.

RESEARCH METHOD FOR
QUALITATIVE RESEARCH

Participants. State the criteria you will use to select participants and how many you are likely to engage in the study (see Chapter 4).

Procedures. A plan for gaining access to the site and participants; gaining permission to interview, record, and observe participants and events (see Chapters 7 and 9); and procedures to ensure participants' confidentiality, and their informed consent to participate in the study (see Chapter 11).

Data Collection. How you will gather information from participants, the site, and artifacts as stated on the worksheets following Chapter 7.

Data Analysis. The techniques you propose to use to organize, analyze, and present the data (see Chapter 10).

Timetable. Some departments require students to plan a timetable for the steps in thesis preparation and writing. Writing a timetable forces the student to think about how much time each step will take and encourages realistic planning for the entire process. In plotting a timetable, include actual dates by which events will happen, rather than merely stating that a literature review will take 3 months, for example. In the introduction to this book, some information was given about estimating time frames for conducting research, and some sample timetables are shown in Appendix O.

Resources. Sometimes students are asked to list the resources they will need to complete their theses. Consider whether you will need assistance with transcribing, typing, editing, or proofreading; the help of a statistician; the use of a computer for statistical computation or for word processing; the use of video or audiotape recording equipment; access to library facilities; access to patients or participants who meet your selection criteria; access to patient records or artifacts in the field; the use of treatment equipment or materials; or assistance from other therapists for carrying out treatment, testing subjects, or interviewing and observing participants.

Reference List. The reference list for a proposal should be written in the style that will be required for the thesis. Find out what that style will be, acquire the appropriate style manual, and study the section on referencing.

Appendices. Include tests, measures, interviews, observation sheets, and other data-gathering instruments; forms to gather subjects' informed consent to participate in the study; and any other forms that may be required by the human subjects committee.

Procedures for the Proposal

You will have been working with your thesis committee members, often known as thesis readers, while preparing the proposal. The completed proposal should be submitted to each committee member at least a week before the scheduled hearing date, so that they have time to review it. Bring your own copy of the proposal to the hearing and be prepared to answer questions about the underlying philosophy and theory, the design and methodology, and the importance and relevance of your proposed study. This is, after all, what you propose to do to meet the department's requirements for a thesis, and your readers will expect that you have thought through the project carefully and that you are able to discuss it knowledgeably.

There will undoubtedly be discussions about certain portions of the proposal, with exchange of ideas about alterations and improvements. There should be no surprises if you have worked with readers ahead of time regarding the preparation of the proposal;

nevertheless, some readers are inspired when involved in discussions with colleagues at the hearing and may well make good suggestions for improvements. Unless you feel strongly that the suggestions would not improve the study, you should make the required changes, resubmit the proposal, and then get the go-ahead to start your research.

Before you can actually start, however, you need to prepare and present materials to the human subjects committee. This procedure was described in Chapter 11, and if you completed the worksheets, you have most of the material you'll need. Some of it may require revising after your proposal hearing. Assuming that the human subjects committee approved your study and all else went well, you may now carry out the study.

Thesis Format

The final step is to write the material in thesis form. Your college may have an idiosyncratic format for thesis writing, but in all probability the form will be similar to those found in Figures 13–1 and 13–2. The basis for the information needed for the thesis can be found on the worksheets you completed at the end of each chapter. The relevant chapter is listed following each topic heading in the two figures. You have probably written a bare-bones statement or two for each component and now need to fill in the details.

Procedures for the Thesis

Most readers prefer to read one or two thesis chapters at a time, as they are written, because in this way they can be sure the student is on track, and necessary changes may be made as the writing progresses. If a reader does not ask you for chapters as you write, it is a good idea to request this type of review to be sure you are using the correct style before getting too far along in the process. Even so, when your readers see the entire manuscript, they will undoubtedly have suggestions for change and will probably want some sections rewritten.

As soon as all the readers are satisfied with the content, a thesis defense should be scheduled. This is a meeting during which you will "defend" your thesis. The defense is often an open meeting that others may attend. It usually takes the form of a summary of the project by you, then a question-and-answer period and a general discussion

```
TITLE PAGE
ABSTRACT
ACKNOWLEDGEMENTS
LIST OF TABLES
LIST OF FIGURES
CHAPTER I    INTRODUCTION
    Background (Chapter 3)
    Purpose of study (Chapter 3 )
    Significance of study (Chapter 3)
    Hypothesis or research question (Chapters 1 & 3)
    Assumptions (Chapter 6)
    Limitations (Chapter 6)
    Definition of terms (Chapter 6)
    Scope of study (Chapter 6)
CHAPTER II    LITERATURE REVIEW (Chapter 2)
CHAPTER III    RESEARCH METHOD
    Research design (Chapter 5)
    Hypothesis
    Procedures:
        Subjects (Chapter 6)
        Instruments (Chapter 7)
        Data collection procedures (Chapter 7)
        Data analysis (Chapter 8)
        Pilot study (Chapter 11)
CHAPTER IV    RESULTS
    Narrative (Chapter 12)
    Tables and figures (Chapter 12)
CHAPTER V    DISCUSSION (Chapter 12)
    Principal findings
    Comparison with findings in related studies
    Interpretation of results/findings
    Implications of the study
    Recommendations for future research
REFERENCES (Chapter 13)
APPENDICES
    Appendix A: Tests and measures (Chapter 7)
    Appendix B: Human subjects materials (Chapter 11)
```

FIGURE 13–1 Format for thesis on quantitative research. Chapter numbers in parentheses indicate where information for each section is located in this book.

about your project. Ask your first reader about the format of the meetings at your college so that you can be prepared.

The outcome of a defense meeting is usually that the thesis is either approved "as is" or approved as long as minor changes are made. A request for major revisions usually indicates that the student did not work closely enough with committee members during the actual writing.

When all the readers are satisfied with the final product, and the approval sheets have been signed (indicating that the student has completed the requirements for the thesis), all that remains is to make the required number of copies and deliver them to the appropriate sites. Colleges usually require copies of theses for the department or college li-

```
TITLE PAGE
ABSTRACT
ACKNOWLEDGEMENTS
LIST OF TABLES (Chapter 10)
LIST OF FIGURES (Chapter 10)
CHAPTER I   INTRODUCTION
   Background (Chapter 3)
   Purpose of study (Chapter 3 )
   Significance of study (Chapter 3)
   Research questions (Chapters 3 & 9)
   Assumptions (Chapter 6)
   Limitations (Chapter 6)
CHAPTER II   LITERATURE REVIEW (Chapters 2 & 9)
CHAPTER III   RESEARCH METHOD
   Research design (Chapter 9)
   Research questions (Chapter 9)
   Procedures:
      Participants (Chapter 9)
      Data collection methods (Chapters 7 & 9)
      Data analysis (Chapter 10)
CHAPTER IV   ANALYSIS AND DISCUSSION
   Results of coding and early analysis (Chapter 10)
   In-depth analysis (Chapters 10, 12, &13)
   Data displays (Chapter 10)
   Checks on the analysis (Chapter 10)
   Hypothesis generation (Chapter 10)
REFERENCES (Chapter 13)
APPENDICES
   Appendix A: Permission forms (Chapter 11)
   Appendix B: Interview outlines (Chapters 9 & 10)
   Appendix C: Start codes (Chapter 10)
```

FIGURE 13–2 Format for thesis on qualitative research. Chapter numbers in parentheses indicate where information for each section is located in this book.

brary; professional association libraries may also request a copy.

Preparing the Thesis for Publication

Students are sometimes interested in submitting their theses for publication. This is an excellent idea and probably should happen more often than it does; however, it is not a simple job because so much cutting and rewriting is necessary. It is difficult to bring oneself to eliminate so much hard-won material! One of the readers might be willing to help and may be more objective about which portions can be ruthlessly discarded while retaining the sense of the work. Generally, the literature review is the chapter that is most massacred. In fact, it must be reduced to about two to four paragraphs for most journals, quite a daunting feat from 15 or 20 pages.

If you plan to rework your thesis for publication, the best plan might be to return to the worksheets you prepared during the project and make a fresh start. Sometimes it is simpler to write something from scratch than to rework material that is written for another purpose. If this sounds like a good idea to you, refer to the first half of this chapter and follow the directions for publishing in a journal.

Stumbling Blocks

Many studies get bogged down when the author receives the article back from the editor and sees that yet more work is needed to get it into publishable shape. Most of us quickly learn that what appears to us to be a flawless piece of work may seem to others to have ample room for improvement.

As soon as you have recovered from the first disappointment, go through the recommendations one by one to get a more realistic feeling for which items will really require more work. You may be surprised at how simple some of the revisions are to make. As the author, you may be too close to the topic to see alternative ways to present ideas. A colleague may help shed a more objective light on things and might have suggestions for the bigger revisions.

Even more discouraging is a case in which some of the requested changes would, in your view, alter the meaning of the writing or misrepresent what you wanted to say. You are under no obligation to make these changes. In such a case, you should write to the editor explaining your concern and stating that you do not believe that altering the text on that particular point would be beneficial. This may lead to a discussion in which you discover that the editor misunderstood your intent because your writing was unclear. Together, you can probably work out a solution acceptable to both of you. If not, however, you should decide how important the point is to you. If it is very important, you may choose to withdraw your article from that particular publication and submit it to another. Always let an editor know if this is what you are doing.

I recommend that you set a deadline by which you will make all the changes, perhaps within 2 weeks. In my experience, if you do not get past this stage quickly, the "rejected" manuscript will sit in a drawer permanently. It would be a loss to you and perhaps to your profession as well to let your manuscript languish and die at this point.

WORKSHEETS

If you are preparing your study for publication in a professional journal:

CHOOSING THE BEST JOURNAL FOR YOUR STUDY

You must decide on the journal of your choice. If this is not immediately clear to you, visit a library and review the journals on display in the journal room. If none of the journals on display look exactly right, look through one of the periodical listings mentioned in this chapter.

List possible journals here:

Appropriate

A. _____ ____ Yes ____ No
B. _____ ____ Yes ____ No
C. _____ ____ Yes ____ No
D. _____ ____ Yes ____ No
E. _____ ____ Yes ____ No

Review the aim and scope, and check off if the journals still seem appropriate.

Pick three of the most promising journals and look through several recent copies of each to see if your study fits the journals' style and content.

Make your first choice of journal:

WRITING STYLE

Review the Author's Guide to find which writing style is used.

State here:

Obtain a copy of this writing style guide.

Review the guide before you start writing.

WRITING

Gather your worksheets from previous chapters and arrange them in sections:

Problem

Background

Purpose

Hypothesis

Method

Results

Discussion

Following the information in this chapter, embellish the material on the **Problem** worksheet, getting it into its final form:

Now write the **Background** section, working from your literature review worksheets.

Statement of Purpose:

Hypotheses:

Describe the **Method,** including:

Subjects:

Instruments:

Procedures:

Give the results:

Now, discuss your **Conclusions:**

Was the hypothesis supported?

Make comparisons with the literature findings:

Your interpretations and conclusions:

Any limitations:

Suggestions for future research:

Compose the reference list:

Write an abstract:

Go back and review your work.

Is it interesting?

Does it tell what was done and what happened, clearly and succinctly?

Are your interpretations and conclusions justified?

PROCEDURES FOR PUBLICATION

Review the Author's Guide again to be sure you have followed all the instructions.

Print the required number of copies of your article.

Write a cover letter to the editor.

References

American Journal of Occupational Therapy. (1996). Author's Guide. *American Journal of Occupational Therapy, 50*(1), 73–74.

American Medical Association. (1995). *Manual of style* (8th ed.) Baltimore, MD: Williams & Wilkins.

American Psychological Association. (1994). *Publication manual of the American Psychological Association* (4th ed.) Washington, DC: Author.

Fetterman, D.M. (1989). *Ethnography step by step.* Newbury Park, CA: Sage Publications.

Katz, B., & Sternberg Katz, L. (Eds.) (1995). *Magazines for Libraries.* New York: R.R. Bowker.

Pasek, P.B., & Schkade, J.K. (1996). Effects of a skiing experience on adolescents with limb deficiencies: An occupational adaptation perspective. *American Journal of Occupational Therapy, 50*(1), 24–31.

The serials directory: An international reference book (10th ed.). (1996). Birmingham, AL: EBSCO.

Stern, E.B. (1996). Grip strength and finger dexterity across five styles of commercial wrist orthoses. *American Journal of Occupational Therapy, 50*(1), 32–38.

Tardieu, C., Lespargot, A., Tabary, C., & Bret, M. (1989). Toe-walking in children with cerebral palsy: Contributions of contracture and excessive contraction of triceps surae muscle. *Physical Therapy, 69*(8), 656–662.

Taylor, L.P. & McGruder, J.E. (1996). The meaning of sea kayaking for persons with spinal cord injuries. *American Journal of Occupational Therapy, 50*(1), 39–46.

Ulrich's international periodicals directory (34th ed.). (1996). New York: Bowker..

Additional Reading

Bates, J.D. (1993). *Writing with precision: How to write so that you cannot possibly be misunderstood.* Sarasota, FL: Acropolis Books.

Carter, J., & Sylvester, P. (1987). *Writing for your peers: The primary journal paper.* New York: Praeger.

Copperud, R.H. (1980). *American usage and style: The consensus.* New York: Van Nostrand Reinhold.

Day, R.A. (1994). *How to write and publish a scientific paper.* Phoenix, AZ: Oryx Press.

International Association of Business Communicators. (1982). *Without bias: A guidebook for nondiscriminatory communication.* New York: John Wiley & Sons.

Ross-Larson, B. (1996). *Edit yourself.* New York: Norton.

Strunk, W., Jr., & White, E.B. (1995). *The elements of style.* New York: Macmillan.

APPENDIX A

Indexes and Abstracts

Abstracts for Social Workers. Quarterly. Abstracts from journals of social work under: social policy and action, service methods, fields of service, the social work profession, history of social work, related fields in the social sciences.

Abstracts of Hospital Management Studies. Quarterly. International abstracts of studies on management, planning, and public policy related to health-care delivery.

Ageline. Produced by American Association for Retired Persons. More than 16,500 documents on all aspects of gerontology. Bimonthly updates.

Bibliography of Bioethics. Since 1975, covers English-language literature on ethical issues related to health care. Includes journals, court decisions, government documents, audiovisuals, newspapers and books. Published annually.

Biological Abstracts. Semimonthly. International abstracts of periodicals including behavioral sciences, bioinstrumentation, environmental biology, genetics, nutrition, and public health.

Child Development Abstracts. Three times per year. Abstracts of articles and books in a wide variety of fields as they relate to infancy and child development.

Combined Health Information Database. Produced by National Institutes of Health. More than 24,000 documents combining four health-related databases: arthritis, diabetes, health education, digestive diseases. Quarterly updates.

Compendex. Produced by Engineering Information Inc. More than 1,102,100 documents on all aspects of engineering and technology including rehabilitation engineering. Monthly updates.

Cumulative Index to Nursing and Allied Health Literature (CINAHL). Print version from 1956 to present; on-line version from 1982 to present. Indexes all major nursing journals and over 125 allied health journals, plus book reviews, pamphlets, films, and recordings. Bimonthly updates.

Current Index to Journals in Education (CIJE). Paper abstracts of education-related journals by subject, author, and journal content. Usually used in conjunction with RIE and ECER; these three form the online version, ERIC.

Dissertation Abstracts. Comprehensive paper abstracts of dissertations by title, author, and subject. Volumes divided into sciences/engineering and humanities/social sciences.

dsh Abstracts. Quarterly from Deafness, Speech and Hearing Publications, Inc., Gallaudet College, Washington, DC. Abstracts articles related to hearing, hearing disorders, speech, and speech disorders. Includes foreign journals.

Education Index. From 1932 to the present. Indexes articles from educational periodicals, conference proceedings, and yearbooks.

ERIC (Educational Resources Information Center). Produced by Council for Exceptional Children. More than 589,000 documents on special education materials. Monthly updates. Compilation of paper indexes: RIE, CIJE, and ECER.

Exceptional Child Educational Resources (ECER). Abstracts education materials related to children with special needs, by subject and author. Usually used in conjunction with RIE and CIJE; these three form the online version, ERIC.

Excerpta Medica. A subsidiary of Elsevier Science Publishing in The Netherlands, first published in 1946. Covers both research and clinical biomedical literature, on a worldwide basis. Fifty-two sections including Rehabilitation and Physical Medicine, Gerontology and Geriatrics, Psychiatry, Occupational Health, and Industrial Medicine.

Hospital Literature Index. From 1945 to the present. Indexes studies on administration, planning, and financing of hospitals and related health-care institutions. All types of health-care facilities are included. Published quarterly and cumulated annually.

Index Medicus. Full and abridged versions available. Documents from approximately 4680 medically related journals. Updated monthly and cumulated annually. Online version is MEDLINE.

Index of Physical Therapy. Indexed by subject and author annually.

Index of the American Journal of Occupational Therapy. Indexed by subject and author, cumulatively from 1972 to 1983, and annually thereafter.

International Nursing Index. From 1966 to present. Indexes 270 international nursing journals and nursing articles from 2600 nonnursing materials listed in Index Medicus. Published quarterly and cumulated annually.

Linguistics and Language Behaviors Abstracts. Produced by Sociological Abstracts, Inc. More than 72,000 documents on language problems, speech and hearing problems, learning disabilities, and special education. Quarterly updates.

MEDLINE. On-line version of Index Medicus. More than 1,600,000 entries on medicine, including biomedicine, and humanities as they relate to medicine. Includes occupational and physical therapy, nursing, social work, biology and physiology, and so forth. Updated monthly and cumulated annually.

PsychINFO. Online version of *Psychological Abstracts.* Entries listed by title, author, and subject; divides psychology into 16 major categories.

PsychLit. On-line database of psychology books, journals, and other materials. Comprehensive. Organized by author and subject.

Psychological Abstracts. Began in 1894 as the *Psychological Index* and changed to *Psychological Abstracts* in 1927. Many journals, serial publications, and dissertation abstracts are scanned for the monthly publication. Cumulative in four volumes per year. Online version is PsychINFO.

REHABDATA. Produced by National Rehabilitation Information Center (NARIC). More than 16,000 documents on rehabilitation including commercial publications, government reports, journals, and unpublished documents. Monthly updates.

Reliable Source for Occupational Therapy. Online information system with literature in database, OT BibSys. Organized by author, subject, and title.

Research in Education (RIE). Paper abstracts of educational reports from 1975 by subject, author, and institution. Available on microfilm. Usually used in conjunction with CIJE and ECER; these two, along with RIE, form the online version, ERIC.

Research Quarterly, American Alliance for Health, Physical Education and Recreation. Covers literature pertaining to physical health, physical education and recreation. Cumulative in 10-year indexes from 1930 to present.

Science Citation Index. Indexes literature from the scientific disciplines including medicine, behavioral sciences, substance abuse, and some nursing journals. Published bimonthly with an annual cumulation from 1955.

Social Planning/Policy & Development Abstracts. Formerly Social Welfare, Social Planning, Policy and Development. From 1979. Also available on-line.

Social Science Citation Index. Since 1969, covers literature in the social sciences including occupational and physical therapy, nursing, educational research, family studies, social work, geriatrics and gerontology, health policy, psychology, and psychiatry. Published three times a year with an annual cumulation.

Sociological Abstracts. Paper abstracts of sociological books and journals by subject and author.

Sport Database. Produced by Sport Information Resource Center. More than 100,000 documents on all aspects of sports, including sports for persons with disabilities. Bimonthly updates.

US Superintendent of Documents, Monthly Catalog of United States Government Publications. 1895 to present. Lists publications issued by all branches of the U.S. government, both the Congressional and the department and bureau publications. Current issues indexed by author, title, subject, and series/report.

Vocational Rehabilitation Index. From 1955 to 1973. Indexes articles from the main vocational rehabilitation journals and government-sponsored reports of vocational rehabilitation projects.

Well-Written Literature Reviews

Case-Smith, J. (1995). The relationships among sensorimotor components, fine motor skill, and functional performance in preschool children. *American Journal of Occupational Therapy, 49*(7), 645–652.

Clark, C., Corcoran, M., & Gitlin, L. (1995). An exploratory study of how occupational therapists develop therapeutic relationships with family caregivers. *American Journal of Occupational Therapy, 49*(7), 587–594.

Croce, R., & DePaepe, J. (1989). A critique of therapeutic intervention programming with reference to an alternative approach based on motor learning theory. *Physical and Occupational Therapy in Pediatrics, 9*(3), 5–33.

Delitto, A. (1994). Are measures of function and disability important in low back care? *Physical Therapy, 74*(5), 452–456.

Eng, J.J., & Pierrynowski, M.R. (1993). Evaluation of soft foot orthotics in the treatment of patellofemoral pain syndrome. *Physical Therapy, 73*(2), 62–68.

Hauzlik, J.R. (1989). The effect of intervention on the free-play experience for mothers and their infants with developmental delay and cerebral palsy. *Physical and Occupational Therapy in Pediatrics, 9*(2), 33–51.

Laflin, K., & Aja, D. (1995). Health care concerns related to lifting: An inside look at intervention strategies. *American Journal of Occupational Therapy, 49*(1), 63–72.

Neuhaus, B.E. (1988). Ethical considerations in clinical reasoning: The impact of technology and cost containment. *American Journal of Occupational Therapy, 42*(5), 288–294.

Stewart, K.B., Brady, D.K., Crowe, T.K., & Naganuma, G.M. (1989). Rett Syndrome: A literature review and survey of parents and therapists. *Physical and Occupational Therapy in Pediatrics, 9*(3), 35–55.

Stratford, P.W., Norman, G.R., & McIntosh, J.M. (1989). Generalizability of grip strength measurements in patients with tennis elbow. *Physical Therapy, 69*(4), 276–281.

Warren, M. (1995). Providing low vision rehabilitation services with occupational therapy and ophthalmology: A program description. *American Journal of Occupational Therapy, 49*(9), 877–883.

APPENDIX C

Hardware Resources

Directory and Buyer's Guide
Available in *Medical Electronics & Equipment News.* Usually in the December issue.

Contains information on equipment for purchase during the upcoming year.

Encyclopedia of Instrumentation and Control. Edited by D.M. Considine.
Available from:
McGraw-Hill Book Co.
New York, NY 10011

A listing of about 700 entries of instruments and equipment.

Informed Consumer Guide to Wheelchair Selection and a series of fact sheets on wheelchairs
Available from:
ABLEDATA
8455 Colesville Road, Suite 935
Silver Spring, MD 20910

The illustrated guide provides an overview of the types of manual and powered wheelchairs currently on the market and explores the selection process and factors to consider when purchasing a chair.

The *Wheelchair Fact Sheet Series* includes specialized fact sheets on children's wheelchairs and powered and manual chairs for adults.

Medical Electronics and Equipment News
Available from:
Reilly Publications Co.
Park Ridge, IL 60068

A semimonthly paper available by subscription. Reports on the availability of instruments including scientific apparatus, electronic devices, laboratory supplies, and material and accessories used in clinical applications, diagnoses, therapy, radiology, surgery, analyses, and research.

Science Guide to Scientific Instruments
Available from:
Science magazine as an annual supplement.
Lists many instruments and manufacturers.

Source of Equipment for Sport Science Laboratories. Edited by R.B. Walker.
Available from:
Canadian Association of Sports Sciences
Guelph, Ontario, Canada

Suppliers of Tests

The Psychological Corporation
757 Third Avenue
New York, NY 10017

One of the largest publishers and suppliers of psychological tests, including aptitude and ability tests, intelligence tests, personality tests, aptitude and interest inventories, reading and vocabulary tests, books on testing.

Stoelting Corporation
1350 South Kostner Avenue
Chicago, IL 60623

Publishers of intelligence tests, form boards, spatial relations tests, coordination tests, motor skill tests, timing and counting devices, biofeedback instruments, sensorimotor apparatus.

J.A. Preston Corporation
60 Page Road
Clifton, NJ 07012

Publishers of sensory-motor equipment, preschool and primary readiness tests, form boards, manual dexterity tests, prevocational skill tests, physical rehabilitation materials, research apparatus and equipment.

Western Psychological Services
12031 Wilshire Boulevard
Los Angeles, CA 90025

Publishers of personality tests, attitudes, traits and leadership inventories, social maturity tests, projective drawing tests, neurological assessments, behavior scales, school readiness tests, special education assessments for learning disabilities, educational achievement tests, perceptual-motor tests, speech and audiometry assessments, health questionnaires, vocational interest and aptitude tests, books on testing, counseling and special education.

Educational and Industrial Testing Service
San Diego, CA 92107

Publishers of personality tests, interest, ability and aptitude inventories, achievement and leadership tests.

Psychological Assessment Resources, Inc.
P.O. Box 98
Odessa, FL 33556

Publishers of achievement and aptitude tests, neuropsychological assessments, personality and intelligence tests.

Institute for Personality and Ability Testing
P.O. Box 188
Champaign, IL 61820

Publishers of personality tests, intelligence tests, and tests of motivation.

APPENDIX E

Bibliographic Sources for Tests

Asher, I.E. (1996). *Occupational therapy assessment tools: An annotated index* (2nd ed.). Bethesda, MD: AOTA.

Contains 200 profiles on all occupational therapy practice areas and reviews over 100 new assessments. Includes revised definitions from AOTA's *Uniform Terminology* (3rd ed.) for evaluation and assessment.

Chun, K.T., Cobb, S., & French, J.R. (1985). *Measures for psychological assessment.* Ann Arbor, MI: Institute for Social Research, University of Michigan.

Title, author, publisher, and description of measures for psychological assessment. A guide to 3000 original sources and their applications.

Kramer, J., & Conoley, J. (Eds.). (1992). *The eleventh mental measurements yearbook.* Lincoln, NB: Buros Institute of Mental Measurement.

The most comprehensive listing of mental measurement tests. Includes index of tests by title, acronym, author, subject, publisher, and a description of most tests in print.

Murphy, L., Conoley, J., & Impara, J. (1994). *Tests in print IV: An index to tests, test re-views, and the literature on specific tests.* Lincoln, NB: Buros Institute of Mental Measurement.

Lists tests in print; indexes by title, acronym, subject, and publisher.

Robinson, J.P. (1991). *Measures of personality and socio-psychological attitudes.* San Diego, CA: Academic Press.

Title, author, publisher, and description of measures of personality.

Robinson, J.P., & Shaver, P.R. (1985). *Measures of social psychological attitudes.* Ann Arbor, MI: Institute for Social Research, University of Michigan.

Title, author, publisher, and description of measures for psychological attitudes.

Sweetland, R., & Keyser, D. (1986). *Tests: A comprehensive reference for assessment in psychology, education, and business* (2nd ed.). Kansas City, KS: Test Corporation of America.

Listing by test and out-of-print tests; indexes for tests for hearing-impaired, physically impaired, and visually impaired; author and publisher indexes.

Software for Qualitative Data Analysis

For further information on choosing computer programs for qualitative data analysis see:

Fielding, N., & Lee, R. (1991). *Using computers in qualitative research.* Newbury Park, CA: Sage Publications.

Miles, M., & Huberman, A. (1994). *Qualitative data analysis: An expanded sourcebook* (2nd ed.). Newbury Park, CA: Sage Publications.

The following list is drawn largely from these two texts. Only programs that are considered user-friendly are included.

ATLAS/ti: Developed by Thomas Muhr, Trautenaustr. 12, D10717 Berlin, Germany.

Distributed by Qualitative Research Management, 73425 Hilltop Road, Desert Hot Springs, CA 92240.

DOS; good for coding, memoing, data linking, theory building.

ETHNO: Developed by David R. Heise, Indiana University.

Distributed by National Collegiate Software of Duke University Press, 6697 College Station, Durham, NC 27708.

DOS; good for data linking, testing links.

ETHNOGRAPH: Developed by John V. Seidel, Qualis Research Associates, Amherst, MA.

Distributed by Qualitative Research Management (address earlier).

DOS; good for coding, memoing.

FOLIO VIEWS: Developed and distributed by Folio Corporation, 2155 N. Freedom Boulevard, Suite 150, Provo, UT 84604.

DOS or Windows; good for coding, database management, memoing, data linking.

HYPERQUAL: Developed by Raymond V. Padilla, Arizona State University, 3327 N. Dakota, Chandler, AZ 85224.

Distributed by Qualitative Research Management (address earlier).

Macintosh; good for coding, database management, memoing, data linking.

HYPER RESEARCH: Developed and distributed by Sharlene Hesse-Biber, Paul DuPuis, Scott Kinder, Boston College, Researchware, Inc., 20 Soren St., Randolph, MA 02368.

Macintosh and Windows; good for coding, theory building from textual, audio and video materials; statistical option.

INSPIRATION: Developed and distributed by Inspiration Software, Inc., 2920 S.W. Dolph Court, Suite 3, Portland, OR 97219.

Macintosh; good for memoing, data linking, theory building.

KWALITAN: Developed and distributed by Vincent Peters, Department of Research

Methodology, Social Sciences Faculty, University of Nijmegen, Th. Van Acquinostraat 4, 6225 GD Nijmegen, The Netherlands.

DOS; good for coding, memoing.

MECA: Developed and distributed by Kathleen Carley, Department of Social and Decision Sciences, Carnegie Mellon University, Pittsburgh, PA 15568.

Macintosh and DOS; good for data linking, theory building.

METADESIGN: Developed and distributed by Meta Software Corp., 125 Cambridge Park Drive, Cambridge, MA 02140.

Macintosh and Windows; good for data linking, network display.

QSR NUD·IST: Developed and distributed by T. Richards and L. Richards, La Trobe University, Qualitative Solutions & Research Pty, Ltd. 2 Research Drive, Bundoora, Victoria 3083, Australia. Also distributed by Scolari, Sage Publications Software, P.O. Box 5084, Thousand Oaks, CA 91359.

2.3 version for Macintosh and Windows, 3.0 version for Macintosh; 2.3 good for coding, search and retrieval, theory building; 3.0 good for coding, search and retrieval, memoing, matrix building, theory building.

QUALPRO: Developed by Bernard Blackman, Florida State University.

Distributed by Qualitative Research Management (address above), and Impulse Development Company, 3491-11 Thomasville Road, Suite 202, Tallahassee, FL 32308.

DOS; good for coding, search and retrieval.

SEMNET: Developed and distributed by Joseph Faletti, SemNet Research Group, 1043 University Ave., San Diego, CA 92103.

Macintosh; good for memoing, data linking, matrix building, theory building.

SONAR PROFESSIONAL: Developed and distributed by Virginia Systems Inc., 5509 West Bay Court, Midlothian, VA 23112.

Macintosh and Windows; good for search and retrieval, database management.

TAP (Text Analysis Package): Developed by Kriss Drass, Southern Methodist University.

Distributed by Qualitative Research Management (address earlier) and Kriss Drass, Department of Sociology, Southern Methodist University, Dallas, TX 75275.

DOS; good for coding, pattern matching, search and retrieval, frequency tables for codes.

TEXT COLLECTOR: Developed and distributed by O'Neill Software, P.O. Box 26111, San Francisco, CA 94126.

DOS; good for search and retrieval, database management.

TEXTBASE ALPHA: Developed by Bo Sommerlund and Ole Steen Kristensen.

Distributed by Qualitative Research Management (address earlier).

DOS; good for coding, search and retrieval, frequency counts, matrix building.

WORD CRUNCHER: Developed and distributed by Johnston & Co., 314 E. Carlyle Avenue, Alpine, UT 84004.

4.5 for DOS, Beta for Windows; 4.5 good for data linking, Beta good for search and retrieval, memoing, data linking.

Principles of the Declaration of Helsinki (World Medical Association)

Adopted by the 18th World Medical Assembly, Helsinki, Finland, 1964, and amended by the 41st World Medical Assembly, Hong Kong, September 1989.

I. Basic Principles

1. Biomedical research involving human subjects must conform to generally accepted scientific principles and should be based on adequately performed laboratory and animal experimentation and on a thorough knowledge of the scientific literature.

2. The design and performance of each experimental procedure involving human subjects should be clearly formulated in an experimental protocol which should be transmitted for consideration, comment and guidance to a specially appointed committee independent of the investigator and the sponsor provided that this independent committee is in conformity with the laws and regulations of the country in which the research experiment is performed.

3. Biomedical research involving human subjects should be conducted only by scientifically qualified persons and under the supervision of a clinically competent medical person. The responsibility for the human subject must always rest with a medically qualified person and never rest on the subject of the research, even though the subject has given his or her consent.

4. Biomedical research involving human subjects cannot legitimately be carried out unless the importance of the objective is in proportion to the inherent risk to the subject.

5. Every biomedical research project involving human subjects should be preceded by careful assessment of predictable risks in comparison with foreseeable benefits to the subject or to others. Concern for the interests of the subject must always prevail over the interests of science and society.

6. The right of the research subject to safeguard his or her integrity must always be respected. Every precaution should

243

be taken to respect the privacy of the subject and to minimize the impact of the study on the subject's physical and mental integrity and on the personality of the subject.

7. Physicians should abstain from engaging in research projects involving human subjects unless they are satisfied that the hazards involved are believed to be predictable. Physicians should cease any investigation if the hazards are found to outweigh the potential benefits.

8. In publication of the results of his or her research, the physician is obliged to preserve the accuracy of the results. Reports of experimentation not in accordance with the principles laid down in this Declaration should not be accepted for publication.

9. In any research on human beings, each potential subject must be adequately informed of the aims, methods, anticipated benefits and potential hazards of the study and the discomfort it may entail. He or she should be informed that he or she is at liberty to abstain from participation in the study and that he or she is free to withdraw his or her consent to participation at any time. The physician should then obtain the subject's freely-given informed consent, preferably in writing.

10. When obtaining informed consent for the research project the physician should be particularly cautious if the subject is in a dependent relationship to him or her or may consent under duress. In that case the informed consent should be obtained by a physician who is not engaged in the investigation and who is completely independent of this official relationship.

11. In case of legal incompetence, informed consent should be obtained from the legal guardian in accordance with national legislation. Where physical or mental incapacity makes it impossible to obtain informed consent, or when the subject is a minor, permission from the responsible relative replaces that of the subject in accordance with national legislation.

Whenever the minor child is in fact able to give a consent, the minor's con-

sent must be obtained in addition to the consent of the minor's legal guardian.

12. The research protocol should always contain a statement of the ethical considerations involved and should indicate that the principles enunciated in the present Declaration are complied with.

II. Medical Research Combined with Professional Care (Clinical Research)

1. In the treatment of the sick person, the physician must be free to use a new diagnostic and therapeutic measure, if in his or her judgment it offers hope of saving life, reestablishing health, or alleviating suffering.

2. The potential benefits, hazards and discomfort of a new method should be weighed against the advantages of the best current diagnostic and therapeutic methods.

3. In any medical study, every patient, including those of a control group, if any, should be assured of the best proven diagnostic and therapeutic method.

4. The refusal of the patient to participate in a study must never interfere with the physician-patient relationship.

5. If the physician considers it essential not to obtain informed consent, the specific reasons for this proposal should be stated in the experimental protocol for transmission to the independent committee (I, 2).

6. The physician can combine medical research with professional care, the objective being the acquisition of new medical knowledge, only to the extent that medical research is justified by its potential diagnostic or therapeutic value for the patient.

III. Non-Therapeutic Biomedical Research Involving Human Subjects (Non-clinical Biomedical Research)

1. In the purely scientific application of medical research carried out on a human being, it is the duty of the physician to remain the protector of the life and health of that person on whom biomedical research is being carried out.

2. The subjects should be volunteers, either healthy persons or patients for whom the experimental design is not related to the patient's illness.

3. The investigator or the investigating team should discontinue the research if in his/her or their judgment it may, if continued, be harmful to the individual.
4. In research on man, the interest of science and society should never take precedence over considerations related to the well-being of the subject.

Available from *World Medical Association, Inc.,* 28 Avenue Des Alpes, 01210 Ferney-Voltaire, France.

Sample of a Consent Form

Electromechanical Games and Exploration Behavior in Profoundly Retarded Adults

Names of investigators: _____

_____ has been asked to take part in a research study on the effect of electro-
(Name of client)
mechanical games on exploration behavior. The purpose of the study is to see if electrome-
chanical games will encourage clients who have diminished interest in their surroundings to
explore and interact with the game.

_____ will be given a battery-powered game for 15 minutes, 3 days per week
for 3 weeks, at the State School. His/her behavior will be recorded in writing by a member of
the occupational therapy staff to see if his/her exploration behavior changes and if the game
interests him/her. Behavior will be videotape recorded on two separate occasions.

_____ will have the choice to interact with the game or not. Participation
is entirely voluntary and _____ has the right to withdraw consent and discontinue participation in the study at any time without prejudice to present or future care at the
State School. There is no cost for any part of the study.

No discomfort or risks are anticipated. It is hoped that _____ will enjoy
interacting with the game and may benefit from doing so by learning more about his/her environment. Information from this study will be anonymously coded to ensure confidentiality
and _____ will not be personally identified in any publication containing the
results of this study. The videotapes and written material from the study will be kept in a
locked cabinet. The videotape recordings will be viewed solely by members of the occupational
therapy department and will be destroyed upon completion of data analysis. The parent/guard-
ian may view any videotape of _____ which is filmed for the study.

_____ OTR, director of the occupational therapy department at the

_____ State School (phone number), will be available to answer any questions you may have concerning the study, the procedures, and any risks or benefits that may arise from participating in the study.

As parent/guardian of the previously named client, I give permission for him/her to participate in the research study described.

A copy of this consent form has been given to me.

Signed _____   Date _____
                Parent/Guardian

_____   Date _____
Principal Investigator's Signature

_____   Date _____
             Witness Signature

APPENDIX I

Sample of Consent Form for Student's Thesis

Hand Therapy Patients' Compliance with Treatment: Therapists' Views

_____ has asked _____ to take part in a study regarding hand
    (Investigator)   (Participant)
therapy patients and their compliance with treatment.

_____ will be asked to tell the investigator two stories, one about a patient
the therapist perceived as successful and one about a patient the therapist perceived as unsuccessful. He/she will also be asked to discuss what elements he/she thinks make a patient
successful or unsuccessful. The investigator will audiotape the stories and all questions and
answers.

Participation in the study is voluntary and _____ has the right to discontinue participation at any time without repercussions. There are no discomforts or risks associated with the study.

Information from the study will be coded to ensure confidentiality and _____
will not be identified in any publication that may result from the study. The audiotapes will
be heard by the investigator, a transcriber, and possibly by another occupational therapy student (who will aid in selecting relevant portions of the tape for transcribing), and the three
faculty advisers to the investigator. The transcribed stories will not be printed for public use,
but short excerpts will be taken from them and included in the investigator's thesis and in
possible future publications.

The investigator will be available to answer further questions regarding any aspect of the study or participation therein (phone). I understand that members of the Human Subjects Committee of the _____ are also available to answer questions (phone).
                                   (Name of Program)

I agree to participate in the study described above. I have been given a copy of this form.

Signed: _____   Date: _____
                   (Participant)

_____   Date: _____
                   (Investigator)

_____   Date: _____
                   (Witness)

APPENDIX J

Sample of Permission Form for Photographs and Other Media Materials

Media Release

I give permission to the Communications Department of the _____

(Name of facility)

to use materials identifying _____ in the following situations:

(Name of client)

_____ External publications (e.g., professional journals, newspapers, magazines)

_____ Radio programs

_____ Television programs

_____ Internal publications (e.g., facility publications)

_____ Internal/residential building displays (e.g., bulletin boards, photo albums)

_____ Conference materials (e.g., slides, overheads)

_____ Other_____

(Specify)

In many cases, the use of the patient's/client's first and last name is not necessary, but can add to the completion of the story or photo. If you do *not* want the last name used, please indicate below:

_____ NO, the use of first and last name is *not* permissible

_____ YES, the first and last names may be used

_____ Only the first name and last initial may be used

I give consent on the condition that the material be used only for the above purpose(s). It is my understanding that I may see the materials before confirming consent or before the material is released. Also, it is my understanding that I will receive verbal notification before any material is used, and that I may place the following restrictions on the material or its use, including time limits:

I give this consent voluntarily, without threat of punishment or promise of special reward. I have been given an opportunity to fully discuss the release and to have my questions answered. I understand that I may withdraw consent at any time prior to release without fear or punishment.

Signature: _____　　Date: _____
(Patient/Client)

Signature: _____　　Date: _____
(Parent/Guardian)

I have fully explained the information above and answered all questions to the best of my ability. It is my opinion that consent has been given knowingly and freely.

Signature: _____　　Date: _____
(Person obtaining consent)

_____
(Title/position)

APPENDIX K

Human Subjects Committee Guidelines for Informed Consent from a Children's Hospital

Informed Consent

One of the most important components of research involving human subjects is that of informed consent.

> For the purpose of these guidelines informed consent will be defined as:
> Consent freely given by a participant in a research project based upon full disclosure of the procedures that the individual will undergo.

General Information

The consent form should be written in terms comprehensible to the lay person and should include all information about the study that any reasonable person would need and want to know. It should, realistically and honestly, express what a participant may expect, and should avoid persuasion by raising false hopes.

Informed consent forms used for research programs are not legal documents, although there have been adverse legal decisions in cases where informed consent was felt to be sufficiently lacking.

Informed consent is to be obtained from every person who agrees to participate in any program falling under the jurisdiction of the Consent Committee. The consent form for each study is to be submitted to the Committee with the approved protocol prior to the beginning of any part of the investigation.

All efforts should be made so that the participant fully understands the information obtained in the informed consent, despite any complicating factors, such as mental incompetence, language difficulties, illiteracy, age, and so forth. If it appears that patients, parents, or guardians are incapable of comprehending this information, the executive officers should be notified and a member of the Consent Committee will be made available. In cases of a language barrier, the executive officer will obtain the assistance of a knowledgeable person in that language to translate the informed consent or interpret during the explanation. Should the participant have questions, and so forth regarding the research once it has begun, the participant will again be provided with an interpreter.

A. Written Informed Consent

A standardized format has been devised in order to facilitate writing of informed consent.

These forms are available from _____. Additional assistance in planning, wording, and developing consent forms may be obtained from _____.

Using the standardized format, the following elements should be included:
1. Description and explanation of procedure
2. Risks and discomforts
3. Potential benefits
4. Alternatives
5. "Consent"

1. *Description and explanation of procedure*

The basic procedures of the research should be stated clearly and concisely in non-technical terms. Special note must be made of any part of these procedures that are experimental. The purpose of the study should be described, and the reason this person is being asked to participate should be explained.

2. *Risks and discomforts*

List in simple terms the most serious risks and those most likely to occur. For each risk or hazard, whenever applicable, answer such questions as: How much will it hurt? How long will it take? What danger will the patient be in? What will be done to counteract adverse effects? Are the side effects reversible? What will be done beforehand to minimize risk or discomfort? Is there inconvenience to the patient regarding time or cost? Could there be psychological harm, invasion of privacy, loss of confidentiality, embarrassment, or social injury?

It is important to state whether risks of experimental procedures or side effects are known.

3. *Potential benefits*

Potential benefits are considered to be either (a) of direct benefit to the subject or (b) of value to future patients or society as a whole. If it is felt that physical or emotional problems might be uncovered during a study, it might be desirable to state that professional services would be offered to help the problem. If appropriate, results of testing, questionnaires, or interviews might be offered to the child's school or physician if the parent or subject requests it.

4. *Alternative*

There are sometimes alternative procedures or medications to the ones described, and these should be listed to give the subject a clear choice. The risks and benefits of each alternative also should be stated. Where there are no alternatives to a particular treatment, this should be noted. If the only alternative is nonparticipation, the section can be omitted. This section has to be carefully worded so as not to make a patient feel pressured into participating because the alternatives are made to sound much less desirable.

5. *Consent*

The following additional items must be contained in every consent form.

1. The assurance that full information regarding the study has been given to the subject.
2. The fact that the physician or investigator is available to answer any inquiries concerning the study.
3. The option of subjects to withdraw from the project at any time without any effect on their treatment or, if hospital employees, their employment.

The following paragraphs are part of the standard format and should be included at the end of the consent document:

I have fully explained to _____ the nature and purpose of the above-
         (Participant/parent/guardian)
described procedure and the risks involved in its performance. I have answered and will answer all questions to the best of my ability. I will inform the participant of any changes in the procedure or the risks and benefits if any should occur during or after the course of the study.

_____
(Investigator's signature)

I have been satisfactorily informed of the above-described procedure with its possible risks and benefits. I give permission for my/my child's participation in this study. I know that

Dr. _____ or his/her associates will be available to answer any questions I may have. If I feel my questions have not been adequately answered, I may request to

speak to a member of the Hospital Consent Committee by calling extension _____.
I understand that I am free to withdraw this consent and discontinue participation in this project at any time and it will not affect my child's care. I have been offered a copy of this form.

_____
(Signature of participant)

_____ _____
(Witness signature)   (Parent/Guardian signature)

Modification of the wording in these paragraphs may be made in certain cases, depending on the nature of the study.

The parent and/or legal guardian must sign the document, as well as the physician or investigator, and witness. The witness is to the signatures only. In cases where witnesses to the explanation are required, a member of the Consent Committee will fulfill this function.

The consent form containing the original signatures must be placed in the medical record. If there is no medical record—as for volunteers, students, and so forth—then the signed copy must be kept in the investigator's files. A copy of the consent form should always be offered to the participant.

If new information occurs during the course of a study, the investigator has the obligation to inform the subject. The consent form should then be revised accordingly and the changes communicated to the executive officer.

B. Other Types of Consent

1. *Letter.* In some instances, the Committee will approve consents in letter form, particularly when they involve questionnaires or other low-risk studies. These generally occur in school populations or retrospective studies of former patients when mailings are sent out to individuals not likely to be at the hospital.

2. *Telephone.* At times, the parents of a child to be considered for a study are not available to sign a consent form. In these rare cases, telephone consent can be obtained. The following phrase is added to the consent form:

Since the parents of the child were unavailable, this information has been conveyed to

_____ by telephone.

_____
(Investigator's signature)

_____
(Witness to telephone conversation)

The investigator should read the consent form to the parent or guardian while a second individual listens to the conversation on another line to witness the fact that consent was given.

3. *Short form.* Occasionally, due to a study's complexity, it is not possible to write a concise consent form. In such instances, the investigator may explain the procedure orally and at length, but present the patients with only a short form to sign. The short form will indicate that all the requirements for informed consent have been met by means of the oral explanation and will include the standard closing paragraphs of written consents. If such form of consent is used, a written summary of what is told the patient should be part of the protocol and must receive Committee approval.

Oral consents should be restricted to extraordinary situations.

C. Participation of Children in Consent Process

Children should be involved in the consent process whenever appropriate or feasible. They should be as fully informed about the research project as is appropriate for the child's age and should be given the right to refuse participation. It is recommended that a child not be used as a subject in research if there is a conflict between parent and child regarding participation.

It is recommended that children younger than 18 years of age who are capable of understanding a procedure and its ramifications and who agree to participate sign the consent form along with the parent or guardian. This process is left to the discretion of the investigator.

APPENDIX L

List of Professional Journals and Their Publishers

Administration

Administration and Policy in Mental Health. Plenum Publishing Corp., 233 Spring Street, New York, NY 10013

Hospital and Health Services Administration. American College of Health Care Executives, Health Administration Press, 1021 East Huron Street, Ann Arbor, MI 48104

Hospitals and Health Networks. American Hospital Association, American Hospital Publishing Inc., 737 North Michigan Avenue, Suite 700, Chicago, IL 60611 (Also available on-line)

Journal of Long-Term Care Administration. American College of Health Care Administrators, 325 South Patrick Street, Alexandria, VA 22314

Journal of Rehabilitation Administration. Journal of Rehabilitation Administration Inc., Box 19891, San Diego, CA 92159

Modern Healthcare. Crain Communications Inc., 740 North Rush Street, Chicago, IL 60611

Aging

Activities, Adaptation and Aging. Haworth Press, 10 Alice Street, Binghampton, NY 13904

American Journal of Geriatric Psychiatry. American Psychiatric Press, Inc., 1400 K Street NW, Suite 1101, Washington, DC 20005

Clinical Gerontologist. Haworth Press, Binghampton, NY

Gerontologist. Gerontological Society of America, 1275 K Street NW, Suite 350, Washington, DC 20005

International Journal of Aging and Human Development. Baywood Publishing Co., Inc., 26 Austin Avenue, Box 337, Amityville, NY 11701

Journal of Aging and Physical Activity. Kinetics Publishers, Inc., Box 5076, Champaign, IL 61825

Journal of Aging and Social Policy. Haworth Press, Binghampton, NY

Journal of Aging Studies. JAI Press, Inc., 55 Old Post Road, Box 1678, Greenwich, CT 06836

Journal of Applied Gerontology. Sage Publications Inc., 2455 Teller Road, Thousand Oaks, CA 91320

Journal of Geriatric Psychiatry. Boston Society for Gerontological Psychiatry International, Universities Press Inc., 59 Boston Post Road, Box 1524, Madison, CT 06443

Journal of Gerontology. Gerontological Society of America, Washington, DC

Journal of Women and Aging. Haworth Press, Binghampton, NY

Physical and Occupational Therapy in Geriatrics. Haworth Press, Binghampton, NY.

Computer Applications

Computers in Human Behavior. Elsevier Science Ltd, Pergamon, PO Box 800, Kidlington, Oxford OX5 1DX, England

Computers in Human Services. Haworth Press, Binghampton, NY

Computers in the Schools. Haworth Press, Binghampton, NY

Health Management Technology. Argus, Inc., 6151 Powers Ferry Road NW, Atlanta, GA 30339.

Health Care

Home Health Care Services Quarterly. Haworth Press, Binghampton, NY

Journal of Allied Health. American Society of Allied Health Professions, 1730 M Street NW, Suite 500, Washington DC 20036

Journal of Home Health Care Practice. Aspen Publishers Inc., 200 Orchard Ridge Drive, Gaithersburg, MD 20878

The Journal of Women's Health Care. Haworth Press, Binghampton, NY

Occupational Therapy in Health Care. Haworth Press, Binghampton, NY

Physical Therapy in Health Care. Haworth Press, Binghampton, NY

Hospice

American Journal of Hospice and Palliative Care. Prime National Publishing Corp., 470 Boston Post Road, Weston, MA 02193

Hospice Journal. Haworth Press, Binghampton, NY

Hospice Letter. Health Resources Publishing, Brinley Professional Plaza, 3100 Hwy. 138, Box 1442, Wall Township, NJ 07719

Occupational Health and Vocational Development

International Journal of Sports Medicine. Human Kinetics Publishers, Inc., 1607 North Market Street, PO Box 5076, Champaign, IL 61825

Job Safety and Health. Subseries of BNA Policy and Practice Series: Environment, Safety and Health Services. Bureau of National Affairs, Inc., 1231 25th Street NW, Washington, DC 20037 (Also available online)

Journal of Health and Social Behavior. American Sociological Association, 1722 N Street NW, Washington, DC 20036

Journal of Occupational Rehabilitation. Plenum Publishing Corp., 233 Spring Street, New York, NY 10013

Occupational Health and Safety. Stevens Publishing Corp., 3630 J.H. Kultgen Freeway, Waco, TX 76706 (Also available on-line)

Occupational Health Nurses Journal. American Association of Occupational Health Nurses, Slack Inc., Thorofare, NJ

Pediatrics and Early Intervention

Child Development. University of Chicago Press, 5720 S. Woodlawn Avenue, Chicago, IL 60637

Infants and Young Children. Aspen Publishers, Inc., 7201 McKinney Circle, Frederick, MD 21701

Journal of Early Intervention. Division for Early Childhood, Council for Exceptional Children, 1920 Association Drive, Reston, VA 22091

Journal of Pediatric Psychology. Plenum Publishing Corp., 233 Spring Street, New York, NY 10013

Pediatric Physical Therapy. Williams & Wilkins, 428 Preston Street, Baltimore, MD 21202

Physical and Occupational Therapy in Pediatrics. Haworth Press, Binghampton, NY

Physical Disabilities—Education and Related Services. Council for Exceptional Children, Division for Physical and Health Disabilities, 1920 Association Drive, Reston, VA 22091

Special Services in the Schools. Haworth Press, Binghampton, NY

Topics in Early Childhood Special Education. Pro-Ed, Inc., 8700 Shoal Creek Blvd., Austin, TX 78757

Physical Medicine and Rehabilitation

Accent on Living. Cheever Publishing Inc., Box 700, Bloomington, IL 61702

American Journal of Physical Medicine and Rehabilitation. Williams & Wilkins, 428 East Preston Street, Baltimore, MD 21202

American Rehabilitation. Rehabilitation Services Administration, US Department of Education, Mary E. Switzer Bldg. Room 3127, 330 C Street NW, Washington, DC 20202

Clinical Laboratory Science. 7910 Woodmont Avenue, Suite 1301, Bethesda, MD 20814

Continuing Care. Stevens Publishing Corp., 3630 J.H. Kultgen Freeway, Waco, TX 76706

European Journal of Physical Medicine and Rehabilitation. Blackwell-MZV, Feldgasse 13, A-1238 Vienna, Austria. (Printed in English)

Journal of Occupational Rehabilitation. Plenum Publishing Corp., 233 Spring Street, New York, NY 10013

Journal of Orthopedics & Sports Physical Therapy. Williams & Wilkins, 428 E. Preston Street, Baltimore, MD 21202

Journal of Rehabilitation. National Rehabilitation Association, 633 S. Washington Street, Alexandria, VA 22314

Physical Medicine and Rehabilitation. Hanley and Belfus, Inc., 210 South 13th Street, Philadelphia, PA 19107

Physical Medicine and Rehabilitation Clinics of N. America. W.B. Saunders Co., Harcourt Brace & Co., The Curtis Center, 3rd floor, Independence Square West, Philadelphia, PA 19106

Physical Therapy Products. Novicom, Inc., 20000 Mariner Avenue, Suite 480, Torrance, CA 91503

Physiotherapy Theory and Practice. Lawrence Erlbaum Assocs., Ltd., 27 Palmeira Mansions, Church Road, Hove, East Sussex BN3 2FA, England

Rehabilitation Administration. Elliot and Fitzpatrick, Inc., Box 1945, Athens, GA 30605

Rehabilitation and Community Care Management. BCS Communications Ltd., 101 Thorncliffe Park Drive, Toronto, Ontario M4H 1M2, Canada

Rehabilitation Counseling Bulletin. American Rehabilitation Counseling Association, 5999 Stevenson Avenue, Alexandria, VA 22304

Rehabilitation Education. Elliott and Fitzpatrick, Inc., Box 1945, Athens, GA 30603

Rehabilitation Index. British Library Medical Information Centre, Boston Spa, Wetherby, W. Yorkshire LS23 7BQ, England

Sexuality and Disability. A journal devoted to the psychological and medical aspects of sexuality in rehabilitation and community settings; Human Sciences Press, 233 Spring Street, New York, NY 10013

Work: A Journal of Prevention, Assessment and Rehabilitation. Andover Medical Publishers, Inc., 15 Terrace Park, Reading, MA 01867

Professional Association Journals

American Health Care Association Provider. American Health Care Association, 1201 L Street NW, Washington, DC 20005

American Journal of Art Therapy. Vermont College of Norwich University, Montpelier, VT 05602

American Journal of Occupational Therapy. American Occupational Therapy Association, Box 31220, Bethesda, MD 20824

AMT Events. American Medical Technologists, 710 Higgins Road, Park Ridge, IL 60068

British Journal of Occupational Therapy. College of Occupational Therapists, Ltd., 6-8 Marshalsea Road, Southwark, London SE1 1HL England

Journal of Allied Health. American Society of Allied Health Professions, University of Illinois at Chicago, College of Associated Health Professions, (M-C518), 808 South Wood Street, Chicago, IL 60612

Journal of Athletic Training. National Athletic Trainers Association, Inc., 2952 Stemmons Freeway, Dallas, TX 75247

Journal of Hand Therapy. American Society of Hand Therapists, Hanley and Belfus, Inc., 210 South 13th Street, Philadelphia, PA 19107

Journal of Rehabilitation. National Rehabilitation Association, 633 S. Washington Street, Alexandria, VA 22314

Journal of Sport Rehabilitation. Human Kinetics Publishers, Inc., PO Box 5076, Champaign, IL 61825

Occupational Therapy International. Whurr Publishers, Ltd., 19b Compton Terrace, London WC1 P4ED, England

Physical Therapy. American Physical Therapy Association, 1111 North Fairfax Street, Alexandria, VA 22314

Physiotherapy. Chartered Society of Physiotherapy, 14 Bedford Row, London, WC1R 4ED, England

Physiotherapy Canada. Canadian Physiotherapy Association, 890 Yonge Street, 9th floor, Toronto, Ontario M4W 3P4, Canada

Public Health Journal. American Public Health Association, Inc., 1015 15th Street NW, Washington, DC 20005

Radiologic Technology. American Society of Radiologic Technologists, 15000 Central Avenue SE, Albuquerque, NM 87123

Rehabilitation Counseling Bulletin. American Rehabilitation Counseling Association, 5999 Stevenson Avenue, Alexandria, VA 22304

Respiratory Care. American Association for Respiratory Care, Daedalus Enterprises, Inc., 11030 Ables Lane, Dallas, TX 75229

Psychiatry and Mental Health

Clinical Supervisor. Haworth Press, Binghampton, NY

Community Mental Health Journal. Human Sciences Press, 233 Spring Street, New York, NY 10013

Hospital and Community Psychiatry. American Psychiatric Association, 1400 K Street NW, Washington, DC 20005

Journal of Family Psychotherapy. Haworth Press, Binghampton, NY

Journal of Organizational Behavior Management. Haworth Press, Binghampton, NY

Occupational Therapy in Mental Health. Haworth Press, Binghampton, NY

Prevention in Human Services. Haworth Press, Binghampton, NY

Residential Treatment for Children and Youth. Haworth Press, Binghampton, NY

Schizophrenia Bulletin. US Public Health Service, National Institute of Mental Health, 5600 Fishers Lane, Rockville, MD 20857

Schizophrenia Research. Elsevier Science B.V., PO Box 211, 1000 AE Amsterdam, Netherlands

Special Services in the Schools. Haworth Press, Binghampton, NY

Research in Health and Education

International Journal of Qualitative Studies in Education. 216 Claxton Bldg. University of Tennessee, Knoxville, TN 37996

Occupational Therapy Journal of Research. American Occupational Therapy Foundation, Slack, Inc., 6900 Grove Road, Thorofare, NJ 08086

Physiotherapy Research International. Whurr Publishers, Inc., 19b Compton Terrace, London WC1 R4ED, England

Qualitative Enquiry. Interdisciplinary journal for qualitative methodology in the human sciences. Department of Sociology, University of Illinois, Urbana-Champaign, 326 Lincoln Hall, 702 S. Wright Street, Urbana, IL 61801

APPENDIX M

Sample Aim and Scope of a Professional Journal

(Reprinted from *The Occupational Therapy Journal of Research* with the permission of the American Occupational Therapy Foundation, Bethesda, MD.)

The Occupational Therapy Journal of Research

Aim and Scope

In 1965 the American Occupational Therapy Foundation Inc. was chartered as a charitable, scientific, literary, and educational society to "advance the science of occupational therapy . . . and increase the public knowledge and understanding thereof." Toward these ends, the foundation has provided support for scholarships, publications, and research. Sponsorship of *The Occupational Therapy Journal of Research* is a further expression of the foundation's commitment to advancing the profession through scientific inquiry.

As its title suggests, the aim of *The Occupational Therapy Journal of Research* is to provide a dynamic medium for the communication of scholarly writings of potential significance to the field of occupational therapy. The Journal seeks to publish original manuscripts pertaining to the impact of activity on the individual, particularly as such activity is applied in a health-related context to prevent disability and to maintain or restore optimal human function or performance.

The Occupational Therapy Journal of Research will consider submitted manuscripts on a broad scope of subjects of potential interest to occupational therapy researchers. Of particular interest are manuscripts that:

- Demonstrate the value and efficacy of occupational therapy procedures or services;
- Describe new occupational therapy assessment or evaluation approaches or address the standardization, reliability, validity, or innovative application of existing measures;
- Advance the conceptual basis for occupational therapy practice through research that bears on the validity of current theories;
- Propose new theories or paradigms that serve to explain or organize existing data in useful ways; and
- Relate to the education of occupational therapy practitioners, particularly as such manuscripts suggest improvements in the educational process on the basis of empirical research.

Additionally, scholarly dialogue is encouraged through Letters to the Editor and invited Commentary. Occasionally, the journal will select discussants to critique accepted manuscripts, and such commentary will be published following designated articles. Readers are welcome to submit thoughtful letters to the editor pertaining to research published in *The Occupational Therapy Journal of Research.* Other features include Briefs, which present amplified abstracts of completed theses or unpublished research projects; Book, Monograph, and Journal Reviews; and Published Elsewhere, a list of recently published articles of potential interest to occupational therapy researchers.

Full-length manuscripts are evaluated through a blind review process, and selection is based on relevance to the profession, scientific merit, timeliness, and scholarly excellence. All contributors are required to assign exclusive copyright to the American Occupational Therapy Foundation Inc., and assurance must be given that manuscripts are not under consideration for publication elsewhere. Potential contributors should consult submission guidelines published in the Journal under Information for Authors.

Sample Author's Guides from Professional Journals

Sample 1: *Physical Therapy: Instructions to Authors*

(Reprinted from *Physical Therapy* with the permission of the American Physical Therapy Association)

Physical Therapy, the official journal of the American Physical Therapy Association (APTA), is a scholarly, refereed journal that contributes to and documents the evolution and expansion of the scientific and professional body of knowledge in physical therapy.

Manuscripts submitted to *Physical Therapy* should address issues of relevance to physical therapy and should do so in accordance with Journal policy and submission guidelines. The Editor reserves the right to return, without review, any manuscript that does not meet these criteria. All submissions accepted for peer review are privileged communications. The identity of the author(s) is kept confidential from reviewers, unless otherwise indicated under "Manuscript Categories."

Physical Therapy accepts manuscripts for consideration with the understanding that the manuscript, including any original research findings or data reported in the manuscript, has not been published previously and is not under consideration for publication elsewhere. Reports of secondary analyses of data sets should specify the source of the data. Manuscripts published in *Physical Therapy* become the property of the APTA and may not be published elsewhere, in whole or in part, without the written permission of the Journal. Send reprint requests to the Editor in care of the Journal Editorial Office.

Manuscript Categories

Manuscripts will be considered for review by the Journal if they fit into one of the following six categories:

Research Report: Any original research, regardless of the methods used. Included in this category are research using quantitative or qualitative methods and research using single-subject designs. *Type of review:* Blind review by two reviewers and one Editorial Board member.

Case Report: Report of the treatment of a patient or a series of patients. These reports are considered appropriate when they provide unique insights into the treatment or natural history of conditions seen by physical therapists. Case reports describing the treatment of multiple patients are especially encouraged. References should be minimal, with emphasis placed on accurate descriptions of the patients, treatments, and outcomes. *Type of review:* Blind review by two reviewers and one Editorial Board member.

Technical Report: An original report that describes and documents the specifications or mechanical aspects of a device used by physical therapists for the purpose of treatment or measurement. Evaluation of the device should be part of the report. References should be minimal, with major emphasis placed on the description of the methods used to evaluate the device. *Type of review:* Blind review by two reviewers and one Editorial Board member.

Literature Review: A critical analysis of literature on a specific topic of interest to physical therapists. Although the review may further a viewpoint or a theoretical approach, this should not be the major purpose of the paper. These reviews are written by acknowledged experts and by invitation only. Persons wishing to write such reviews may nominate themselves through communication with the Editor. *Type of review:* Nonblind review by two reviewers and one Editorial Board member.

Clinical Perspective: A scholarly paper expounding on a specific clinical approach to patient care, either on a theoretical or practical basis. References should be sufficient to support opinions put forward in the paper. These papers are written by acknowledged experts and by invitation only. Persons wishing to write such papers may nominate themselves through communication with the Editor. *Type of review:* Nonblind review by two reviewers and one Editorial Board member.

Professional Perspective: A scholarly paper addressing professional issues in physical therapy, health care, and related areas. The author should expound on a specific point of view. References should be sufficiently extensive to support the opinions put forward in the paper. These papers are written by acknowledged experts and by invitation only. Persons wishing to write such papers may nominate themselves through communication with the Editor. *Type of review:* Nonblind review by two reviewers and one Editorial Board member.

Other Types of Editorial Material

Commentaries: Commentaries on articles are invited by the Editor and are intended to provide dialogue on controversial issues or to provide discussion of implications of issues raised in an article. *Type of review:* The Editor determines whether a Commentary will be forwarded to the article author(s) and whether it will be published. The Editor also reviews the author response and determines whether this response is acceptable for publication. Author responses to Commentaries that are not submitted within the set time limit will be treated as Letters to the Editor.

Abstracts: Brief synopses of articles relating to the practice or science of physical therapy. The Associate Editor for Abstracts and Reviews is responsible for maintaining a list of abstracters and for the coordination, selection, and assignment of articles to be abstracted. Abstracters may not abstract an article to which they contributed or in which they were in any way recognized. *Type of review:* All abstracts are reviewed by the Associate Editor for Abstracts and Reviews. The Editor has final responsibility for decisions regarding publication of abstracts. Unsolicited abstracts will not be accepted.

Reviews (Books, Software, Videotapes): Critical reviews of books, commercial software, and videotapes of interest to physical therapists. The Associate Editor for Abstracts and Reviews is responsible for maintaining a list of reviewers and for the coordination, selection, and assignment of materials to be reviewed. Reviewers may not review any material to which they contributed or in which they were in any way recognized. *Type of review:* All reviews are reviewed by the Associate Editor for Abstracts and Reviews. The editor has final responsibility for decisions regarding publication of reviews. Unsolicited reviews will not be accepted.

Reviews of Computer Programs: Critical reviews of noncopyrighted, basic-language computer programs either for MS-DOS operating systems or for Apple computers. The programs must be of value to physical therapists and must represent a unique or utilitarian contribution. The Associate Editor for Abstracts and Reviews is responsible for maintaining a list of program reviewers. Persons submitting computer programs must submit two floppy disks with the program on them and three copies of the program code listings, along with a brief description of the program and a set of instructions. The description, instructions, and program code will be published with the review. *Type of review:* All reviews of computer programs are reviewed by the Associate Editor for Abstracts and Reviews. The editor has final responsibility for decisions regarding publication of reviews.

Letters to the Editor: Letters to the Editor should relate specifically to articles published in *Physical Therapy* or to issues of relevance to the physical therapy profession. To be considered for publication, letters must be received within 8 weeks of publication of the article. Letters must be submitted double-spaced, with two copies provided. Receipt of Letters to the Editor is not acknowledged; however, correspondents will be notified if the letter has been accepted for publication. Authors of any article discussed in a letter will be invited to respond. Accepted Letters to the Editor will be printed with the author response whenever possible. Letters and responses should be signed by all authors. *Type of review:* Decisions regarding publication of letters are made by the Editor.

Permissions

Protection of Subjects: For Research Reports, authors must include a written statement documenting informed consent of subjects and approval of the study by an institutional review board or similar body. The statement should indicate that the rights of human and animal subjects were protected.

Photograph Release: Authors must obtain and submit written permission to publish photographs in which subjects are recognizable. This statement must be signed by the subject, parent, or guardian. To conceal a subject's identity, the subject's eyes may be obscured in the photo with a black bar.

Reprinting Tables and Figures: Authors must obtain and submit written permission from the original sources, in the name of APTA, to publish illustrations, photographs, figures, or tables taken from those sources.

Copyright Release

All manuscripts must be accompanied by the following statement, signed by all authors:

In compliance with the Copyright Revision Act of 1976, the undersigned author or authors warrant that they have sole ownership of the work submitted, that the work is original and has never been published, and that the author or authors have full powers to grant such rights.

In consideration of APTA's journal, *Physical Therapy,* taking action in reviewing and editing my (our) submission, the author (authors) undersigned hereby transfer(s), assign(s), or otherwise convey(s) all copyright ownership to APTA, in the event that such work is published by APTA in *Physical Therapy.*

In addition, the author or authors hereby grant APTA's journal, *Physical Therapy,* the right to edit, revise, abridge, condense, and translate the foregoing work.

For these purposes, the editors define "work" as the actual manuscript submitted and any original research findings and data reported in the manuscript.

Conflict of Interest

Authors are expected to disclose in a cover letter any commercial/financial associations that might pose a conflict of interest in connection with the submitted article. All funding sources supporting the work should be acknowledged in a footnote on the title page. The information will be held in confidence by the Editor during the review process.

Prior Disclosure

Prior disclosure of the contents of any manuscript in a widespread and substantive form may make the manuscript ineligible for publication in *Physical Therapy. Note:* Published abstracts and presentations at meetings do not constitute prior disclosure. Authors seeking clarification of this policy must contact the Journal Editorial Office *before* releasing to the media information from their manuscripts and *before* allowing distribution of portions of a manuscript in any form.

Manuscripts that have been presented orally at a scientific meeting or at a professional forum should include a footnote alerting readers to that fact. Authors should notify the Editor in a letter of transmittal of any such oral presentations.

Key Words

Authors may suggest up to five key words that they believe best represent the manuscript content. Editorial staff will use this list, along with subject headings from *Index Medicus* and the *Sixty-Five-Year Index to Physical Therapy,* to choose key words if that article is accepted for publication.

Manuscript Preparation

Authors and reviewers should use their judgment in determining whether statements of hypotheses are necessary in a manuscript.

The Journal welcomes papers that contribute to the literature, even if they report statistically nonsignificant findings. Authors of such papers should pay particular attention to the need to (1) justify the study, (2) make a case as to why the alternative hypothesis was viable before data were collected, and (3) address the possibility of a Type II statistical error.

Authors should specifically define all variables in articles. Titles of articles should not be general or vague and should reflect measured variables.

Whenever probabilistic statistics are used in a study, statements of the probability should be included in the Results section. The use of p values in abstracts, in introductions to papers, and in discussions of the literature should be avoided.

Physical Therapy requires identification of statistical programs in articles. Authors should include this information in manuscripts.

All manuscripts must be submitted double-spaced.

Papers should include the following:

Title page with the title, the author name(s), and footnote of biographical data about the author(s). (See recent issues for examples.) The Journal lists author credentials in the following sequence: terminal academic degree (e.g., PhD), professional degree (e.g., PT), professional certification (e.g., ATC), and honorary degree (e.g., FAPTA). Include a notation in the footnote if work was supported by a grant or other funding sources or was adapted from a conference presentation.

Abstract of 150 words or fewer. Research Report and Technical Report abstracts should have a structured format that includes the following major headings: Background and Purpose, Subjects, Methods, Results, and Conclusion and Discussion. Abstracts for other types of papers should include purpose, summary of key points presented, and conclusions or recommendations.

Text (15 pages or fewer preferred). Use 2.54-cm (1-in) margins and 21.6- by 27.9-cm (8½- by 11-in) bond. State purpose in the introduction. Refer to recent issues for examples of acceptable headings.

Manufacturer's information in a footnote for all equipment and products mentioned in the text. Place at bottom of the page on which the item is mentioned, include full address with ZIP code, and use consecutive symbols (*, , , , #, **, , , , , ##). Use International System of Units (English units may be given in parentheses).

Acknowledgment of important contributors (optional). Place in a separate paragraph at end of text.

References indicated by superscripts numbered consecutively in the text and presented consecutively on a separate sheet after the text. Follow AMA style for references, except for the following: In the reference list, include all authors' names for works with up to four authors; if five or more authors, list the first three names followed by "et al." Reference authors in the text each time they are mentioned. Use *Index Medicus* for journal abbreviations.

Tables numbered consecutively and placed after the references. Refer to recent issues for acceptable tabular format.

Figures numbered consecutively and placed after the references and tables. Provide one original and four copies of each figure. Provide all legends on one sheet. Submit camera-ready material for line drawings, graphs, and charts. Lettering should be large, sharp, and clear, and abbreviations used within figures should agree with journal style. Send only black-and-white photos in sharp focus and with good contrast. Size 12.70 cm by 17.78 cm (5 in by 7 in) preferable. Write first author's last name and figure number on a gummed label, and place on back of the original set of figures. Copies of figures should not be labeled. Use arrow to indicate top of figure if not obvious. Do not write directly on the back of camera-ready material. Do not use paper clips or staples.

Send figures protected between two pieces of cardboard. *Note:* The Journal does not return artwork to authors. Authors should retain copies for their files.

Appendixes numbered consecutively and placed at the end of the paper. Use appendixes to provide essential material not suitable for figures, tables, or text.

The style manual for *Physical Therapy* is the *American Medical Association (AMA) Manual of Style, 8th ed.,* published by Williams & Wilkins (Baltimore, MD). For acceptable format and reference style, authors should consult this reference. Do not use AMA style to format tables; instead, refer to recent issues of *Physical Therapy*.

All correspondence will be sent to the first author named on the manuscript unless otherwise requested.

When submitting a new manuscript, include the following:

- Five copies of the paper
- One original and four copies of each figure
- Permission statements (protection of subjects, photograph release, permission to reprint tables and figures)
- Copyright release statement, signed by all authors
- Cover letter stating category of article being submitted; any potential conflict of interest; and corresponding author's address, day and evening phone numbers, and FAX number

When submitting a revised manuscript, include the following:

- Three copies of the revised paper
- One original and two copies of each revised figure
- Cover letter stating that the manuscript is a revision (provide manuscript number) and including any changes in corresponding author's address, phone number(s), and FAX number
- Authors of accepted manuscripts will be asked to provide, if possible, a computer diskette from an IBM or compatible PC in WordPerfect ASCII file format.

Author Approval, Reprints

The Journal reserves the right to copyedit manuscripts accepted for publication in accordance with its style and format. All material submitted to the Journal is also edited to improve readability. Authors will be given an opportunity to review the edited manuscript before publication.

Abstracts; Reviews of Books, Software, and Videotapes; and Letters to the Editor are also copyedited by Journal staff. Unless extensive editing is required, the abstracter, reviewer, or correspondent will not be sent a copy of the edited version to review.

Authors are invited to order reprints of their articles that appear in *Physical Therapy*. A reprint order form will be sent to the corresponding author at the time of publication, along with a copy of the issue in which the article appears. Readers should contact the corresponding author of the article to obtain reprints.

Send all submissions and other editorial communications to

The Editor
Physical Therapy
American Physical Therapy Association
1111 North Fairfax Street
Alexandria, VA 22314-1488

Sample 2: Author's Guide from the *American Journal of Occupational Therapy*

(Reprinted from the *American Journal of Occupational Therapy* with the permission of the American Occupational Therapy Association.)

The American Journal of Occupational Therapy welcomes manuscripts that pertain to occupational therapy. Feature-length manuscripts (12–18 pages) may include (a) reports of research, educational activities, or professional trends; (b) descriptions of new occupational therapy approaches, programs, or services; (c) review papers that survey new information; or (d) theoretical papers that discuss or treat theoretical issues critically. Short manuscripts (3–6 pages) may be (a) descriptions of original therapeutic aids, devices, or techniques; (b) case reports that describe occupational therapy for a specific clinical situation; or (c) opinion essays that discuss timely issues or opinions and are supported by cogent arguments. In addition, the journal publishes letters to the editor, book reviews, and software and technology reviews. All copy is subject to editing. Important considerations are interest to the profession, originality, timeliness, validity, readability, and conciseness.

Submission

Manuscripts must be submitted with the author's explicit assurance that they are not simultaneously under consideration by any other publication. To permit anonymous peer review, send three copies (including three copies of tables, photos, drawings, etc.) to the Editor, Elaine Viseltear, 616 Tanner Marsh Road, Guilford, CT 06437. In your letter of transmittal, designate the senior author or another person as correspondent. The journal cannot assume responsibility for the loss of manuscripts.

Preparation

The entire manuscript, including the abstract, quotations, tables, and references must be typed double-spaced on 8½ × 11-inch white paper, with 1-inch margins.

Title page. Titles should be short and specific and should summarize the main idea of the paper. List three key words or phrases (not mentioned in the title) that highlight important aspects of the material presented in the article. Provide author's names, degrees, job titles, and current affiliations at the bottom of the page or on a separate sheet. (Include previous work affiliation if the article was written during the time of that affiliation.) Please include city, state, and zip code for workplace, as well as a telephone number for the corresponding author.

Abstract. Every feature-length manuscript must have an abstract (maximum of 150 words). The abstract should be factual, succinct, and sufficiently complete to enable the reader to grasp the essence of the paper quickly. A structured abstract includes a statement of the objectives, method of study, results, and conclusions reached. A descriptive type of abstract indicates the subjects covered, central thesis, sources used, and conclusions.

Text. The introduction should include a statement of purpose (why the manuscript topic is being presented to occupational ther-

apy readers at this time) or an indication of the topic's importance or relevance to the field. The literature reviewed should be limited to those citations of primary relevance to the topic and should emphasize the more recent publications.

Acknowledgments. Acknowledgments must be brief. They should be typed double-spaced and appear after the text but before the reference page. Acknowledgments to people precede those for grant support. If the article is based on a thesis or on a presentation at a meeting, state this fact following the acknowledgments of people and grants.

References. References must also be typed double-spaced. Follow the style shown in the fourth edition of the *Publication Manual of the American Psychological Association* (1994), listing references in alphabetical order at the end of the article and providing authors' names and year of publication for in-text citations.

Personal communications or other nonretrievable citations are described in the text. Provide name and date if the information was obtained from a person; provide name, date and address if the information was obtained from an organization. Articles accepted for publication but not yet published can be included as references if you provide the name of the journal or book publisher.

Authors are solely responsible for the accuracy and completeness of the references. You should review and check them thoroughly. See the examples below for commonly used reference listings.

Journal article:

Ottenbacher, K., & York, J. (1984). Strategies for evaluating clinical change: Implications for practice and research. *American Journal of Occupational Therapy, 38,* 647–659.

Book With Individual Author:

Ayres, A.J. (1973). *Sensory integration and learning disorders.* Los Angeles: Western Psychological Services.

Edited Book:

Hopkins, H.L., & Smith, H.D. (Eds.). (1978). *Willard and Spackman's occupational therapy* (5th ed.). Philadelphia: Lippincott.

Book with Corporate Author and Author as Publisher:

American Psychiatric Association. (1980). *Diagnostic and statistical manual of mental disorders* (3rd ed.). Washington, DC: Author.

Tables. Tables should be self-explanatory and can be used if they supplement, rather than duplicate, the text. Type tables double-spaced, one on a page. Provide titles for each, and cite them in numerical order in the text.

Figures. Figures can be line drawings, graphs, charts, or photographs. Omit figures that repeat information given in the text or that do not enhance the understanding of the article.

Line drawings, graphs, and charts should be done professionally. Submit photographs as glossy black-and-white prints. Tape photographs onto a white piece of paper and write only on the paper. Do not use paper clips on photographic material. Symbols, abbreviations, and spellings should be consistent with those given in the text. Each figure must be labeled: Specify the figure number and the name of senior author and indicate the figure's orientation (top) with an arrow.

Figures are cited in numerical order in the text. They must have captions, which should be typed double-spaced on a separate sheet of paper and numbered in consecutive order.

A letter of permission to publish (in duplicate) from the subjects must accompany the photographs of all identifiable subjects.

Abbreviations. The use of abbreviations is discouraged. If they are used, they are spelled out on their first appearance.

Patents

AOTA's copyright of the *American Journal of Occupational Therapy* only protects articles or works of authors published in the journal from unauthorized copying. It does not protect any items or products mentioned in such articles or works of authors.

Any device, piece of equipment, splint, or other item described with explicit directions for construction in an article submitted to the *American Journal of Occupational Ther-*

apy for publication is not protected by AOTA copyright and can be produced for commercial purposes and patented by others, unless the item was patented, or its patent is pending, at the time the article is submitted.

Copyright

Authors are required to convey copyright ownership of their manuscripts to AOTA. Manuscripts published in the journal are copyrighted by AOTA and may not be published elsewhere without permission. Permission to reprint journal material for commercial or other purposes must be secured in writing from AOTA's Periodical Publications Department.

Manuscript Review

All accepted manuscripts are subject to copyediting. Authors will receive a photocopy of the edited manuscript for review and final approval, as well as reprint order forms. The manuscript must be returned to AOTA by first-class mail within 72 hours. The author(s) assume(s) final responsibility for the content of the manuscript, including the copyediting.

Style/Style Manual

We have adopted the *Publication Manual of the American Psychological Association* (4th edition, 1994) as our style guide. Consult the manual for all style questions.

If you have questions about the paper you contemplate submitting, refer to similar papers published in the journal. Alternatively, contact the Editor for writing guidelines regarding the following: Brief or New articles, Case Reports, Program Descriptions, Scientific Papers, Review Papers, and Procedures on Special Issues.

Sample Timetables from Students' Theses

Sample 1

This timetable is based on the fall semester of 1995 and the spring semester of 1996.

Pilot study conducted and any necessary amendments made to the rating scale.	Fall semester, 1995
Pre-test on students using the Leadership Skills and Responsibilities Rating Scale.	Second week of Spring semester, 1996
Students will colead ILS groups.	Weeks 3–13; Feb–Apr
Results of pre-test tabulated.	Week 3; Feb 5
Post-test students using the rating scale.	Week 12; Apr 2
Results of post-test tabulated.	Week 13; Apr 9
Results and Discussion sections written.	Weeks 14–16; Apr–May
Chapter 1 written	Nov
Chapter 2 written	Sept 1995–Jan 1996
References and Appendices written	Jan 1996
Meet with readers	Every 4 weeks

Sample 2

Sequence of procedures and time frame:

1. Pilot study to evaluate appropriateness of questions	2 weeks
2. Revise survey	1 week
3. Printing of survey and cover letter	1 week
4. Obtain list of pediatric occupational therapists in Massachusetts	2 weeks
5. Address, stamp, and stuff envelopes	1 week
6. Response time	3 weeks
7. Send follow-up post cards	1 week
8. Response time	2 weeks
9. Tabulate and evaluate data	2 weeks
10. Analysis of data	1 week
11. Write up results and discussion	4 weeks
TOTAL	20 weeks
Ongoing review of literature	Weeks 1–16

Sample 3

Timetable:

Oct–Nov 1995	Thesis proposal to committee
Dec 1995	Approval of human subjects committee
Nov 1995–Jan 1996	Review of the literature
Dec 1995–Feb 1996	Data collection and analysis
Feb 1996–Mar 1996	Write up results
Mar 1996	Final draft to readers
May 1996	Ready for hearing

Sample 4

Timetable:

Late December to mid-January	Complete thesis proposal
Mid-January to early February	Thesis proposal hearing
February	Human Subjects Committee review
February to mid-April	Collect data and work on literature review
End April to end May	Complete data analysis
June to August	Complete writing of thesis
September	Thesis hearing
End September	Make revisions

Index

An "f" following a page number indicates a figure; a "t" indicates a table. Page numbers in bold are those where the topic is discussed most fully.